Alzheimer's Solved

To order additional copies, please contact us.
BookSurge, LLC
www.booksurge.com
1-866-308-6235
orders@booksurge.com

HENRY
LORIN

ALZHEIMER'S SOLVED

(CONDENSED EDITION)

www.AlzheimersSolved.com

2005

Alzheimer's Solved
(Condensed Edition)

TABLE OF CONTENTS

Please note that all diagrams and references are located at the end of the book.

CHAPTER 5 Alzheimer's Disease Processes   51
(Average readers may wish to skip this somewhat technical chapter.)

CHAPTER 6 The Conditions That Lead to Most
Cases of Alzheimer's   61

CHAPTER 7 Characteristics of Semi-Starvation   69
(Average readers may wish to skip this somewhat technical chapter.)

ACKNOWLEDGEMENTS

I would like to thank my editor, TerriRhnee Pippin Grannis.

I would also like to thank Ann Hutson, Janet Lorin, and Rebecca Lorin for the initial computer preparations of this manuscript.

I am grateful to Janet Lorin, Rebecca McSwain, Sally Fallon and Richard Cote for their advice.

I appreciate the help provided by Katie Thompson, Sharon Crocker, and Kyra McGowan, my publishing consultants at BookSurge Publishing.

Finally, I would like to thank Harriet Reavis and Hedy Sladovich for their helpful suggestions.

Many years of evenings and weekends went into this effort, time that would otherwise have been spent with my family. I sincerely thank my wife, Janet Lorin, and our two children, Rebecca and Douglas Lorin, for their patience and understanding during this time.

IMPORTANT NOTE

The information in this book is intended solely for education purposes only. This book should not be used as a substitute for qualified, professional medical advice. Do not change any medical treatment or therapy without consulting your personal physician. The conclusions and opinions expressed in this book are based on review by the author of medical and scientific literature that the author believes is reliable. The reader should understand that others may disagree with the author's views.

This Book Is Dedicated To The Memories Of Vance Wolff, My Wife's Father; Rudy Lorin, My Own Father; And Colonel Don Conroy, A Friend Known To The World As The Great Santini. These Three Veterans Of World War Two Are Resting Eternally In The Beaufort National Cemetery In Beaufort, South Carolina.

CHAPTER 1
Introduction

1-1   This Condensed Edition

I began studying the published scientific literature related to Alzheimer's disease in 1996. Within a year or so it became obvious that cholesterol was the key that unlocked the door to understanding this disease. In my studies, cholesterol also revealed itself to be a key that unlocked the door to other medical conditions, as well.

In 1999 and 2000 I wrote *Alzheimer's Solved*. Its pages contained all the things I had learned regarding cholesterol's connection to Alzheimer's disease and some other medical conditions.

Alzheimer's Solved, which was copyrighted in October, 2000, contained over 360 (eight by eleven inches) pages of text, much of it very technical in content. I self-published copies of the book, and spent the years 2001 and 2002 getting those copies into the hands of a dozen or so well-respected national and international Alzheimer's researchers. In return, I received some positive comments, despite the fact that my conclusions regarding the cause of Alzheimer's seemed somewhat radical.

In preparing this version of *Alzheimer's Solved* for the general public, I chose to do two things. First, to shorten its length, and secondly, to make it more "reader friendly." I also decided to leave out discussions of medical conditions that were without a direct connection to Alzheimer's disease.

Alzheimer's Solved (Condensed Edition) contains no new conclusions, and no revisions of previous conclusions. The statements and conclusions made in the original 2000 text still hold true today. There was not even a need to add additional, newer references to the several thousand references already cited. It is my opinion that relevant scientific journal articles published from 2001 on, when studied objectively and judiciously, do not convincingly contradict the conclusions made in my 2000 text.

It will take time, but gradually more and more members of the medical and scientific communities will reach conclusions similar to those found in this 2005 condensed version of my 2000 text. Several researchers already appear to be headed in the right direction, though they have yet to piece together all the parts of the puzzle.

Readers of this book will be far "ahead in the game." They will be able to make adjustments in their lifestyle that will help to avoid developing Alzheimer's disease.

1-2   Two Men Born in 1918

Vance Wolff was a Halloween baby. He was born October 31, 1918 in a farming community on Maryland's Eastern Shore region. The Eastern Shore is the flat countryside that runs from the Chesapeake Bay to the western boundary of Delaware. There were always farming chores for young Vance to do during the times he wasn't in school. He liked to play soccer and also developed a musical talent on the trombone.

Rudolph Lovrekovich was born eleven days after Vance Wolff on November 11, 1918. This was the day that World War One officially ended. Rudolph's birthday was known for many years as Armistice Day. Today we call it Veteran's Day. Rudolph was born in Detroit, Michigan and grew up in the shadows of the great automobile factories. He was a star athlete in high school, playing football, baseball and basketball.

Vance Wolff served as an enlisted man in the Ninth Army Air Corps during World War Two. Rising to the rank of sergeant, his duties included intelligence work, interpreting aerial reconnaissance photographs and analyzing films taken by gun sight cameras. On at least two occasions he was forced to parachute out of transport airplanes when his unit made rapid location changes. He had never received any parachute training prior to his two jumps, but one had to do as one was ordered. On another rapid location shift the transport plane he was a passenger in was forced to make a landing in an area without a runway. He and the other men aboard were told to hang by their hands from the ceiling of the plane as it crashed. The underside of the plane tore away. Vance and the others were unharmed, thanks to their not being seated during the plane's impact.

Rudolph Lovrekovich served during World War Two in the U.S. Army's 28th Division. Rudolph rose to the rank of sergeant and was a combat engineer. Combat engineers used explosives to demolish obstructions that hindered friendly troop movements, as well as buildings and bridges that could be of benefit to the enemy. They were also trained in the use of construction equipment for the building of roads and bridges. The activities of combat engineers would many times depend on whether their units were advancing or retreating.

Rudolph Lovrekovich received the Bronze Star medal for leading his squad of engineers into the Siegried Line during the advance into Germany in the fall of 1944. Under heavy fire and carrying dynamite charges strapped to their backs, Rudolph and his men crawled up to concrete tank obstacles and placed the explosives in strategic locations. They detonated the charges while still being fired upon by the enemy. The explosions created a roadway through the lines into German territory. U.S. tanks and troops were then able to advance successfully during this battle with fewer casualties.

In December, 1944, Rudolph was captured during the Battle of the Bulge and spent the last five months of World War Two as a P.O.W. in a German prison camp.

When the war was over, Rudolph returned to the U.S. and worked as a carpenter, doing all phases of residential construction and repair work in the areas around Detroit. Though his carpenter jobs were physically demanding, he steadily gained weight through the years. At times he carried over 300 pounds on his 5-foot, 10-inch frame. Rudolph's sister and two brothers also became obese as well. His three siblings died of diabetes and heart disease ailments.

Rudolph and his wife Carol raised four children. After the children were on their own, Rudolph and Carol retired and moved to South Carolina in 1981. He was never able to lose weight; and, gradually, he developed symptoms of diabetes and heart disease. Rudolph was later diagnosed as having colon cancer. The cancer caused his death in 1993, at the age of 74. Though his overweight body had failed, his mind was still sharp as ever, right up to the end.

After World War Two, Vance Wolff found employment with a major food product company. He worked as an accountant and manager at various company plants in Pennsylvania, New Jersey, New York, and Washington, D.C. The combination of a desk job and the limitless eating of all types of food resulted in a large gain in weight. Vance weighed over 310 pounds at one point. Though he stood slightly over six feet in height, his body frame was very narrow. The 310 pounds he carried was truly excessive.

Vance and his wife Grace raised two children. After the children were on their own, Vance and Grace retired and moved to South Carolina in 1979. In the mid-1980's Vance developed a blockage in a heart artery that was due to atherosclerosis. He underwent balloon angioplasties to open the artery on two separate occasions. With the help of his wife, Vance set out to religiously do all the diet and lifestyle changes necessary to try to halt the atherosclerosis that was surely leading to a shortened lifespan.

Vance successfully lost all the excess weight he had been carrying by following a strict low-fat, low-cholesterol diet combined with exercise. His weight went from over 300 pounds down to 160 pounds. His doctor placed him on a new (at the time) drug that lowered blood cholesterol levels. This was the first of what are now known as statin drugs, and his blood cholesterol measurements gradually fell to less than 200 mg/dl (from 354 mg/dl in 1986 to 194 mg/dl in 1990). Vance could have been classified as the cardiologist's perfect patient, for he followed all of his doctor's rules faultlessly. His heart disease symptoms subsequently disappeared by 1990.

Vance began to develop memory and concentration problems in late 1990 and early 1991. In 1992 his physician began to suspect that he was developing Alzheimer's disease. By the mid-1990's, Vance was exhibiting all of the signs of the disease. He was not remembering the names of people he had known all of his life, including close family members. He would get lost very easily. It became impossible for him to do simple mathematical tasks (remember that he had been an accountant before retiring).

Vance eventually reached the point where he did not know his own daughter's name. He had to be watched continuously and could not attend to his own basic needs. He occasionally showed signs of physical aggression.

Through the heroic efforts of his wife, Grace, he was cared for at home until shortly before the end. Vance Wolff died in July of 1999. The cause of death was pneumonia and the complications of Alzheimer's disease.

Vance was my father-in-law. My wife was able to help her mother care for Vance on a daily basis throughout the years of his illness because we lived only three miles away. I helped as much as I could.

Vance Wolff was a wonderful man. I have many great memories of him and our children doing things together. I try to not think about the difficult years near the end.

Regarding Rudolph Lovrekovich, he and his family had their last name changed to Lorin in 1967. He was my father. He was also my neighbor for the last years of his life, living next door. I think of him every day and I miss him.

From 1981 on, my family, my wife's parents, and my own parents all lived in the same small

Southern town. Our fathers were the same age and very similar medically up to one point in time. My wife's father developed Alzheimer's disease after that one point in time, a time when he and my father differed with respect to a key health factor. This book begins with my analysis of that factor.

1-3   About the Author

What are my qualifications in writing a book about Alzheimer's disease? First, I had daily contact with a man who developed this mind-stealing disease. From 1981 up until his death, my wife, Janet, and I had been closely involved with his health situation. Janet had been trained and worked as a cardiology technologist, so she was very familiar with what it means for people to have heart disease.

Secondly, I am a health professional in that I am a dentist, having graduated from the Medical University of South Carolina in 1981 with a Doctor of Dental Medicine Degree (DMD). Though I do not pretend to have the training that a physician (MD) has, we in the dental school did receive what many would consider to be a high level of training regarding the anatomy, physiology, and "workings" of the human body.

Thirdly, before dental school, I graduated from college as a chemistry major. I have an understanding of the scientific method when it comes to medical research.

In my searches of the literature I refused to be fenced into reading only the scientific journals that were limited to the brain and nerves. All fields of medicine were open for investigation as far as I was concerned. My only rule was that the journals had to be legitimate, peer-reviewed publications that were available in the library of the Medical University of South Carolina in Charleston, South Carolina, or could be retrieved by loan from another medical school's library. The only "anecdotal" evidence in this book is from my observations of the changes in Vance Wolff over the years.

I alone performed all research and reviews of the medical/scientific literature in the years 1996 to 2000.

Those individuals reading this book who are not health professionals may want to purchase a medical dictionary of the type found in popular bookstores. The medical dictionary I used was *Mosby's Medical Dictionary, Fourth Edition,* Published by Mosby-Yearbook, Inc. in 1994.

I also used the *Merck Manual, Sixteenth Edition,* published in 1996.

The following textbooks were used as references in the writing of this book.

Biochemistry, Fourth Edition by Lubert Stryer, published by Freeman and Company, 1995.

Textbook of Medical Physiology, Ninth Edition by Guyton & Hall, published by Saunders, 1996.

Human Anatomy and Physiology, Second Edition by Elaine Marieb, published by Benjamin/Cummings, 1992.

Molecular and Genetic Basis of Neurological Disease, Second Edition, edited by Roger Rosenberg, published by Butterworth-Heinemann, 1997.

Neuroanatomy by Richard Snell, published by Little, Brown, 1992.

Williams Textbook of Endocrinology, Eighth Edition, edited by Jean Wilson, published by Saunders Company, 1992.

Encyclopedia of Neuroscience, edited by George Adelman, published by Birkhauser, 1987.

Desk Reference for Neuroscience, Second Edition, edited by Isabel Lockard, published by Springer-Verlag, 1991.

The references listed at the end of the book are all available in the libraries of medical schools in the United States and throughout the world. Many are available over the Internet on Medline and similar services.

1-4   Watching Alzheimer's Develop in a Man

It should be obvious to the reader that we did not know at the time that Vance was beginning to develop Alzheimer's disease. Older people are supposed to be forgetful, aren't they? We were thrilled at his accomplishments: weight loss, increased exercise capability, lowering of blood pressure, increased energy, and last but not least, the dramatic lowering of his blood cholesterol levels.

The incidences of memory lapses and confusion became more prevalent as the months passed. Vance experienced fainting spells due to low blood pressure (hypotension) and a heart arrhythmia (irregular heartbeat). He eventually had a heart pacemaker surgically implanted in his chest. He developed strange (to us) skin rashes, experienced pain in his joints, and suffered from muscle cramps, especially in the large muscles in his hip and leg areas. Vance developed cataracts in both eyes. He also began to exhibit epileptic seizure activity.

Despite Vance's memory and thinking problems, low blood pressure problems, cataracts, seizure activity, heart arrhythmia, and the problems with his muscles, skin, and joints, we were happy about one thing; he kept his blood cholesterol levels low and never experienced another blockage in a heart artery.

Looking back, Vance Wolff did everything right in order to beat heart disease. With the help of his wife, he became the cardiologists' perfect patient. He lost weight to the extent that he actually became underweight for his frame. Vance eliminated practically all fat and cholesterol from his diet. He exercised every day. He faithfully took every medication prescribed by his cardiologist, including his statin drug.

Today I believe that Vance, unknowingly, went too far in the quest to defeat heart disease. It was not easy to accept this conclusion. Readers may not agree with me. Most in the medical community will not agree with my conclusions. In this book I will demonstrate to both the average person and the medical/scientific professional that my conclusions are backed by sound evidence.

What is my primary conclusion? That it is indeed possible for a person to have blood cholesterol levels that are too low. There are illnesses, including Alzheimer's disease, that are the direct result of having low blood cholesterol levels over extended periods of time.

CHAPTER 2
Introduction to Alzheimer's Disease

2-1   What is Alzheimer's?

The following definition for Alzheimer's disease is one that I prefer: Alzheimer's is a dementia in which the cognitive functions of the human brain steadily decline over time. The cognitive functions are memory, learning, perception of surroundings, and judgment or reasoning ability. Alzheimer's disease is incurable.

In the early stages of the disease the patient exhibits short-term memory loss, while still remembering events that may have occurred forty or fifty years earlier. There is a problem for the patient in finding the appropriate words when speaking. He or she may sense a problem, and think that something in their mind is not working correctly.

The next stages are ones where memory worsens and tasks involving abstract thinking, such as balancing a checkbook, become difficult. The patient does inappropriate things, such as pouring hot soup into a glass of iced tea. Driving an automobile becomes hazardous. Even getting dressed in appropriate clothing is difficult. Time of day and day/date confusion occurs. The patient gets lost easily, even in his or her own house.

In stages near the end, the patient may wander around continuously and at all hours of the day and night. Writing becomes unreadable. Familiar faces become unfamiliar. Some patients become verbally abusive and use curse words, even if they have never been known to do it before. They may even engage in acts of physical aggression to those around them. Shocking personality changes occur.

In the very last stages of Alzheimer's the patients become unable to communicate or take care of themselves. They require 24-hour attention. Even the previously spared distant memory is lost. The patient becomes incontinent. Eventually, the body fails. Patients are said to die *with* Alzheimer's, not *of* it. (The actual causes of death in Alzheimer's cases are discussed in a later chapter.)

Two things must be pointed out before continuing. First, the signs and symptoms just described are not the same in every patient, and there is a great deal of overlapping of the stages. Secondly, the time frame varies greatly from patient to patient. In some cases the process may be as short as two to four years. In others, patients may still be functioning even after fifteen years following the initial diagnosis.

It has been said, and I have seen it firsthand, that the patient with Alzheimer's disease dies two times. The mind dies first, followed later by the death of the body.

I have been describing the signs, symptoms, and stages of Alzheimer's disease. Unfortunately, there is no perfect diagnostic medical test that will absolutely determine whether or not a person has the disease. Several different tests are utilized in cases of suspected Alzheimer's. A detailed history is an important first step. Blood tests and a comprehensive neurological examination with several mental measurement exercises are performed. The patient undergoes brain-imaging tests in order to provide a picture of the brain. The reasons for obtaining pictures of the brain in suspected cases of Alzheimer's will be discussed in a later section.

The physician must rule out other possible causes for the dementia that a patient may exhibit. These include such things as a thiamine deficiency, long-standing alcoholism, a reaction from medications that the patient may be taking for another condition, or a number of other possible causes of mental difficulties.

The patient may have vascular dementia, which is not the same as Alzheimer's. The differences between the two dementias will be covered in a later chapter.

The only way to absolutely confirm a diagnosis of Alzheimer's in a patient is by examining samples of brain tissue taken after death has occurred. An accuracy rate of 80 to 90 percent is possible before death by utilizing the various diagnostic tests that are currently available, but only if an experienced physician is overseeing the tests. *Patients are sometimes mistakenly diagnosed as having Alzheimer's, when they actually have some other condition.* I cannot stress that enough. Be wary of any physician or nurse who immediately puts forth the opinion that your loved one has Alzheimer's, because there's a very good chance that their quick opinion is wrong.

Alzheimer's disease is the primary cause of 60 to 70 percent of all dementia cases. Vascular dementia is suspected in about 10 to 30 percent of the others.

Here are some of the "numbers" of Alzheimer's disease:

-four million Americans have Alzheimer's

-in the next thirty years that number will grow to 14 million (hopefully, that will not occur after the publishing of this book)

-it is the fourth leading cause of death, following heart disease, cancer, and stroke in people aged 65, up to 40 or 50 percent of those around the age of 90 or older

-Alzheimer's disease affects more women than men.

It usually takes between two and five years after the first symptoms occur before the physician is able to reasonably diagnose the patient as having Alzheimer's disease. Two or three years after a definite diagnosis, patients may begin to require specialized care, perhaps in an institution. Three or four years later the patients usually expire.

The typical time frame, therefore, between initial symptoms and the eventual death of the patient is about eight to ten years.

The financial cost of Alzheimer's to the U.S. healthcare system is now well over $100 billion each year.

There is a significant emotional cost of Alzheimer's as well. I am speaking of the family members of each patient who must make drastic changes in their own lifestyles in order to deal with all the aspects of their loved one's illness.

We will now discuss some of the things that are occurring in the brain of an Alzheimer's victim. The primary working cells of the brain are called neurons. In Alzheimer's the neurons are gradually dying. All brain areas are usually suffering the changes associated with neuronal death, but the parts of the brain that are affected the most in Alzheimer's are those in what is called the limbic system. The mental changes seen in the patient are directly connected to the deaths of the neurons in the limbic system. Please keep in mind, however, that brain cells are usually dying throughout the brain of a patient with Alzheimer's.

Neurons are one of the few types of cells that do not reproduce. They are supposed to last a lifetime. Those neurons that are dying in the brain of an Alzheimer's victim are not replaced. This is the reason why the disease is presently incurable.

The structures in the brain's limbic system are responsible for the "thinking processes" that we perform. The term we use is cognitive function. Memory, perception, learning, reasoning and judgment are the cognitive functions based in the limbic system. In other words, the intelligence capabilities that have placed humans at the top of the animal kingdom's evolutionary ladder are found in the limbic system.

In Alzheimer's, these limbic system structures suffer neuronal death, which then results in the symptoms seen in the patient. Remember, however, that cells are usually dying throughout the patient's brain.

The structures associated with the limbic system are the hippocampus, the parahippocampal gyrus, the cingulated gyrus, the amygdala, the hypothalamus, and the anterior thalamic nucleii. The fornix is the main fiber that connects these structures. It is important to know that the connections between the parts of the limbic system and other areas of the brain are very complex and beyond the scope of this book. We will, therefore, concentrate on just those structures in the limbic system in our discussions.

Let me remind the reader that diagrams illustrating these parts of the human brain can be found at the end of this book.

Two structures closely associated with the parts of the limbic system are the olfactory bulbs, located at the base of the brain. Our senses of smell and taste are centered in the olfactory bulbs, which are close to the area behind the bridge of the nose. We will discuss the olfactory connection to the limbic system in greater detail in a later section.

The limbic system structures as a whole are associated with the temporal lobes of the brain. There are two temporal lobes, one on each side. They extend downwards and wrap underneath the brain.

In the next section we will discuss the brain structures again in relation to the changes seen in Alzheimer's disease. Do not panic, however. I am not a neuroanatomist. We will, therefore, narrow our focus and keep our discussion as "uncomplex" as possible.

2-2   Plaques, Tangles, and Brain Shrinkage

When speaking of Alzheimer's the following terms mean the same thing: senile plaques, amyloid plaques, and Alzheimer's plaques.

When the brain tissues of someone who has died of Alzheimer's disease are examined under a microscope, there is seen a material called beta amyloid. This material is found between the neurons in the brain. Therefore, when speaking about the beta amyloid plaques of Alzheimer's, or the senile plaques of Alzheimer's, we are talking about accumulations of a protein material outside of the neurons.

Beta amyloid is also found along the walls of blood vessels that serve the brain of an Alzheimer's victim. It is laid down in a continuous pattern alongside these vessels.

Early in the course of the disease, beta amyloid begins accumulating as small fragments, a little at a time. Gradually, these small fragments build up into large deposits, which we call plaques.

There is also a formation inside of the neurons that are dead or dying that is said to resemble tangled fibers. They are termed neurofibrillary tangles. The important things to remember at this point are that in the brains of people who have died with Alzheimer's disease there are found two distinguishing features. Beta amyloid plaques are present outside of neurons and alongside the walls of blood vessels. Neurofibrillary tangles, or simply tangles, are found inside of neurons that are dying or already dead.

The outer surface of the brain is called the cerebral cortex or gray matter. The cerebral cortex consists mainly of neurons, which again are the primary "working cells" of the brain. Also found in the cerebral cortex are unmyelinated nerve fibers, blood vessels, and supporting cells. "Unmyelinated" means that the nerve fibers that provide the connections between neurons in this area do not have very much insulating coating (myelin) around them. There are many fissures and sulci (plural of sulcus) that the cerebral cortex follows beneath the outline of the brain. The gray matter of the cerebral cortex can account for up to 40 percent of the total weight of the brain. Therefore, the bodies of neurons, the primary working cells of the brain, make up almost 40 percent of the total weight of the brain.

Internal to the gray matter of the cerebral cortex is the white matter. The white matter consists of myelinated nerve fibers that run in bundles, providing the connections between all of the gray matter (which contains the neurons). The white color is due to the myelin insulating coatings surrounding these fibers.

In the diagrams for this section are seen the general outer structure of the brain and the approximate locations of the parts of the limbic system. The hippocampus is the one structure most identified with the brain tissue changes seen in Alzheimer's disease.

It is now time to discuss a third finding common to Alzheimer's patients. It is atrophy of their brains. Simply put, the brains of Alzheimer's patients exhibit shrinkage. Remember, there are other terms for this that mean the same thing. They are brain atrophy, cerebral atrophy, cortical atrophy, and ventricular widening.

This brain shrinkage involves the structures of the limbic system, so we also speak of hippocampal atrophy when discussing Alzheimer's.

If studies demonstrated that the brains of Alzheimer's patients are shrinking, then something is gradually being lost or taken from these brains. The obvious question is, just what is that "something"?

2-3   The Things That Do Not Cause Alzheimer's

Over the years there have been many theories put forth as to the cause or causes of Alzheimer's disease. I found no theories in the medical/scientific literature that consistently revealed a definite cause-and-effect relationship. We will now review some of the things that do not cause this disease.

The herpes virus was found to not be a cause of Alzheimer's. Other common viruses and bacteria, such as those causing flu and measles, were also not implicated.

Blood transfusions have not been shown to play a role in the disease.

Various allergic conditions are no more prevalent in Alzheimer's patients when compared with non-Alzheimer's control patients.

The season of birth does not play a role in the later development of the disease.

The chronic inhaling of possibly harmful odors is not related to the development of Alzheimer's. As we will see in a later section, there is an olfactory deficit present in many cases of the disease. We will explore it fully in that later section.

Alzheimer's is not caused by being exposed to the electromagnetic fields surrounding any electric motors, large or small.

Workplace exposures to the following agents are not connected to Alzheimer's disease: lead, asbestos, organophosphates and hydrocarbon solvents. Occupations with exposure to constant vibrations are not implicated, either.

Deficiencies of vitamin E were not more likely to be found in Alzheimer's patients in comparison with people who did not have the disease.

Thyroid function was found to be within normal limits in Alzheimer's patients.

Some researchers have noted that there may be increased levels of iron in the brains of Alzheimer's patients, especially in the areas of brain cell tissues. Iron is known to cause the oxidation of various molecules in tissues. However, the reason that excess iron seems to be found in the areas of cell damage is based on the fact that to begin with, there is a large amount of it in the human brain. The iron levels in a healthy brain are equal to or higher than the levels found in the liver.

Aluminum was thought at one time to be the cause of Alzheimer's, but the vast majority of researchers in this field have, by now, dismissed it. The idea of a link between Alzheimer's and aluminum began almost thirty years ago when some kidney dialysis patients developed dementia. It was found that the solutions used in the dialysis treatments were causing increased aluminum build-up in the brains of these patients. When dialysis solutions not containing aluminum were substituted, the type of dementias found earlier were no longer developing in these folks. In addition, it was found that the tissue damage in the brains linked to excessive aluminum did not match the type of damage seen in Alzheimer's disease.

Some researchers believe that exposure to mercury is the cause of Alzheimer's disease. It is indeed true that pure mercury can cause neurological damage, just as is the case with some of the other heavy metals.

Mercury is found in many places in the Earth's crust, though it is not quite as common as aluminum or some of the other metals. It is found in fish and other seafood.

There are some researchers who find no link between Alzheimer's and mercury, and a few who claim there is. A group of scientists at a large Midwestern university concluded the mercury is released in small traces from amalgam tooth fillings, and that this is the cause of Alzheimer's disease. However, there is another group of scientists at this very same university who studied older women ranging from 75 to 102 years. These researchers concluded from their studies of the elderly women that there were no differences in mental status between the women based on their having or not having dental amalgam fillings.

There is a research team based in Switzerland which concludes that Alzheimer's patients have higher blood levels of mercury, but that it has no connection to either the presence of dental amalgam fillings or to the eating of seafood containing mercury. In fact, 71 percent of the Alzheimer's patients in their study had no amalgam fillings. The authors of this study state that they do not know why there were increases in blood mercury levels in the Alzheimer's patients.

What were the statistics upon which they based their conclusions? There were a total of 33 Alzheimer's patients in the study and 110 people acting as healthy controls. Only 4 of the 33 Alzheimer's patients had blood mercury levels that were clearly higher than the healthy controls. I do not believe that 4 out of a group of 33 can justify making a conclusion about the entire group.

I looked for research concerning actual measurements of mercury in brain tissues. I found a recent report where researchers studied actual brain tissue specimens taken from diseased patients. They found no increases of mercury in Alzheimer's patients.

Some researchers believe copper causes Alzheimer's, but their evidence is far from conclusive.

Finally, there are some individuals who believe that Alzheimer's disease results from eating beef hamburger meat tainted with an infectious agent called a prion. We know that Mad Cow disease is spread by eating beef products that contain one of these very rare prions. But is Alzheimer's caused by eating beef products that contain a harmful prion?

The answer is a most definite no.

First, let us cover some brief background information. Prion proteins themselves are normal proteins found in tissues throughout our bodies. They associate with cell membranes, and are numerous in the brain. Though it can be confusing, prion proteins are not the same as the harmful prions that cause disease.

Prion diseases, of which there are four, are characterized by the fact that they cause holes in the brain. This is why they are known as spongiform encephalopathies (sponge-like holes). In Mad Cow disease, for example, harmful infectious prions cause the normal prion proteins to change into a destructive form, called scrapie prion proteins. It is these scrapie prion proteins that cause the tissue damage, resulting in holes in the surrounding brain tissue.

The initial symptoms of someone with a prion disease may resemble those of Alzheimer's. And it is true that the brain tissues of someone dying of a prion disease will exhibit amyloid plaques. However, neurologists and neuroscientists can readily tell the difference between these illnesses. What follows are some of these differences.

Alzheimer's is a disease of the elderly in the vast majority of cases, as we all know. Victims of Mad Cow disease can be almost any age. The other prion diseases can also occur in folks that are not necessarily elderly.

The amyloid plaques that form in the brain tissues of prion disease patients are not the same kind of amyloid plaques found in Alzheimer's brains. A special tissue stain used by pathologists is able to show the differences.

Finally, because of these holes, prion disease brain tissues look very different from Alzheimer's brain tissues.

Alzheimer's brain tissues can show remnants of prion proteins in damaged areas, but that is simply because prion proteins are normally found in these tissues anyway.

The brain tissues from people dying with Alzheimer's disease have been undergoing close examinations for many years. The scientists performing these examinations are very well aware of the concept of prion diseases. They recognize that Alzheimer's is not caused by a harmful prion or anything else found in beef products.

Let us look at this issue from a larger, common sense perspective. If Alzheimer's is caused by eating beef products, such as hamburger, a question to ask is, do vegetarians ever get Alzheimer's?

The answer is a most definite yes.

In addition, let us think of couples who have lived together for many years. Typically, they will have eaten the same foods for all those years. If Alzheimer's results from eating beef products tainted with a harmful prion, then couples should be developing the disease simultaneously. This clearly is not happening.

As you will read in a later chapter, people with Down syndrome will always develop Alzheimer's damage in their brains if they live long enough. It is simply not logical to think that the thousands of individuals with Down syndrome somehow all managed to eat beef hamburger made from infected cattle.

Finally, in reading this book you will learn the true cause of Alzheimer's, and it does not involve prions or any other agents supposedly lurking in beef meat products. And the same can be said for pork, turkey, chicken, lamb and any and all other meats. You can not get Alzheimer's disease from eating meat or meat products.

2-4   Studies of Twins

Many researchers believe that Alzheimer's is a "genetic disease," and those people later developing the disease were destined to their fate from the time of birth. If Alzheimer's were a purely genetic disease, then studies of identical twins would show that if one twin developed the disease, then the other one should, too. Reviews of the medical literature showed that this was not the case.

Some people may have a genetic make-up that is said to predispose them to develop a particular disease, but that another factor plays a part in whether or not they actually develop the disease.

Do the studies of Alzheimer's in twins show the disease to be purely genetic in origin? The answer is definitely no. Do studies show that there is some predisposition towards developing the disease? Some studies say yes and some say no. There definitely are some identical twins where both developed Alzheimer's. Most large studies show rates for identical twins to be in the ranges from 18 to 40 percent. One study showed a rate of 83 percent, but it was a very small study.

If Alzheimer's were a purely genetic disease, then the rates in all of the identical twin studies would approach 100 percent.

The rates of 18 to 40 percent for Alzheimer's in identical twins may in fact be exaggerations of the true situations, because studies of this type can sometimes be subject to an unconscious bias on the part of those conducting the research.

Is Alzheimer's disease caused purely by one's genetic make-up? No. Are some people more likely than others to develop the disease? Yes, but the genetic influences are not major ones, except in a very few families spread around the globe.

There is a category of people who are definitely genetically programmed to develop Alzheimer's. These are people born with Down syndrome.

For everyone else who does not have Down syndrome, the conclusion drawn from this section is that Alzheimer's does not have a pure genetic cause. We, therefore, need to look elsewhere in the pursuit of the real basis for the disease.

2-5   Other Dementias

Alzheimer's disease is the cause of almost 70 percent of all dementia cases. Vascular dementia is responsible for about 10 to 30 percent of the cases. There is a third type of dementia called Lewy Body disease that is probably another type of Alzheimer's. In Lewy Body disease, the patients have memory loss, but they also experience visual hallucinations, tremors, and are more prone to wandering. In this book, we will concentrate on Alzheimer's disease.

In vascular dementia, strokes in particular regions of the brain cause the problems involving lost memory. The patient frequently has high blood pressure (hypertension) and atherosclerosis, and may have had a heart attack in the past. The strokes in vascular dementia are caused by blood vessels in the brain being blocked or bursting open. The brain area served by the affected blood vessel does not receive adequate blood flow, and that area suffers damage as a result.

In vascular dementia the mental deficits occur in a stair step fashion. A stroke causes a worsening of the patient's mental status, but he or she will then remain at that plateau. If the factors leading to the stroke (usually hypertension) are then controlled with treatments and medications, the patient's mental status my not get any worse.

This is in contrast to patients with Alzheimer's, for their mental condition progressively gets worse in a steady fashion over time.

In vascular dementia, brain shrinkage does not often occur. In Alzheimer's, however, brain shrinkage is a universal finding.

Some researchers believe that a person can have both kinds of dementia. Some patients may indeed have properties of both dementias, but I will also show that the conditions did not develop at the same time.

Patients can be easily misdiagnosed as having the wrong dementia. The medicines used in the treatment of Alzheimer's are different from those used in vascular dementia, where hypertension is a contributing cause.

For example, Alzheimer's patients usually have low blood pressure and decreased blood clotting activity. Vascular dementia patients are given blood thinners and medicines to lower blood pressure, which if given to an Alzheimer's patient can actually cause bleeding to occur in the brain.

What are the observed differences between these two dementias?

An Alzheimer's patient usually cannot do simple mathematical problems. Someone with vascular dementia can probably still do simple mathematical problems.

A vascular dementia patient may ask the exact same question several times in a row but will quit when your same answer finally registers. An Alzheimer's patient will ask different questions, one right after another, and they all will be somewhat inappropriate and nonsensical. You will never be sure if your answers were satisfactory.

Vascular dementia patients will usually be aware of their current surroundings. Alzheimer's patients will not, and they may totally forget where the bathroom or kitchen is, even if they have lived in the same place for years.

A vascular dementia patient can decide to call someone, then dial the number correctly and converse normally with the person they called. An Alzheimer's patient cannot do the phone call tasks just described.

Finally, vascular dementia patients usually know the names of family members and friends to whom they may be talking. Alzheimer's patients will not, unfortunately, know the names of people to whom they are talking, including brothers, sisters, daughters, sons, husbands or wives. This is one of the cruelest aspects of the disease.

CHAPTER 3
Introduction to Cholesterol

3-1   The First Clues About Cholesterol and Alzheimer's

In 1996, I happened to see a broadcast of a 1994 program about Alzheimer's on television. In the program, Dr. Allen Roses, one of the world's foremost authorities on the disease, said two things that caught my attention. First, he said that the typical Alzheimer's patient's brain weighs two-thirds of a normal person's brain. Second, he said something about a protein called apolipoprotein E that is involved in the process of Alzheimer's disease. Apolipoprotein E is normally a protein that transports cholesterol.

A day or two later I happened to read in a medical magazine, that in Alzheimer's disease there is a protein called apolipoprotein E associated with the accumulation of something called beta amyloid in these patients.

In the library of the Medical University of South Carolina in Charleston, I looked up information regarding cholesterol and the brain. I learned that cholesterol molecules constitute 40 percent of the molecules in some areas of the brain. The rest of the brain is protein, water and fats of various kinds.

Back in the mid-1980s, Vance was overweight and had undergone heart artery procedures in a battle against atherosclerosis. He embarked on a successful campaign of weight loss, exercise and a very rigid diet. Fat and cholesterol intake was reduced greatly. He won the battle against atherosclerosis in that he never suffered a heart attack and never had to undergo any further artery procedures.

Based on my knowledge of Vance's history, I thought of a way to test for a connection between cholesterol and Alzheimer's.

Vance developed Alzheimer's after several years of an extremely low intake of cholesterol and the use of a medicine that inhibited cholesterol formation in his body. It may have been a pure coincidence, but maybe it was not. The way to test it was to find a group or category of people who almost never have low cholesterol and see if they have a low incidence of Alzheimer's disease. Such a group, by consistently having high blood cholesterol levels, probably would also have high rates of heart disease and obesity.

The group that came to mind consisted of people with maturity onset diabetes. These are people who develop diabetes as adults after decades of eating more food than their bodies require. Maturity onset diabetics are overweight, suffer from heart disease and similar ailments, and cannot regulate their glucose (blood sugar) levels in an ideal manner. To help with glucose regulation, many of them have to take an oral medication. Eventually, they may have to take insulin injections. Many maturity onset diabetics do not require insulin injections, and for this reason they are said to have non-insulin dependent diabetes mellitus, or NIDDM. The other term used is Type 2 diabetes.

Of course, there are always exceptions to every rule. Some people with NIDDM have always been slender, have never had high cholesterol, and do not have classic heart disease. Their diabetic problem usually is one of insulin resistance, which means that cells in their body will not allow the insulin already present to escort glucose across the membranes and into the cells' interiors. As a general rule, however, NIDDM (or Type 2 diabetes) is associated with obesity and high blood cholesterol levels. NIDDM is the more common form of diabetes. Although there is some genetic basis for the development of the diabetes, many of the patient's diabetic symptoms will resolve if the patient can manage to lose the excess weight and become physically fit.

NIDDMs are afflicted with atherosclerosis/heart disease, circulation problems, eye problems, and numbness in the hands or feet. Gangrene can be a problem in the feet of some long-term NIDDMs and this can lead to amputations.

I set out to investigate if NIDDMs, a group with universally high cholesterol levels, would, therefore, have a low rate of Alzheimer's disease.

It was not difficult to find the published research that showed that NIDDMs do not seem to get Alzheimer's disease. Some investigators discovered this relationship (low rate of Alzheimer's in NIDDMs) a long time ago.

There are a small number of researchers who mistakenly think that NIDDM patients may be at an elevated risk for developing Alzheimer's. However, if they read all the research available on this particular topic, they would understand their error. There are 18 million people with diabetes in the U.S. It's obvious that we do not have 18 million cases of Alzheimer's.

I found research stating that the Cree Indians of Canada have a low rate of Alzheimer's. I also found research that said the Cree have high rates of diabetes!

This was my first confirmation that high blood levels of cholesterol, which NIDDMs possess, would probably offer a protective effect against the development of Alzheimer's disease. (The NIDDMs are at risk for developing vascular dementia.)

Could it really be that simple? Could Alzheimer's simply result from having low blood cholesterol levels over a long period of time? The next step was to find out the whole story of cholesterol and its relationship to our bodies.

3-2   Making Cholesterol Molecules

What is cholesterol? Is it some type of parasite that hides seeds of future disease in the foods we eat? Is cholesterol a tool used to punish people for having the desire to eat things that taste good to them?

Pure cholesterol is a waxy substance that can, under the right conditions, form crystals. In humans and other animals, however, it is not normally found in a pure, concentrated state. It may be helpful to think of the term "cholesterol molecules" rather than the word cholesterol. Cholesterol molecules are in the walls of every cell in your body and also in the walls of every smaller compartment found inside of those cells. We use the term cell membrane instead of cell wall. From now on, think of cholesterol molecules as being one of the several building blocks that make up the cell membranes of every type of tissue in your body.

Cholesterol molecules are also used as the basic structure for several hormones and vitamins.

Cholesterol molecules are not proteins, not carbohydrates, and not a source of energy. Cholesterol is a sterol. Sterols are molecules in which the atoms are arranged in rings. Cholesterol molecules have a four-ringed structure with several other atoms attached. This four-ring structure is very stable and extremely resistant to breaking up once it is formed.

Though cholesterol is not a fat, it is grouped together with fats in a category called lipids. Lipids, as a rule, do not dissolve easily in water or water-based solutions, such as blood. Alcohols, ether, and several other substances can act as solvents on lipids and lipid structures. Oils are fats in liquid form. Fats consist of three straight chains of carbon atoms that are linked together. The term triglyceride means three chains. The reason cholesterol and fats are in the same group (lipids) is because they share the property of not easily dissolving in water.

How are cholesterol molecules made? The four-ringed structure and attachments consist of twenty-seven carbon atoms. The entire cholesterol molecule is made with two-carbon building blocks called acetate molecules. These two-carbon acetates are linked together to make longer carbon chains that are then twisted and folded into the four-ringed basic sterol structure. To make each molecule of cholesterol requires the use of at least thirty enzymes and a considerable input of energy. And each cell needs hundreds or even thousands of cholesterol molecules for its membranes.

The two-carbon acetates are usually derived from glucose, a carbohydrate. They can also come from fats (fatty acids). Both glucose and fats provide energy, too. Thus, both the energy needed and the two-carbon acetates can come from glucose or fatty acids.

Of the thirty enzymes needed to make a cholesterol molecule, one of them is said to be a rate-limiting enzyme. This means that this enzyme is the key to whether the construction of a cholesterol molecule goes forward to completion or is stopped. This enzyme is called 3-hydroxy-3-methyl-glutaryl-CoA reductase. The name is usually shortened and called HMG-CoA reductase.

Therefore, one way to limit the production of cholesterol molecules is to inhibit this key enzyme called HMG-CoA reductase. The new drugs called "statins" do just that. Statin drugs that lower cholesterol are called HMG-CoA reductase inhibitors.

Cholesterol molecules do not dissolve in water. One part of the cholesterol molecule will get close to water molecules quite readily. At the end of the basic four-ringed structure of the cholesterol molecule is a hydroxyl group, which consists of an oxygen atom and a hydrogen atom. This hydroxyl group part of the cholesterol molecule is "friendly" to water or water-based solutions (such as blood and the solutions found inside of cells). This end that likes water molecules will be called the water-loving end.

The other end of a cholesterol molecule, containing the rings, dislikes water molecules (water-blocking). This end likes fats and oils.

This is the key to why cholesterol molecules are important components of cell membranes. When arranged in a membrane, water-based solutions can get close to the membrane (because of the hydroxyl groups sticking out), but the water cannot get through the membrane due to the rest of the structure of the molecules (the water-blocking ring ends).

The parts of the cell involved in making cholesterol are the endoplasmic reticulum and the Golgi apparatus. All cells can make some cholesterol, but the sites of major cholesterol manufacturing are the liver and the intestines.

To summarize, cholesterol molecules are critical for cell membranes in every cell in your body. Making cholesterol molecules requires significant amounts of carbon-building material, significant amounts of energy, and thirty enzymes. The enzyme that can control the production process of cholesterol molecules is called HMG-CoA reductase. The statin drugs that interfere with the process of making cholesterol molecules act by inhibiting this enzyme.

3-3   Cholesterol is Essential for Life

The cell is the basic unit of all the tissues of the body. The cells of one organ or tissue are different from the cells of other organs and tissues. The cell's basic parts consist of a nucleus, mitochondria, lysosomes, endoplasmic reticulum, and Golgi bodies. The cell is covered with a cell membrane, which contains the cell's interior fluid, cytoplasm. Each of the basic cell parts just listed is also covered with membranes.

The cell membrane on the outside of the cell and the membranes covering the interior components are made up of cholesterol molecules and phospholipid molecules. Phospholipids are long-chain fatty acids that do not have any ringed structures in them, in contrast to cholesterol molecules. They are similar to cholesterol in that they have one end that likes water molecules (water-loving) and another end that dislikes water (water-blocking). This water-blocking end likes oils and fats. Thus, phospholipids act as barrier molecules to water and water-based solutions such as blood and cell cytoplasm fluid.

The cell membrane is called a lipid bilayer, because it is only two molecules thick over the entire surface of the cell. One layer of cholesterol molecules and phospholipid molecules are arranged with their water-loving ends pointed outward, and the second is arranged with their water-loving ends pointing inward. This means that their water-blocking ends are up against each other in back-to-back fashion. This arrangement provides the water-barrier property of the cell membrane.

The cholesterol molecules fit neatly into the two layers of the cell membrane. The term used to describe this is "lipid packing." The integrity of a cell membrane is determined by the degree of lipid packing. The health status of a cell depends on the integrity of the membrane. Thus, if the amount of lipid packing is not at the ideal level, then harmful things can get into the cell and good things can leak out. This is a way of defining what disease is at the level of the cell. A healthy cell is one that has a healthy cell membrane that can control what comes into the cell and what goes out of the cell. A diseased cell, or sick cell, is one that is losing the ability to control what goes in and what goes out of the cell.

The cells of one organ or tissue are different from the cells of other organs or tissues. This also holds true for their membranes. Different types of cells possess different types of cell membranes. One of the ways in which cell membranes differ from one another is in the types of phospholipids that reside within the membrane. However, no matter what kind of phospholipid is in the cell membrane, <u>all cell types share one specific common ingredient: cholesterol molecules.</u>

Large proteins of various kinds are spread apart in the cell membranes. The proteins provide for the transport of various things into and out of the cell. Food for the cell, typically carbohydrate chains of glucose, is brought into the cell via a protein in the cell membrane. Wastes are ushered out of the cell by a different protein.

What holds the cell membrane together? Is there a "glue" that bonds the cholesterol and phospholipid molecules together? The answer is no. The lipid bilayer remains intact because the water-blocking parts of cholesterol and phospholipid molecules have a natural attraction between each other. This helps stabilize them in their side-to-side and back-to-back arrangement in the lipid bilayer.

If there is only this attraction property and no "glue," does that mean that the molecules and phospholipids could move around in the bilayer? The answer is yes.

These cholesterol and phospholipid molecules cannot turn upside down in relation to the bilayer arrangement, but they are free to move around.

The lack of a "glue" also means that readily inserted into the cell membrane or removed from it are phospholipid and cholesterol molecules.

What holds the large proteins in place? And what keeps the entire cell from simply collapsing, if the membrane has no rigid properties? The answer is that each cell has a stabilizing cytoskeleton. The cytoskeleton provides the shape and form of a cell in spite of the non-rigid aspect of the cell membrane.

When a greater amount of cholesterol is in the lipid bilayer, the cell membrane is said to be "less fluid." The membrane becomes more rigid and also has better qualities as a barrier or wall to things trying to get into or out of the cell.

If a lesser amount of cholesterol is in the lipid bilayer, the cell membrane is said to be "more fluid." The membrane becomes less rigid and is a weaker barrier or wall to things trying to get into the cell or things getting out of the cell. In summary:

1. More cholesterol results in less fluidity, which produces a better barrier.

2. Less cholesterol results in increased fluidity, which leads to a poorer barrier that can allow leakage of things into or out of the cell.

This concept of "membrane fluidity" is discussed again in a later chapter.

The health of cells depends on the integrity of their cell membranes. Therefore, cholesterol molecules, common to all the different cell types in your body, can be considered to be the most important molecule in your body.

3-4   Plants Do Not Have Cholesterol

Cholesterol molecules are found only in animals. No plant contains cholesterol. Cell membranes of plants and cell membranes of animals must both fulfill the task of providing a barrier to water-based solutions. Animals' cell membranes must be flexible to allow for movement while still maintaining the integrity of the cell membrane barrier.

Plants are not designed to be flexible, nor do they move around. On a microscopic level, the cell membranes of plants are rigid. You can see this for yourself by doing a little experiment. Take a fresh leaf from any tree, bush, or flower. Bend the leaf. At some point it will snap and at the line of leaf breakage you will see liquid begin to seep out.

Now use your thumb and finger and pinch some of your own skin. Then let it go. There is no seepage of liquids. You cannot even see where you did it unless you pinched yourself really hard.

The unique structure of cholesterol molecules makes them perfect for slipping into membranes to prevent leakage of cell components when the membranes are flexed.

Cholesterol can, therefore, be thought of as nature's "water-proofing" molecule for animal cell membranes. Cholesterol molecules allow cell membranes to flex while maintaining barrier integrity.

Skin contains cholesterol in great quantities. In addition to cholesterol, some of the other components of skin are ceramides, phospholipids, and fatty acids (fats). There also are significant amounts of water held in healthy skin. The layers of membranes containing cholesterol, fats, phospholipids, etc., keep the water trapped in the skin.

3-5   Hormones and Vitamins From Cholesterol

Cholesterol molecules are used as "construction" elements in the membranes of all cells. The four-ringed sterol basic structure is durable and resistant to alteration. What can be altered are the arrangements of atoms attached to the four-ringed basic structure. Changing these attachments can convert a molecule used as a building block into a molecule used as a chemical messenger. A hormone is a chemical messenger that can initiate and regulate various activities of organs and tissues of the body. Changing and rearranging the atoms attached to them turn cholesterol molecules into some of the most important hormones in the body.

The hormones that start as cholesterol molecules are produced in the adrenal glands, and in the male and female sex organs. There are five classes of steroid hormones that begin as cholesterol molecules: progestagens, androgens, estrogens, mineralocorticoids, and the glucocorticoids.

The main progestagen is progesterone. Progesterone participates in the female menstrual cycle and in the maintenance of the uterine tissues during a pregnancy.

One of the important androgens is testosterone. Testosterone provides for the development of secondary male sex characteristics and aids in the development of skeletal muscles.

Estrogens are required for the development of secondary female sex characteristics. Estrogen participates in the menstrual cycle along with progesterone. Estrogen has a tremendous ability to promote cell and overall tissue growth. During pregnancy, when cell and tissue growth proceed at maximum rates, the placenta is producing large quantities of estrogen.

The primary mineralocorticoid is aldosterone. Aldosterone works in the kidneys to regulate the balance of sodium, potassium, and hydrogen ions. This in turn affects blood volume and blood pressure.

The primary glucocorticoid is cortisol. Cortisol has many actions throughout the body. It promotes the breakdown of fat and protein tissues. It promotes the formation of glucose (the primary fuel for cells), utilizing the products of fat and protein breakdown. Cortisol is very important for the body's ability to deal with stress of all kinds: mental, surgical, traumatic injury, temperature, etc.

The length of time that these hormones last in the body is short. New hormone molecules must be made continuously, depending on the various physical conditions and situations to which the body is being subjected.

Next we will discuss something of which very few people are aware. We all know vitamin D is essential for the development of strong bones. Vitamin D is required for the absorption of calcium and phosphorus in the intestinal tract. Few people are aware that vitamin D molecules start out as cholesterol molecules! The ultraviolet rays of the sun act on cholesterol molecules in the skin to cause this transformation. Vitamin D molecules are necessary for the health of adults as well as children. Because of this need, vitamin D is added to milk and other foods. In the past, children in northern climates without sufficient sun exposure would develop a disease called rickets. In rickets the bone is soft and abnormal, and as a result the leg bones may bend outward.

Cholesterol molecules are also the starting points in the creation of bile salts. Bile salts are necessary for the absorption of fats from our intestinal tract. There are several important vitamins including A, E, and K that are absorbed along with the fats. It is important that we have fats in our diet and sufficient bile salts to absorb them.

3-6   Making Cholesterol for Cell Membranes

Nature has provided three methods in order to help insure that enough cholesterol molecules are available for use in cell membranes.

First, each cell has the capability to manufacture cholesterol. Energy, materials, and thirty enzymes are required for this task. The manufacturing of cholesterol takes place in the endoplasmic reticulum. Then, the molecules go to the Golgi apparatus where they are either stored for future use or immediately inserted into the cell's membrane.

Second, cells that are unable to make enough cholesterol themselves can depend on the liver for help. The liver makes significant amounts of cholesterol and also derives it from the foods passing through the intestines.

Third, cells can obtain cholesterol from other cells in the body through a type of "forced contribution" system. One of the actions of cortisol is to force cells to give up cholesterol (also protein and fats), and thus cells in need can fulfill their requirement.

There is a daily pattern of cholesterol synthesis in the human. Cholesterol synthesis is highest in the middle of the night when you are sleeping. During the day, the manufacturing of cholesterol molecules slows down.

This pattern is the result of two influences. First, the timing of when meals are eaten has an effect. If the body had not received sufficient food, then the making of cholesterol slows down.

Second, cortisol output by the adrenal glands reaches a peak around 11:00 a.m., just when daily physical activities are traditionally going strong. Cortisol forces cells to contribute cholesterol (also proteins and fats) to other cells that may temporarily have a greater need. Cortisol has another effect. It stops cholesterol production by blocking the actions of HMG-CoA reductase. Cortisol stops the production of cholesterol molecules so that foods will be used for energy production instead.

For the cells that have been forced by cortisol to contribute cholesterol, fats, and proteins, they will have the opportunity to replenish themselves at night, when cortisol levels go down and cholesterol synthesis goes up.

What are some of the factors that control cholesterol synthesis? In an individual cell, for instance, the process continues until the cell membrane and interior parts have more than enough. At some point, there is a sense of an excess of cholesterol, and it forces the enzyme we are now familiar with, HMG-CoA reductase, to stop working.

The liver slows down cholesterol synthesis whenever it senses that food passing through the intestine contains cholesterol that can be gathered for free.

3-7   Transporting Cholesterol

Cholesterol and fats (triglycerides) are collectively called lipids, because of the property they share; they do not dissolve in water or water-based solutions, such as blood.

A fatty acid does not have any ring structures. A fatty acid is simply a long string of carbon atoms with an acid group at one end.

Three of these fatty acid chains can be linked to a molecule of glycerol. This large molecule is called a triglyceride. "Triglycerides" mean the same thing as "fats."

Now, if only two fatty acid chains connect to a three-carbon glycerol group and on the third carbon is attached a phosphorus group, you then have a phospholipid.

All three of these molecules, the triglyceride fats, the phospholipids, and cholesterol, are called lipids.

It is necessary to have cholesterol, phospholipids, triglyceride fats, and fatty acids transported in blood. How is it done?

Nature has devised a system during evolution to transport these things using lipoproteins. A lipoprotein is a combination of a protein and a lipid. Most lipids being transported in the blood, either to or away from cells, are connected to lipoproteins.

Lipoproteins are classified according to their composition, size, and density.

They are all shaped like a ball or sphere, more or less. These lipoprotein spheres vary greatly in size. A chylomicron that carries mostly triglycerides may be 60 times larger than an HDL, which consists of cholesterol, phospholipids, and protein.

CHYL means chylomicron, VLDL stands for very low-density lipoprotein, LDL is low-density lipoprotein, and HDL is high-density lipoprotein.

COMPOSITION OF LIPOPROTEINS IN BLOOD PLASMA

Lipoprotein	Protein %	Cholesterol %	Phospholipid %	Triglyceride %
CHYL	1	4	7	88
VLDL	8	22	16	54
LDL	21	46	22	11
HDL	50	20	26	4

The protein of the lipoprotein particle is on the outside of the sphere. The protein will link up with special "receptors" on the surfaces of cells.

The protein part of a lipoprotein is called an apoprotein. It can also be referred to as an apolipoprotein.

We will mainly be concerned with three lipoproteins in this book. We will also be primarily concerned with the transport of cholesterol, because it is common to all membranes of the body. Just be aware that the different phospholipids and triglycerides are also moved via lipoproteins.

The three lipoproteins important to us in this book are low-density lipoprotein, or LDL; high-density lipoprotein, or HDL; and apolipoprotein E, or apo E. All three are intimately involved with transporting cholesterol molecules.

These proteins are designated with a specific letter. This helps clarify which apolipoprotein goes with which lipoprotein.

LIPOPROTEIN	APOLIPOPROTEIN	MOLECULAR WEIGHT
LDL	B-100	549,000
HDL	A	17,500
APO E	E	34,000

The low-density lipoprotein (LDL) has an apolipoprotein (B-100) that is much larger than the other two. LDL normally carries cholesterol molecules to the cells of the body from the liver.

High-density lipoprotein (HDL) has a much smaller apolipoprotein (A). It has a molecular weight of only 17,500, as compared to the B-100's weight of 549,000. HDL normally carries cholesterol molecules from cells to the liver, the reverse of LDL.

Apolipoprotein E is actually a type of high-density lipoprotein, or HDL, in most people. Rather than call it HDL-Apo E, it is referred to just by the name given to its protein, apolipoprotein E, or apo E in the shortest version.

Apo E is the primary lipoprotein that transports cholesterol in nervous tissues. By nervous tissues we mean the brain, the spinal cord, and the nerves throughout the body. In all tissues other than nervous tissues, cells receiving cholesterol get it from LDL.

3-8   LDL and Apo E

In this section we will briefly discuss the delivery of cholesterol molecules to cells. Remember cells possess the ability to manufacture some cholesterol molecules, but most cholesterol comes from lipoproteins transported through the blood.

Low-density lipoprotein (LDL) is the major carrier of cholesterol to the cells. It starts out in the liver as very-low density lipoprotein (VLDL), which contains a large amount of triglycerides as well as cholesterol.

When the liver sends off a VLDL, which subsequently becomes an LDL, it does not know which cell in which body tissue will get cholesterol from the LDL. The system works with a mechanism, whereby, those cells in the body that need cholesterol molecules will display a special receptor protein on the surfaces of their cell membranes. This receptor is a large protein and is called the low-density lipoprotein receptor. It is abbreviated as LDL-receptor.

Cells that are not in need of cholesterol molecules do not express (make visible) any LDL-receptors on their exterior cell membrane surfaces. Cells that do need cholesterol will express LDL-receptors. The B-100 protein portion of an LDL that may be passing by will fuse with the LDL-receptor and then be brought inside the cell, where the cholesterol molecules can be utilized. The LDL-receptor then cycles back to the membrane surface, ready to catch another LDL. If the cell has a satisfactory amount of cholesterol, it will stop expressing the LDL-receptor.

Each LDL-receptor can bind LDL because the B-100 protein fits neatly into it. The B-100 protein is a giant protein. Only one at a time can fit into the LDL-receptor.

Apolipoprotein E (apo E) carries cholesterol too, but it is smaller than an LDL. It also will bind to an LDL-receptor and donate cholesterol molecules. Because it is smaller, several apo E's can bind at the same time to one LDL-receptor.

Remember also that apo E is actually classified as a high-density lipoprotein (HDL) in most people. We normally think of HDL's as bringing excess cholesterol away from tissues and back to the liver. Here we have a type of HDL (apo E) doing the opposite—delivering cholesterol to the cells. Remember also that apo E is the lipoprotein that delivers cholesterol to the brain and other nervous tissues.

Let us review what we have covered:

1. If a cell is in need of cholesterol, it expresses an LDL-receptor on its cell membrane.
2. The large B-100 protein of a passing LDL binds to the LDL-receptor in a one-to-one ratio.
3. The LDL is brought into the cell where the cholesterol is utilized.
4. If the cell needs more cholesterol it expresses the LDL-receptor again.
5. Apo E also can bind to an LDL-receptor. Because apo E is much smaller than an LDL, each LDL-receptor can bind several apo E's at one time.
6. Apo E delivers cholesterol to the cells, in spite of it actually being classified as an HDL in most people. HDL's normally carry cholesterol away from cells.
7. Apo E's are the main carriers of cholesterol in brain and other nerve tissues.

3-9   Antioxidants and Cholesterol

Oxygen is necessary for life. The energy cells need is produced when oxygen is combined with carbon-based molecules in a specific, controlled manner. We call this process oxidation. Oxygen plus iron produces the red powder we call rust. The examples are endless.

In our bodies, oxygen atoms are transported from the lungs to our tissues in red blood cells. The oxygen atoms combine with carbons from glucose or fat. Not only is energy the result of the combination, but a significant amount of heat is also produced. Our body temperature is maintained through this process.

There is an unfortunate downside to this. Oxygen will also combine with molecules in our bodies in harmful ways. The heat we just mentioned serves to increase the rate of non-beneficial oxidation of molecules in our cells. Just how is this oxidation harmful to cells?

An intact cell membrane barrier is necessary in order to keep harmful things from getting into the cell and good things from leaking out of the cell. The cell membrane is made up of cholesterol molecules and phospholipid molecules.

If a membrane molecule, especially a cholesterol molecule, had an oxygen atom combine with it on another place on one of its rings, then it would be pulled out of the membrane by the attraction of the water-based solution. Multiply this by the hundreds of cholesterol molecules in a cell's membrane and you will have the death of the cell.

Oxygen atoms can be found to exist in several forms that are harmful to cells. The "superoxide anion radical" is oxygen with an extra electron that readily combines with molecules in tissues. When people talk of damage caused by "free radicals," it is usually the superoxide anion to which they are referring.

Another harmful form of oxygen is found in hydrogen peroxide. Hydrogen peroxide is very injurious to cell membranes.

Our bodies do not just sit idly by and let oxidation processes occur. There is a constant battle going on to counteract the damaging effects of oxidation. Several vitamins have antioxidant properties that our bodies try and utilize. Vitamin C, also known as ascorbic acid, is a water-soluble vitamin that protects against oxidation, especially the oxidation of cholesterol. A deficiency of vitamin C causes the disease called scurvy. In the past, sailors on long sea voyages would develop scurvy. Their symptoms were bleeding gums around the teeth. They would be unable to eat, especially if the gum sores got so bad that bone became exposed around the roots of their teeth. To prevent scurvy, sailing ships would stock up at every port with fruit, which contains vitamin C.

Vitamin E is a fat-soluble antioxidant vitamin that also protects cholesterol molecules from oxidation. In fact, the primary antioxidant vitamin found in brain and other nerve tissues just happens to be vitamin E. However, vitamin E deficiency alone does not cause Alzheimer's.

What is the best antioxidant for the protection of cell membranes against oxidation processes? The answer is a fresh supply of cholesterol molecules. Why else would our bodies have such an elaborate production and distribution system for cholesterol molecules?

3-10   Stop Using the Terms "Good" and "Bad" Cholesterol

In the 1950's and 1960's the notion that cholesterol and heart disease were linked became prevalent in scientific circles.

First, it was said the measurement called total cholesterol indicated who would and would not have a heart attack. Then it was said a "high" LDL measurement would indicate someone who would have a heart attack, since LDL was cholesterol going to the tissues. Then it was thought a ratio of some measurements, either LDL to HDL, or total cholesterol to HDL, etc., would pinpoint who would have a heart attack. Why are new theories constantly being developed as to the cause of heart attacks? Because there is still no dependable way of telling ahead of time those who will have a heart attack.

Back when it was thought a high LDL measurement would supposedly pinpoint who would have a heart attack, it was some researcher's idea to start calling LDL the "bad" cholesterol because of this. Since HDL carried cholesterol away from cells, including cells in arteries, it was decided to call HDL the "good" cholesterol. Now as I briefly pointed out in the earlier paragraphs, the research of heart disease theory has evolved far past the point of using just an LDL measurement to determine those at highest risk. However, the "bad" and "good" cholesterol labels for LDL and HDL are still being used today.

There are plenty of people with "high" levels of LDL cholesterol who do not suffer heart attacks, and there are people with "low" or "safe" LDL cholesterol levels who do have heart attacks. The relationship between cholesterol and heart disease is just not that simple.

For those rare people born with familial hypercholesterolemia there is a connection that is simple to see. But these are people with blood cholesterol levels of 500, 600, or 700 mg/dl or more, measurements that are far above the average person.

I suggest that the scientific and nutrition communities stop using the simplistic labels of "good" and "bad" for HDL and LDL cholesterol.

3-11   Measuring Blood Cholesterol Levels

What are "normal" cholesterol levels? The short answer is, it depends on with whom you are talking. Scientists associated with the National Cholesterol Education Program (NCEP) recommend the optimal adult level of total cholesterol should be under 200 mg/dl. An adult with total cholesterol between 200 and 240 mg/dl is said to be at risk for heart disease. Over 240 mg/dl and you fall into the high-risk category.

The NCEP recommends that the total cholesterol measurement be used as an initial screening tool only. Before any actual treatment therapy is begun, the patient should have a total lipoprotein profile. The blood levels of total cholesterol (TC), high-density lipoprotein (HDL), and triglycerides (TG) are measured.

The use of the TC, HDL, and TG's levels calculates the amount of low-density lipoprotein (LDL). The NCEP recommends basing treatment decisions on the calculated level of LDL. Also to be considered along with the LDL level is the presence of any risk factors such as smoking, high blood pressure, family history of heart disease, etc.

The levels of LDL are said to be "healthy" at less than 130mg/dl, "risky" between 130 and 160 mg/dl, and if over 160, then drug treatment to lower the levels should be considered. There are some in this field who think people should try to lower their LDL level to less than 100mg/dl in order to be "safe."

The official recommendations are that diet and exercise should be the first therapies for people with "high risk" LDL levels. If after a period of time the LDL and total cholesterol levels do not decrease, then drug therapies are to be considered.

We will now discuss the numbers in cholesterol testing, since so much emphasis and medical decision-making are based on them.

A fasting level of cholesterol is used in attempts to standardize the measurements. A "morning samples only" may add some consistency. Cholesterol values can change as much as eight percent in the same patient depending on what time of day the sample is taken. This means a patient's theoretical true cholesterol of 200 mg/dl might test to anywhere from 184 to 216 mg/dl.

From one day to the next may mean an even greater variation in measurements, up to fifteen percent. A potential fifteen percent variation means that on Monday, Mrs. Smith's total cholesterol value may read 200 mg/dl, and on Tuesday may read 230 mg/dl.

The patient's position may also have an effect, believe it or not. Blood samples drawn when a patient is lying down may read up to fifteen percent lower than when the patient is upright. So which cholesterol measurement should be used? Upright, lying horizontally, or at an angle somewhere in between?

With cholesterol variations ranging normally from 8 to fifteen percent, due to such things as time of day, patient position, and even the particular day of the week, it becomes important to consider these factors.

Returning to my earlier question about what constitutes "normal" cholesterol values, not only does it matter who you ask, it depends on whether or not the person you are asking happens to be aware of the potentially large variations possible when measuring blood cholesterol levels.

3-12   Your Skin and Hair Must Have Cholesterol

The cell membrane consists of cholesterol and phospholipid molecules "floating in a bilayer." There are attractions between the parts of the molecules, but they are not rigidly "glued" to one another.

Skin is made up of epithelial cells, which are produced by keratinocytes. But what holds these epithelial cells together? To me, "floating" bilayer of cholesterol and phospholipid molecules does not sound strong enough to perform the task of holding our skin cells together. Is there some type of "glue" in our skin cells?

The answer is yes. A sulfur group is attached at the sterol end of the cholesterol molecule to create cholesterol sulfate. These cholesterol sulfate molecules make up a significant percentage in the deeper layers of our skin. These deeper layers provide the strong attachment properties that hold our skin to the connective tissues underneath.

Cholesterol sulfate is the glue that holds our skin together. However, we know our skin is continuously sloughed off. If cholesterol holds the skin together, how can layers be lost at the same time?

The answer is, cholesterol sulfate molecules are able to freely migrate through epithelial cells. Other molecules in skin such as plain cholesterol, ceramides, and fatty acids, stay with the epithelial cells as they progress in an external direction, until they reach the top layer where they are sloughed off as dead cells. It may be more accurate to say that the growing epithelial skin cells are migrating while the cholesterol sulfate molecules are staying in the deeper layers of cells.

Not only are cholesterol sulfate molecules key to the skin's adhesive properties, they are also important for the maintenance of the waterproof, germ-proof, and solvent-proof properties of the skin.

By solvent-proof, I mean various substances with the ability to dissolve some things that will not readily dissolve on our skin. The first ones that come to mind are soaps and detergents, however, there are many others. An especially good example is dishwashing detergent. Here is something that will dissolve baked-on grease, yet our skin seems to be unaffected by it. Why, your hands may even end up feeling softer!

Hair is very durable in spite of its non-rigid character. Of what does hair consist? Plain cholesterol, ceramides, free fatty acids, fatty alcohols, and of course, cholesterol sulfate. Hair maintains its properties under normal washing techniques, time after time. Think of all the chemicals used in hair products. To me, hair is amazing in its ability to withstand everything that is done to it in the name of beauty.

Remember that one of the most important "glues" in our body is made from cholesterol molecules. Our skin and hair depend on it.

CHAPTER 4
Introduction to the Brain

4-1   Neurons, Cholesterol and Glucose

The cells that are the functional units in brain tissue are neurons, which are similar to other cells in the body. The cell membrane of a neuron is made up of cholesterol and phospholipid molecules arranged in the familiar bilayer pattern, two molecules in width.

Neurons are responsible for sending and receiving messages. Each neuron has a branch projecting away called an axon. The axon transmits signals from the neuron to other neurons, body organs, or muscles. Each neuron has just one axon.

Neurons receive signals through branches called dendrites. In contrast to the one axon per neuron arrangement, each neuron can have many dendrites.

The signals neurons send and receive are called nerve impulses. It takes a large amount of energy to generate and transmit these nerve impulses. The fuel used by the brain to provide this energy is glucose (blood sugar), just like in other body tissues. However, the neurons of the brain are different in that very large amounts of glucose are required. It must be supplied via the blood circulation in an uninterrupted stream.

The connecting points between axons and dendrites are called synapses. The axon from one neuron and the dendrite from another do not physically touch in the synapse. There is a small space between them. The nerve impulse must "jump" across this space. A neurotransmitter molecule is released when the signal reaches the synapse. When released, these molecules cause the nerve impulse to continue on through the dendrite side of the connection and on to the next neuron.

The membranes on either side of the space in a synapse are no different from other cell membranes. However, the bilayers of cholesterol and phospholipid molecules in the membranes of a synapse are subject to a significantly greater amount of stress than in other cell membranes. It is critical for healthy brain functioning that the membranes in synapses are replenished adequately.

4-2   Myelin and Cholesterol

The signals that flow through nerves are electrochemical impulses. The impulse is a wave formed by the movement of ions in and out of the membrane of the nerve fiber. These ions are charged atoms of sodium and potassium.

Just as a wave travels along the surface of the ocean, nerve impulses flow by wave action through our nerve fibers. In an ocean wave the water molecules move in relation to the ocean's surface, but they do not move along horizontally with the wave onto the shore. In nerve fibers, the ions move in relation to the nerve membrane, but they do not move along with the nerve impulse wave to the end of the nerve fiber.

In electricity, electrons flow through the metal at the speed of light, which is 186,000 miles per second. In our bodies, nerve impulse speeds are measured in feet per second, not thousands of miles per second. Nerve impulse speeds vary from one foot per second up to 300 feet per second. There are different types of nerves in our body, which account for the different speeds of impulses.

The nerve fibers we are speaking of are axons. The impulse flows through the axon and as it does some of the ions leak into the surrounding tissues. Permanent leakage of ions out of the membrane results in a slower and less efficient impulse.

To improve the speed and efficiency of nerve impulses, nature has developed an insulating cover for some nerve fibers. This insulating covering is called myelin. Myelin prevents the leakage and wasting of ions into the tissue around a nerve fiber. As a result of myelination, the impulse wave travels much faster. It also travels in a more efficient manner because less energy is wasted.

Myelin is structured the same way a typical cell membrane bilayer is structured, with a few differences.

The major difference between the regular cell membrane bilayer and the myelin bilayer is in the percentage of lipids that make up each bilayer. The regular cell membrane bilayer is about 50 percent lipid (cholesterol and phospholipids). The myelin bilayer is almost 80 percent lipid.

This, then, is the reason why myelin is white in color and flexible-it is almost 80 percent lipid. Thus, the internal areas of our brain are called white matter because the areas consist of myelinated fibers.

Myelin is wrapped around nerve fibers in what is referred to as "jellyroll" fashion. In the central nervous system (CNS), which consists only of the brain and spinal cord, the myelin is supplied and maintained by cells called oligodendrocytes. In the peripheral nervous system, which consists of the nerves of the body in all areas outside of the brain and spinal cord, the myelin is supplied and maintained by Schwann cells.

In myelin, 40 percent of the lipid molecules are cholesterol molecules. Nature invented myelin to wrap around and around nerve fibers. The only way to maintain barrier integrity while wrapping in concentric layers is to have a large number of cholesterol molecules. Remember also that nerves themselves need to be flexible and resistant to damage from physical movements. Myelin, with its high cholesterol content, is ideal for these functions.

It is interesting also to note that between the concentric wrappings of myelin layers are trapped deposits of a salt-and-water solution. This trapped water does at least three things. First, it adds to the electrical insulating capability around the nerve fibers. Second, it helps provide a cushion against abrupt physical movements. The "fatty" nature of myelin provides a cushion. Third, the water helps to stabilize the temperature of myelin and nerve fibers. Water has a great capacity to absorb heat. This protects against heat build-up. Research has shown that heating above normal body temperature causes myelin to become thinner, which in turn affects nerve impulse conduction.

In the peripheral nervous system (the nerves of the body outside the brain and spinal cord), Schwann cells provide a nerve's myelin. There are hundreds and even thousands of Schwann cells on each nerve fiber, depending on how long the fiber is. Some fibers are three or more feet in length. Each Schwann cell provides a myelin wrapping of one small segment of nerve fiber.

In the CNS (the brain and spinal cord) there are billions of neurons and their nerve fibers. These fibers are arranged in bundles. The oligodendrocytes provide the myelin for these CNS fibers. The neurons and their bundled fibers are in a limited amount of space in the brain and spinal cord, and everything is squeezed closely together. Each oligodendrocyte supplies the myelin wrappings for 20 to 40 nerve fibers of neurons. An oligodendrocyte has branches called "processes" that connect to the 20 to 40 nerve fibers.

The speed of nerve impulses depends on two things. This first one is the diameter of the fiber. The larger the fiber, the faster the impulse will travel. Secondly, the thicker the coating of myelin, the faster and more efficient will be the nerve impulse.

This concept may be summarized in a few sentences:

1. Small, unmyelinated nerve fibers have the slowest nerve impulse speeds.
2. Large nerve fibers with thick myelin coatings have the fastest nerve impulse speeds.
3. A small nerve fiber with a thick myelin coating has a fast nerve impulse speed, and also consumes less energy, making it efficient as a result. This third category describes what we find in the human brain. Our brain has billions of neurons and small myelinated nerve fibers, all in a confined space.

In humans, myelination of nerves begins before birth and is completed by the second to third year of life. In situations of extreme starvation in early childhood, myelination may not occur properly. The child may develop a mental retardation. This mental retardation from starvation or malnutrition cannot be corrected, even if a healthy diet is provided later in childhood.

Cholesterol is the most important molecule found in myelin. How do we know this? There was an experiment performed in which developing laboratory animals were given a chemical that inhibits the body's production of cholesterol molecules. The animals were fed a healthy diet. The other components of myelin (phospholipids, proteins, etc.) were still produced in a normal amount. Only cholesterol molecules were limited. The result was that decreased amounts of myelin were produced in direct proportion to the decreased amounts of cholesterol molecules. Again, this was in spite of normal production of the other components of myelin.

It has traditionally been assumed that once myelin forms around nerve fibers, it will remain basically stable and unchanged forever. There is research, however, which shows that myelin is not as inactive and stable as many in the medical community believe. There is a measurable amount of cholesterol turnover in myelin in the brain. By turnover, I mean the removal of oxidized and damaged cholesterol molecules and their replacement with "fresh" cholesterol molecules. This turnover rate is slower in myelin than in other tissues of the body, but it does occur.

As evidence of this need for "fresh" molecules of cholesterol in myelin throughout life, let me discuss briefly a disease called abetalipoproteinemia. In this disease, the patients have very few low-density lipoproteins (LDL's) in the blood. In these patients it has been demonstrated that there are defects in myelin in the brain and loss of nerve fibers that normally have large myelin coatings.

This is a book about Alzheimer's disease, so it would be fair for the reader to ask if there is evidence of defects in myelin in this disease. The answer is yes. There is specific evidence of damage to myelin in Alzheimer's disease. As for general evidence of myelin problems in Alzheimer's, remember these things:

1. In the human brain, 33 percent of its dry weight is made up of myelin.
2. The most abundant molecule found in myelin is cholesterol.
3. In Alzheimer's disease the brain shrinks in size and weight and there is found the condition called "myelin pallor."

Myelin pallor is the descriptive term that means the myelinated fiber tissue of the brain, specifically the white matter areas, are pale, and it is due to there actually being less amounts of myelin in these areas.

On a brain MRI, the difference between the whiter and darker (gray) areas of the image of the brain has been shown to be due to the cholesterol content of the tissues. The whitest areas on an MRI are the areas with the most cholesterol.

4-3   Other Cells of the Brain

There is a vast network of supporting cells in the brain that are not directly involved in nerve signal transmissions. These supporting cells are known as glial cells or glia. They are smaller than neurons. There are almost ten times as many glial supporting cells as there are neurons in the human brain.

Oligodendrocytes make the myelin that covers the nerve fibers in the central nervous system.

Oligodendrocytes have a high rate of metabolism, especially during active myelination. In humans, this occurs in the first two or three years of life.

Oligodendrocytes make cholesterol molecules, but they also receive apolipoprotein E (apo E) particles from the bloodstream. Apo E transports cholesterol molecules (and lipids) in the nervous system. I interpret this to mean that at least in the mature nervous system, oligodendrocytes rely to some extent on outside sources of cholesterol molecules for the maintenance of myelin coverings.

Astrocytes are related to oligodendrocytes, but they do not produce myelin. Astrocytes provide a structure for the brain. I think of it as a soft skeleton. However, they also serve many other functions.

Astrocytes cover the synapses between neurons. They can capture and recycle neurotransmitters for use by neurons. Astrocytes provide a chemical buffer zone for the protections of neurons. They store glucose for use by neurons.

Astrocytes make cholesterol molecules because they must maintain cell membrane integrity, which in turn maintains the strong supporting structure. Astrocytes also receive apo E, the transporter of cholesterol in the brain. This means that astrocytes, like oligodendrocytes, must rely on the bloodstream as a source of cholesterol, in addition to the cholesterol molecules they make themselves.

Microglia are small cells with spike-like projections. Microglia move around and have protective functions.

Microglia react to brain trauma by scavenging up dead neuron fragments.

In normal healthy states, the microglia are at rest.

In Alzheimer's disease the microglia are activated, proving there is some type of inflammatory process occurring. In addition, microglia produce amyloid during these confrontations with inflamed brain tissues. We will discuss this in a later section.

4-4   The Cell Skeleton

In the human body, bones are arranged in a skeleton to act as the basic support structure. Muscles act on the bones to produce movement. In cells there are components with similar properties. Instead of muscle and bones, we use the terms filaments and microtubules in speaking of the cell's cytoskeleton. The word cytoskeleton means both the rigid components of a cell and the parts that act like muscles and tendons in a cell.

There are two types of filaments inside cells, microfilaments and intermediate filaments. Both types function as elastic support structures in a cell. They can change the outer shape of a cell.

Microtubules are hollow, cylindrical tube structures of various lengths. They have the unique properties of being able to assemble or disassemble in an instant. The job of the microtubules is to move things around in the cell. Nutrients need to be moved into the cell, wastes need to be moved out, and inner structures need to be moved.

Microtubules are formed when proteins called tubulins are arranged into long, hollow, cylindrical tubes. Small phosphoproteins are in control of the process of arranging tubulin proteins into microtubules. These phosphoproteins are referred to as tau proteins. Without tau protein, tubulins cannot be formed into microtubules.

In the brain, neurons have abundant amounts of tau protein, and it is concentrated in the axon part of each neuron. This is the hardest-working part of a neuron, thus it is understandable that tau protein and microtubules would be abundant there.

Tau protein with extra phosphorus groups is said to be hyperphosphorylated. When tau is hyperphosphorylated, it not only stops binding to microtubules, but it begins to bind with other tau protein segments that are also hyperphosphorylated.

The microtubules disassemble when tau protein is no longer binding to them, and as a result the moving processes inside the cell slow down and eventually stop. The health of the cell is then at risk.

When hyperphosphorylated tau protein segments bind to each other instead of the microtubules, they do so in pairs. As the two tau protein segments bind to each other, they assume a twisted formation.

When clusters of tau are seen in neurons, they are called neurofibrillary tangles. The presence of these neurofibrillary tangles means that the neurons were either dying or were already dead at the time of the patient's death.

These neurofibrillary tangles are one of the two microscopic findings in the brains of Alzheimer's patients. The other finding is the presence of amyloid plaques.

What causes this hyperphosphorylation of tau protein? It is through the action of an enzyme that is already found normally in the cell.

The enzyme most likely to cause tau protein to become hyperphosphorylated is glycogen synthase kinase three-beta. We will refer to it as glycogen synthase kinase.

(There are representative drawings of tau protein, microtubules, etc. at the end of the book.)

4-5   The Blood-Brain Barrier

The most complex part of our body is the brain. The neurons and other cells need a constant supply of oxygen and glucose. Carbon dioxide and waste products must be removed quickly. The ability of the neurons to transmit signals is affected by the contents of the bloodstream.

To protect the brain's nerve signals from being affected by certain substances, there is a "shield" called the blood-brain barrier. The blood-brain barrier is not a separate membrane layer. Capillaries (tiny blood vessels) are slightly different in the brain as compared to other capillaries in other parts of the body. The cells that make up the walls of capillaries are called endothelial cells. In the brain's capillaries, the endothelial cells hold each other more tightly than do the endothelial cells of capillaries in other body areas. They are said to exhibit tight junctions.

Because of these tight junctions between the endothelial cells in brain capillaries, there is limited access from the bloodstream to brain tissue. Substances that readily pass from the blood into muscle or liver tissue may be stopped by this blood-brain barrier.

Some of the substances that pass readily through the blood-brain barrier into brain tissues are oxygen and glucose. The brain cannot go without oxygen for more than about ten seconds. Neurons in the brain have only enough stored glucose to last two to three minutes at the most. Water, carbon dioxide, and essential amino acids readily pass through the blood-brain barrier. Substances that dissolve lipids, such as alcohol and various medical anesthetics, can easily pass through.

There are some substances that have a slight ability to pass through, not as easily as those mentioned in the previous paragraphs. These slightly permeable substances include electrolytes such as potassium, sodium, and chloride.

Substances that do not pass across a healthy, functioning blood-brain barrier include large proteins and things that do not dissolve lipids. Many wastes from other tissues, such as urea, are prevented from entering the brain.

The blood-brain barrier is present in most, but not all the areas of the brain. For instance, the hypothalamus, which monitors the chemical make-up of the blood, has no blood-brain barrier in the capillaries that serve it. The hypothalamus checks for the build-up of toxins and waste products. It also regulates the amount of water in the body and the temperature of the body.

The brain uses several different kinds of molecules as neurotransmitters, which are chemical signals. Many of these neurotransmitters are plentiful in the general circulation of the body. The blood-brain barrier keeps the ones from the general circulation separate from those in the brain. This prevents neurons from being overloaded with chemical signals, which can result in uncoordinated and even dangerous nerve electrochemical firings.

This book is about Alzheimer's disease. Alzheimer's patients have been shown to exhibit an altered blood-brain barrier.

This book is also about cholesterol. Remember that the cell membranes of these capillary endothelial cells are just like all other cells in that they have cholesterol molecules in them. Do the tight junctions keep cholesterol that is circulating in the bloodstream from entering the brain tissue? The answer is no. There are low-density lipoprotein receptors on the endothelial cells of brain capillaries. Brain capillaries allow the brain to take up LDL's that are carrying cholesterol molecules by using these LDL-receptors. You will remember that apolipoprotein E is the major carrier of cholesterol in the brain, and that apo E readily binds to the LDL-receptors, also.

Not only is cholesterol transported across the blood-brain barrier into the brain, cholesterol levels in the bloodstream can affect the degree of permeability of the barrier. In animal experiments it has been shown that high blood cholesterol levels can lead to a decreased ability for various things to cross the blood-brain barrier. You will recall from an earlier section that higher cholesterol levels lead to decreased membrane fluidity. Lower cholesterol levels lead to higher membrane fluidity. The research leads one to conclude that if high cholesterol levels cause decreased blood-brain barrier permeability (fewer things can cross), then the opposite should also be true. That is, that lower cholesterol levels cause increased blood-barrier permeability (more things can cross as the blood-barrier becomes "leaky").

The blood-brain barrier also effectively keeps various medicines from entering the brain. This has been a problem for people with illnesses such as brain tumors. Fortunately, a way was found to treat these people. The solution was to connect the anti-tumor drugs to cholesterol molecules in chemical preparations called liposomes. As the brain tissue takes up the cholesterol/liposome preparation through the blood-brain barrier, it is also taking up the beneficial anti-tumor medicine.

4-6   Apo E Transports Cholesterol in the Brain

Apolipoprotein E is the major carrier of cholesterol in the brain and other parts of the nervous system. It is also found throughout the body and is produced by the liver, spleen, and kidneys. Apolipoprotein E is usually referred to as apo E.

Apo E is technically classified as an HDL in most people. Apo E binds to the LDL-receptor, and several can fit at the same time, because it is smaller than an LDL.

Apo E has been found to be very important for healthy nerve (neuron) development and maintenance. This includes the growth and maintenance of the myelin coverings around nerve axons.

Neurons use the same mechanism that other cells in the body use regarding cholesterol. If a neuron needs cholesterol it displays an LDL-receptor on its membrane. An apo E carrying cholesterol binds to it. Neurons not in need of cholesterol keep their LDL-receptors hidden inside of their membranes.

Apo E has been shown to be important when neurons are damaged by trauma, disease, or what can best be described as normal wear-and-tear, especially at the synapses. In areas of nerve injury there are found high amounts of apo E. It has a great ability to scavenge cholesterol molecules in areas of nerve injury. By picking up cholesterol, apo E acts much like HDL's. The salvaged cholesterol is then directly used for repair and regeneration of nerve cell axons and the rebuilding of myelin sheaths.

What is the proof that cholesterol is a key ingredient in the repair of nerve axons? In experiments performed with neurons in laboratory cultures, apo E of two different types was added to the cultures. Axon regeneration and remyelination were measured. One type of apo E that contained cholesterol was shown to promote regeneration and remyelination of axons. Another type of apo E was added in which the cholesterol molecules had been removed. In these cultures there was no growth or remyelination of the nerve axons.

The synapses of neurons are the critical components in the nervous system. Problems at synapses are devastating to the functional processes of the brain. Synapses are active and stressful places and the cell membranes of the terminals on each side of the synaptic space require adequate amounts of cholesterol molecules. In experiments with animals that were specifically bred to be deficient in apo E, there was degeneration of the animals' central nervous systems. The damage was severe at the terminals. The degeneration of the synapses leads to the loss of nerve signal transmissions and eventually to the death of the neurons.

In similar experiments, laboratory animals lacking apo E were subjected to head and brain injuries. The animals did not recover very well when compared to injured animals with normal levels of apo E.

The hippocampus is the part of the limbic system that is critically involved with learning and memory. The hippocampus must have adequate amounts of cholesterol as was just pointed out. Proof of this was also found using animals specifically bred to be lacking in apo E. These animals were unable to learn and memorize ways of getting out of a maze that was set up in the laboratory. These animals continuously bumped into the walls of the maze. This was in contrast to the animals with normal amounts of apo E. These normal animals had no trouble learning and memorizing ways to escape the maze.

Apo E is said to possess antioxidant effects. It is also said to have beneficial immune system influences. Both of these properties are directly related to the delivery of cholesterol molecules by apo E. The best antioxidants are "fresh" cholesterol molecules.

It is important to study apo E because it binds to and transports beta amyloid almost the same as it binds to and transports cholesterol. Beta amyloid is the substance that accumulates in the brains of people with Alzheimer's disease.

4-7   Apo E, Microtubules, and Tau Protein: Summary

Apo E is the primary carrier protein of cholesterol molecules in the brain and other nervous system tissues. Apo E delivers cholesterol to neurons by binding to the LDL-receptors on the cell membranes. Apo E is found inside the neuron as well. Tau protein segments are important for the assembly of microtubules, which are the movers of substances (including cholesterol) inside the neuron. When tau binds to itself it begins the process of becoming a neurofibrillary tangle.

Obviously the tau protein in a neurofibrillary tangle is not stabilizing the formation and function of microtubules. If microtubules are not forming, then substances(including cholesterol) are not being moved around in the neuron. The health of the neuron suffers. Damage and death will eventually occur. This is the real significance of seeing neurofibrillary tangles in a neuron.

4-8   The Human Brain is Different

Under a microscope, human brain tissue looks like the brain tissue of other mammals. The neurons, astrocytes, oligodendrocytes, etc., from horses, mice, rats, dogs, and humans are remarkably similar in appearance; they also function in similar ways. How is the human brain different from brains of other mammals? It is different in two respects: relative size and degree of encephalization. The term encephalization means the amount of grooves and fissures present in the brain. The more grooves and fissures present, the greater the surface area of the brain, and the higher the degree of intelligence.

In relation to body size, humans have the largest brains of all the mammals. In fact, the larger the body size of a mammalian species, the smaller the brain in relation. The only full-size mammals that come close to humans regarding brain size and degree of encephalization are the dolphins.

A typical human brain weighs about 3.3 pounds (we can use the weight of brains as a good indicator of brain size). If we compare this to a typical human body weight of 155 pounds, we get a comparison ration of 0.021, or 2.1 percent. Therefore, a typical human brain makes up 2.1 percent of total body weight.

This is about the same percentage as that found in small animals such as rats and squirrels. But when the human brain measurement of 2.1 percent is compared to all mammals larger than a dog, the human brain is the largest by far in relation to body size.

In comparing the full-size mammals' ratios to the ratio of human brains, an elephant has a brain-to-body ratio of 0.55 percent, while the typical gorilla ratio is less at 0.24 percent. Again we find that the human's ratio of 2.1 percent is much larger.

There are two reasons why I am discussing the fact that humans possess a relative brain size far greater than other full-size mammals. First, the number of neurons and their connections to other neurons increase geometrically when the absolute volume of brain tissue increases. Volume increases according to the following progression: 1,8,27,64,125, and so forth. The geometric increases in number of neurons and their connections to other neurons are directly related to geometric increases in degrees of intelligence.

The result of this huge difference in the intellectual capability of humans over other animals is that humans are at the top of the evolutionary ladder. Humans do not run fast, they are not strong, they do not hear or see the best, they do not possess the sharpest sense of smell, and they do not withstand weather extremes without the help of clothing. It is the intelligence that goes along with having the largest brain relative to body size that has placed humans at the top.

The second reason why I am discussing the large brain size of humans is that there is a drawback to this situation. This drawback is based on the fact that brain tissue is a hot bed of activity in terms of metabolism. Generating and sending electrochemical signals consumes high amounts of fuel (glucose) and oxygen. Much heat is produced, and this heat, along with oxidation, causes damage that must be repaired in a never-ending manner. The relatively large brains in humans indicates that it is a big job to keep the "thinking machine" going and in good shape. The human brain constitutes only 2 percent of the total body mass, yet the brain's operation and upkeep accounts for 15 percent of the body's total metabolism!

4-9   The Human Brain and Evolution

There is a simple diagram of the human brain at the end of this book.

Olfactory is the term that pertains to the sense of smell. Olfactory nerve endings in the upper nasal/sinus region are connected to the brain via the two olfactory bulbs and the olfactory cortex. The olfactory cortex is part of the temporal lobe of the brain.

From an evolutionary standpoint, the sense of smell is very important. In most mammals, a functioning olfactory system can mean the difference between life and death. Many aspects of mating also depend on the use of the olfactory system.

The olfactory areas of the brain are very active metabolically. High metabolic activity means high rates of energy production from glucose, high oxygen requirements, and high production of wastes that must be removed. It also means that higher amounts of harmful byproducts of oxidation, such as free radicals, are also produced. This means there is a higher need for replenishment of various required substances, including cholesterol. One of the references listed at the end of the book details the activity of an enzyme called G6PD. It is involved in the production of energy that is, in turn, used for the production of cholesterol and fatty acids. In the olfactory bulbs, this enzyme has an activity level that is four times greater than in other parts of the brain.

If one part of the brain typically has a higher metabolic rate than other parts of the brain, then a condition of chronic malnutrition or semi-starvation and/or chronic low cholesterol levels may lead to damage to or at least a deficit in that area.

Is there evidence of damage or a decrease in function of the olfactory system in patients with Alzheimer's disease? The answer is yes. Often one of the earliest signs of Alzheimer's disease is an altered sense of smell.

The olfactory cortex is part of the temporal lobe of the brain. This is where the conscious awareness of an odor occurs. How we humans react to an odor originates here. However, the area in a human brain taken up by the olfactory cortex is small compared to the brains of other mammals, even though the human brain overall is much larger.

If you stop and think about it, humans do have a smaller capability in the area of smell sensation compared to most other mammals. Humans cannot track another animal by smelling the ground, cannot mark the boundaries of a territory and detect those boundaries using odors, and cannot tell if a bear or lion is sneaking up in an effort to have a human for a meal.

If we as humans now have less capability for smell sensation because of a smaller olfactory apparatus, what became of the structures of our ancestors' brains that were part of a larger olfactory system? In other words, evolutionary processes in the human brain have changed parts of the olfactory structures over time. What have ancient olfactory tissues been changed into? If we cannot smell as well as our prehistoric ancestors, what did we get in return as an evolutionary trade-off?

Researchers have determined that the olfactory structures of prehistoric humans evolved over time into new structures. The name given to the area at the base of the brain where these changes have taken place is rhinencephalon, which means, "nose-brain." Over time, evolutionary processes turned the ancient nose-brain structures (used only to detect smells) into structures that humans now use for complex memory, learning, thinking, and emotions. These modern human structures, derived from the primitive nose-brain, include the hippocampus, the hypothalamus, the amygdale, and the anterior nucleus of the thalamus. As we learned earlier, they comprise the limbic system.

The anatomical connections of the limbic system are very complex; and the system interacts with almost every other area of the brain. The limbic system governs our emotions, logic, reasoning, personality, behavior, and the interactions of food and hunger. The hippocampus plays an important role in memory, along with the amygdala. Information—its recognition, storage, retrieval, and usage, are all functions of the hippocampus. Most of the regions of the cerebral cortex are connected in one way or another with the hippocampus.

Although the limbic structures started out in prehistoric human ancestors as simply part of an odor-recognition system, they now function in ways that make the human brain the most advanced brain on the planet.

If parts of the olfactory system have been determined to have a high metabolic activity rate, then it is safe to presume that the limbic system, which evolved from olfactory structures, also has a high rate of metabolism. It follows that more nutrition, oxygen, waste removal, and fresh cholesterol are needed. Also needed is more neutralizing of harmful free radicals by the antioxidation mechanisms in the brain.

What would happen if all of the beneficial processes were not maintained? Damage to the neurons of the limbic system, and specifically the hippocampus, may result. Damage to the hippocampus results in memory problems.

The limbic system is what makes humans different from other animals. It is the hardest working part of the brain. Humans can out-think any other animal on Earth.

As we age, our capability to provide maintenance slows down. The limbic system is, over a long period of time, vulnerable to shortcomings in nutrition, antioxidant activity, and fresh cholesterol supplementation.

In conclusion, the hippocampus and other structures of the limbic system are what separate humans from other mammals. The limbic system is an area of high metabolic rates, which means a high level of maintenance is required. As we get older, it becomes more difficult to provide this high level of maintenance. Oxidation of the cell membranes' components is going to occur. If maintenance, which includes the supplying of fresh cholesterol molecules, does not keep up, then neurons will die. Dying neurons in the limbic system (and cortex) are, in fact, the definition of Alzheimer's disease.

4-10   Human Brain Metabolism

The human brain has a very high concentration of cholesterol and fat molecules confined in a relatively small area. All lipid tissues in the body, including the brain, are subject to being damaged by oxidation processes. In the various places on the human body where fat is deposited, the actual measurements of metabolic activity are low. The processes involved with keeping the human organism alive are actually taking place in other parts of the body, such as the heart, skeletal muscles, lungs, brain, and the various organs. Since the body's fat deposits are relatively less active metabolically, the exposure to oxidation processes is much lower.

As an example of the susceptibility of lipid tissue to oxidation, trim some fat off of a refrigerated cut of meat. Leave the fat in an open place, at room temperature or above (remember that body temperature is 98.6 degrees Fahrenheit). Within a short time, the fat will show signs of becoming rancid. Rancid means the same thing as being oxidized. The fat inside our bodies would get rancid if it were not relatively insulated from exposure to the oxygen and tissues that are very active metabolically.

The brain is one place where a high concentration of lipid tissues must coexist with a very high concentration of metabolic activity. It takes a great amount of energy to send nerve impulses, and consequently, high amounts of fuel (glucose) and oxygen must be provided to supply this energy. The chemical burning of glucose produces heat as well as energy. Oxygen is carried to the brain using atoms of iron in the blood, and iron has been shown to promote oxidation processes.

Let's add up all these variables. There is an abundance of heat from the burning of glucose, there is ample oxygen, there are great quantities of iron atoms, and the huge amounts of cholesterol and other lipid molecules are in close proximity. This has to be considered as a setting for a potential disaster.

Some tissues of the body can go without oxygen for long periods of time, up to 30 minutes in some instances. In active skeletal muscles, anaerobic activity (non-oxygen consuming) can continue for 30 seconds or more. However, in the brain, denial of oxygen after only five or ten seconds results in unconsciousness.

As far as energy supply is concerned, most neurons in the brain have the capability to store only two minutes' worth of glucose.

There is a consensus of opinion in the medical community that cholesterol and the other lipids in the adult brain are inert and unchangingly stable.

There is evidence, however, from as long as 30 or more years ago, which shows there is a turnover of cholesterol in the brain—though it might be at a slower rate of turnover than that found in other tissues.

Researchers have shown that oxidation of cell membranes in synapses occurs, and oxidation results in higher fluidity in the membranes. This higher fluidity damages the ability of synapses to conduct nerve impulses.

Oxidized cholesterol molecules have been shown to damage the endothelial cells found inside blood vessels throughout the body, including those in the brain. The brain depends on capillaries to continuously supply the nutrients and oxygen it needs.

It should be obvious that you cannot put processes with high rates of metabolism and large quantities of cholesterol and other lipids close to each other without oxidation taking place. However, as stated earlier, our bodies have systems that combat these damaging processes of oxidation, and the brain is the location of several of these systems.

Three well-known antioxidants in our bodies are vitamin E (alpha-tocopherol), vitamin C (ascorbic acid), and beta-carotene. There is medical evidence that people with higher levels of these antioxidants tend to have better memory performances over time. Vitamin E happens to be the most prevalent antioxidant vitamin in the brain, and vitamin C is effective in layered tissues reached by blood (skin-type tissues). Blood vessels and all epithelial tissues derive antioxidant benefits from vitamin C.

As previously mentioned, there is no evidence (to my knowledge) showing that Alzheimer's disease is caused simply by low levels of vitamin E.

4-11   Respirator Brain and G-Lock

There is a balancing act between 1) the very active metabolic processes that occur in the large human brain (unique in the animal world) and 2) a protective system that protects lipids in the brain from damage by these active metabolic processes.

What happens if, over a relatively short amount of time, the protective systems fail? For an example, we can look at a condition known as "respirator brain."

There are times when someone may experience a severe drop in blood pressure. A massive heart attack, heart seizure, or trauma in an accident, are just a few of the incidents that can cause a drop in blood flow to the brain resulting in unconsciousness. The person's heart resumes or continues beating, but they are not breathing adequately on their own. The person is placed on a respirator—a machine that breathes for them.

Over a period of time the person is tested for signs of electrical brain activity. If there is no sign of electrical brain activity, then a decision may be made to discontinue the artificial breathing support.

Usually what happens is, in the initial stages of the low or absent blood pressure period, the person's brain stops functioning. The maintenance processes, including those that protect against oxidation, slow down or stop, due to the inadequate blood flow to the brain. From that point on, the brain undergoes oxidation and massive tissue breakdown occurs, even if an adequate flow of oxygenated blood is restored.

At the autopsy, the person's brain is no longer a brain as we think of it. The process of oxidation and tissue breakdown that occurred at 98.6 degrees F. has turned the brain into a liquefied "soup." It can actually be poured out of the skull through a hole.

Respirator brain is an example (albeit a gruesome one) of what can happen to the human brain if not for all the protective systems in our bodies.

If blood flow to the brain is slowed down or stopped for a period of even five or ten seconds, the person is at risk. An example of this occurs when high-performance jet pilots suffer "G-lock."

Some maneuvers performed by jet fighters can subject the pilot to positive G forces. During these maneuvers, the pilot's blood is pulled away from the head and down toward the feet. The pilot attempts to keep the blood up towards the head using exercises involving tightening the leg and abdominal muscles. A special flight suit (called a G-suit) worn by the pilot assists by squeezing the legs, which also helps keep blood flowing towards the head.

If the exercises and the G-suit are not able to maintain blood flow to the brain, the pilot begins to suffer symptoms within ten seconds. The first symptom is tunnel vision, then there is a loss of color—everything appears gray. Then a full blackout occurs. This is known as "G-lock."

If the pilot does not escape G-lock and regain consciousness, the resulting plane crash is almost always fatal. All the events described can occur within just 15 seconds.

4-12   Where Does Human Brain Cholesterol Come From?

The human brain has the greatest concentration of cholesterol of any organ in the body. From where does the cholesterol in the human brain originate? There are two answers to this question, depending on the age of the person. The answers can be found in experiments and research performed over the last 30 to 40 years.

Regarding the research reports of these experiments that I have reviewed, all but one have used laboratory animals in providing the information about cholesterol and the brain. In most of these experiments, radioactive isotopes are used to label various carbon and hydrogen atoms in glucose, cholesterol, and two-carbon acetate molecules. At different stages in the experiments, the animals are sacrificed. The locations and amounts of the "radio-labeled" substances are recorded.

Because experiments like these involve sectioning and analyzing brain tissues, it should be obvious to see why humans cannot be used in these types of experiments. This is perhaps the main reason why the details of the relationship between cholesterol and the human brain have not been widely studied, and also why the subject still remains mysterious to many in the medical field.

Cholesterol molecules for the developing brain of a fetus are synthesized (made) in the brain area. The neurons and the myelin insulating coatings around axons all utilize cholesterol molecules made locally. Cholesterol molecules from the mother are used in the developing organs of the fetus. None of the cholesterol from the mother is used by the developing brain structures. Cholesterol molecules made by the developing liver of the fetus are not used in brain development, either. The time frame covered in this answer is the prenatal period, but it extends into the neonatal (newborn) period as well. This answer is derived from experiments performed with mice, rats, sheep, and humans.

How do we know that the <u>developing</u> human brain synthesizes all the cholesterol molecules it needs? How do we know that it does not take cholesterol molecules from LDL's circulating in the bloodstream?

Over thirty years ago there was an experiment performed involving women scheduled for therapeutic abortions due to serious maternal medical complications.

The women were given radioactive compounds that would label different components of the brains of their developing fetuses. This experiment determined that human fetal brain synthesizes (makes) all the cholesterol molecules for neurons and myelin within its own brain area, and does not use cholesterol molecules from the mother or even from its own liver.

In other experiments, brain cells and cells from the brain capillaries were taken from newborn rats. The cells were placed in culture liquids that contained ample amounts of nutrients. The cells synthesized cholesterol molecules. When the cells were placed in culture liquids containing abundant LDL cholesterol (like that found in the bloodstream), the cells used these cholesterol molecules instead of making their own. This demonstrates that brain cells and cells from brain capillaries possess the ability to utilize cholesterol molecules from the bloodstream, even though the cells synthesize them, for the most part.

HMG-CoA reductase is the key enzyme governing the rate of cholesterol production. In rats, the activity levels of HMG-CoA reductase reach a peak at four days of age. Thereafter, the activity levels decrease as the levels of LDL-receptor activity increase. This means that after birth, the rat brain slows down the process of making cholesterol molecules while it increases the taking of cholesterol from the bloodstream.

The cholesterol used by the fetal brain neurons and myelin was synthesized locally in the brain area, as was just explained. Glucose from the mother's maternal blood was the source. Glucose also provided the energy for the synthesis of the cholesterol molecules by the fetal brain.

In the adult human brain, the usual source of carbon atoms for making cholesterol is two-carbon acetate groups from fatty acids. The adult brain usually reserves glucose for energy production only.

The milk of mammals, including human breast milk, contains abundant amounts of cholesterol. Newborn animals (neonates), however, utilize these cholesterol molecules for development of organs and muscles, not for brain development. The brains of neonates continue to synthesize the cholesterol molecules they need locally in their own brains, and this includes human newborns. Glucose provides the carbons and the fuel.

Human breast milk contains cholesterol, while many infant formulas do not, but they contain glucose.

Does the human brain follow the same cholesterol pathways as other mammals?

The answer is no. In most other mammals, the brains are almost fully developed within a short time after birth. In humans, however, brain growth continues for a long time. It takes several years for myelination to be completed. After the completion of the myelination phase, the thinking processes of the brain are able to begin functioning at a higher level.

Are the cholesterol pathways of the brains of fully mature animals (including adult humans) different from the cholesterol pathways of the brains of prenatal and neonatal offspring?

Yes. In adult animals, including humans, cholesterol in the brain exchanges with cholesterol in the circulating blood. At some point in human growth, possibly puberty or shortly thereafter, brain cholesterol levels become connected to body cholesterol levels. The human brain cells still retain the ability to make cholesterol molecules. However, the evidence also shows that the brain gets cholesterol from the general circulating bloodstream as well. This will be discussed in detail later.

The myelin pathways of cholesterol are the same as for neurons, astrocytes, and other brain cells. The cells that make myelin are oligodendrocytes. During prenatal and early childhood periods, the myelination process is very active. After adulthood is reached, two things occur that can be demonstrated scientifically. First, the activity of the enzyme HMG-CoA reductase is shown to decrease to lower levels in oligodendrocytes. Second, the oligodendrocytes begin to display LDL-receptors on their cell membranes. In summary, this means that 1)during growth and development periods, the oligodendrocytes make the cholesterol molecules for myelin, and

2) in adulthood, the oligodendrocytes rely on cholesterol from the bloodstream for repair and maintenance of the myelin coatings.

What are the effects of poor nutrition on the developing brain with regards to cholesterol?

There is abundant literature available on conditions such as caloric malnutrition. The reader should look up the terms "marasmus" and "kwashiorkor" in an encyclopedia or medical dictionary. A type of mental retardation is associated with children who have these conditions.

Let us consider a condition of "cholesterol-starvation" that was artificially induced in an experiment. A chemical that inhibits cholesterol synthesis was added to developing mouse brain tissues in a culture. Nerve growth was retarded and damage was evident in the myelinated axons, dendrites, and nerve terminals in synapses. The culture contained all the other nutrients needed. Only cholesterol synthesis was affected.

The tissues were then placed in a culture, with nutrients, that did not contain the anti-cholesterol chemical. The tissues recovered to a healthier condition, but not to the same level as the tissues that were not subjected to the anti-cholesterol chemicals at any stage of growth.

In an experiment opposite to the one described with mice, two groups of 16-week-old baby pigs were used. One group consumed milk without cholesterol, while the other group consumed milk with cholesterol. The baby pigs receiving milk with cholesterol grew faster and had better brain development than the pigs in the non-cholesterol group.

Once an animal is an adult and brain development has been completed, is the cholesterol in the brain stable, inert, and "unchanging," or is it dynamic and "changing"? Is the status of cholesterol molecules in neurons different from those in myelin?

It is now recognized that cholesterol in the adult brain is not inert or "unchanging." Brain cholesterol molecules are dynamic and in constant turnover.

There is no "storehouse" of inert cholesterol in the brain. Structures in the adult brain share cholesterol molecules. They also obtain cholesterol molecules from the general blood circulation.

In the turnover process, all cholesterol molecules eventually end up in the bloodstream, usually after being oxidized. Brain cholesterol molecules that are not oxidized can also end up in the bloodstream if there is an excess of them in the brain.

Cholesterol turnover in the brain is faster than the turnover of other membrane molecules, such as phospholipids and proteins, though it is still slow compared to the turnover in other body tissues.

Using radioactive isotopes in rat brains, researchers found that after six months' time, there was only 8 percent of the radio-labeled cholesterol still remaining in the brain. In other words, 92 percent of the cholesterol in neurons, astrocytes and other cells in the brain, will be gone in six months, having been replaced by "fresh" cholesterol molecules. In myelin, 30 percent of the radio-labeled cholesterol is still present after six months, or stated the other way, "fresh" cholesterol molecules replace 70 percent of the cholesterol molecules in myelin. One can conclude from this, that cholesterol turnover in myelin is slower than the turnover in neurons and in other brain cells and structures.

This research demonstrates that cholesterol molecules in myelin take part in a turnover cycle, also. Myelin is definitely not inert or "unchanging" in the adult brain.

Within one month of the administration and uptake of radio-labeled cholesterol molecules by both young and adult rats, the marked cholesterol uniformly distributes throughout the brain. All parts of the brain can exchange cholesterol molecules with other parts of the brain.

Cholesterol turnover is more rapid in the areas of the brain that are involved the most with specific thinking functions. The neurons that do the most thinking and are, therefore, the most metabolically active, seem to have the greatest need for "fresh" cholesterol molecules. In the human brain, what area is responsible for the heaviest burden of thinking functions? The limbic system.

It was found that over a mouse's lifetime, the brain cholesterol content increased until the last stages near the end of its lifespan, when cholesterol levels decreased. Similarly, researchers determined that in humans at age 70, the average person has 11 percent less cholesterol in their brain as when they were 40 years old.

What role does the blood-brain barrier play in brain cholesterol metabolism? In adult humans, the blood-brain barrier is a barrier to many things, but it is not a barrier to cholesterol molecules. From experiments conducted 20 and 30 years ago, it was demonstrated that cholesterol from the circulating bloodstream crosses the blood-brain barrier to be used in brain tissues in adult animals. Cholesterol molecules also cross the barrier from the brain into the bloodstream.

Brain tumors, like other cancers, grow at uncontrollable rates and therefore have an unending need for cholesterol. It has been demonstrated that brain tumors obtain their cholesterol molecules from the general circulating blood by bringing them across the blood-brain barrier.

Blood-brain barriers posed a problem to doctors who wanted to deliver anti-cancer drugs to brain tumors. The barrier stopped the potentially life-saving drugs from reaching the brain tumors. It was discovered that by placing the anti-cancer drugs in small man-made particles called liposomes, it would be possible to move the drug across the blood-brain barrier. Liposomes are tiny "capsules" made of cholesterol and phospholipid molecules. This is further evidence that in adult human brains, cholesterol molecules readily cross the blood-brain barrier from the blood into the brain tissues.

It has been shown that there are low-density lipoprotein receptors on the endothelial cells of the brain capillaries. Their purpose is to bind LDL's and apo E's in order for cholesterol to be carried across the blood-brain barrier. Astrocytes can control the numbers of LDL-receptors in the capillaries, depending on the need of the neurons.

It has been demonstrated that LDL-receptors associated with capillaries, astrocytes, and neurons are displayed at higher frequencies (meaning more cholesterol is needed from the bloodstream) in the following situations: tissue repair, growth of cancerous tumors, and in Alzheimer's disease brains.

Where does human brain cholesterol come from? In the developing fetus, the brain makes almost all of its own molecules from glucose molecules. In the adult brain, however, some molecules are made in the brain from two-carbon acetates and some are taken from the general bloodstream. In adult humans, the brain's cholesterol levels are directly related to the blood's cholesterol levels. All cholesterol molecules in the brain undergo turnover, though it is slower than in other body tissues.

In the years 1995 through 1997 at least four scientific papers were published concerning the source of cholesterol in the human brain. Each paper concluded that the brain makes all the cholesterol it needs locally, and it does not utilize the bloodstream as a source of cholesterol.

The problem with these papers is that they used young, developing animals in their experiments and then made conclusions about cholesterol metabolism in adult brains. <u>You now know that it is incorrect to do this.</u> I encourage researchers, health professionals and others to review the references at the end of the book, drawing on experiments conducted over a span of 30 years by different researchers. In mammals, including humans, the fetal brain and developing brain do not depend on the bloodstream for cholesterol molecules. The adult (mature) brain does. Adult blood cholesterol levels do indeed have an influence on brain cholesterol levels, though it is not an instantaneous relationship, due to the fact that brain cholesterol metabolism is slow.

4-13   Cholesterol is Continuously Lost From the Brain and Other Body Tissues

After acknowledging that cholesterol is used in making bile salts, most health professionals would say that the only alternate destination of cholesterol would be the adherence to the walls of arteries, creating the clogging which leads to heart disease. Therefore, the purpose of this section is to demonstrate what actually happens to most of the cholesterol in our bodies.

All cholesterol molecules are lost, sooner or later. Many become oxidized. These oxidized cholesterol molecules will no longer fit inside cell membranes, so they are gathered up and excreted. Most cholesterol molecules, however, are lost because the tissue the molecules are in is lost.

Our skin is totally renewed every 39 to 48 days. This means that all of the skin's cells are lost within seven weeks, and with them go great quantities of cholesterol.

Our intestines, the inside surfaces of which are a type of skin, also lose great quantities of cells (and, therefore, cholesterol). As food is forced through intestines by a rhythmical contraction-relaxation motion, the cells lining the intestines are scraped off. These cells end up in the feces and are excreted.

Muscle cells lose cholesterol, too. The rates of cholesterol loss depend upon how active the muscle is. Heart muscle loses a large amount of cholesterol that must be replaced within a given time. This should not be surprising, since the heart is working 24 hours a day. Another type that is very active and exhibits high cholesterol turnover is the muscle in the tongue. The actions of both eating and talking keep the tongue very busy.

Most cholesterol molecules in the brain probably end up being oxidized. The brain makes up only 2 percent of body weight, but accounts for 15 percent of the body's metabolic activity. The high oxygen flow, the heat, the iron present, and the transmitting of nerve impulses through billions of nerve connections, all add up to an environment where oxidation of cholesterol molecules is common.

The brain excretes oxidized cholesterol molecules. Oxidized cholesterol is readily moved across the blood-brain barrier for disposal. Some researchers believe that cells in the brain can intentionally oxidize cholesterol molecules in an effort to dispose of excess cholesterol. They would be oxidized eventually anyway.

What happens to the oxidized cholesterol molecules from the brain after they are moved across the blood-brain barrier and into the bloodstream? Oxidized cholesterol from the brain ends up in urine.

A situation in which normal non-oxidized cholesterol molecules can be lost from the brain is as a result of the action of cortisol. Cortisol will be discussed in detail later.

4-14 Brain Atrophy (Shrinkage)

There are several terms that mean shrinkage of the tissues of the brain: brain atrophy, cortical atrophy, cerebral atrophy, and ventricular widening.

Some amount of brain atrophy can occur in many people purely as a consequence of getting older. Most of the time these measurable amounts of brain atrophy are not accompanied by any mental impairment. In cases of severe brain atrophy, symptoms of mental problems are found.

Loss of brain tissue can occur quite rapidly in cases of cerebral infarction, also known as a stroke. In the area where the stroke has occurred, the interruption of blood flow causes the tissue to die, and the immediate area shrinks during the healing process. Though this technically is a form of brain atrophy, it is not the same thing as the overall brain atrophy that occurs throughout the brain of someone with Alzheimer's disease.

It was found that in a study of ten people, ages 100 and older, that there were considerable variations in the degree of brain atrophy. All ten were mentally alert. This study points out that mild stages of brain atrophy, even at the age of 100, do not mean they will necessarily affect mental abilities. There is a point, however, where the degree of brain atrophy is accompanied by changes in mental conditions.

Again, a hallmark sign of Alzheimer's disease is atrophy of the hippocampus. The hippocampus is a structure that is critical to memory processing and many other functions of learning, thinking, and emotional responses. In Alzheimer's, however, the entire brain exhibits degrees of atrophy, not just the hippocampus and other structures in the limbic system.

CHAPTER 5
Alzheimer's Disease Processes

(Average readers may wish to skip this somewhat technical chapter.)

5-1   Neurons are Dying in Alzheimer's: Amyloid

Amyloid begins as a long-stranded string of amino acids in a repeating sequence. The longer amyloid strand is cut into smaller pieces, called fibrils. Amyloid fibrils are not all the same length, depending on the cells and tissues involved.

The amyloid fibrils of Alzheimer's derive their name according to the numbers of amino acids present in their chains. The more common fibrils are beta-amyloid (1-40) and beta-amyloid (1-42). Simply remember that it starts as a very long strand and then is cut into shorter segments. These shorter segments of amyloid are what accumulate in the brains of Alzheimer's patients.

Beta amyloid can bind to cholesterol or phospholipids and become inserted into the cell membrane. They may also remain in the solution around neurons and astrocytes. If enough of the soluble amyloid fibrils accumulate and begin to condense, they are said to be in aggregated (accumulated) form. As the accumulation progresses, they evolve into dense plaques.

They are more commonly referred to as senile plaques, and may also contain cells that are part of the inflammatory response of the body and parts of dead cells.

Accumulations of amyloid can cause the death of neurons that are touching or are close to the plaques. The neurons associated with amyloid plaques show the hyperphosphorylation of tau protein that results in the production of neurofibrillary tangles. This leads to disorganized microtubules, which in turn affects the cell's ability to function. Neuron deaths eventually occur.

There are several theories as to how beta amyloid actually causes the neurons to die. One is that significant amounts of beta amyloid in cell membranes, or next to cell membranes, will cause the cell to allow too many calcium ions to move inside of the cells. This "calcium channel hypothesis," however, does not explain all of the neuron deaths found in Alzheimer's.

Another theory is that beta amyloid itself causes oxidation of the molecules in the cell membranes of neurons, and this causes the death of neurons. The "oxidation hypothesis," however, does not explain all of the neuron deaths found in Alzheimer's.

Neurons require a constant supply of glucose. It is possible that beta amyloid accumulation in the cell membrane and around the cell interferes with glucose absorption. But the "low-glucose hypothesis" does not explain all the neuron deaths found in Alzheimer's.

Deposits of beta amyloid accumulate in and around the capillaries and eventually damage occurs to the vessels. Since these blood vessels are part of the blood-brain barrier, support for neurons suffers when there is damage to these vessels.

Research shows that accumulations of beta amyloid may trigger the body's inflammatory response mechanism. Another theory, therefore, is that amyloid build-up causes a state of chronic inflammation to occur.

There is evidence that beta amyloid can be broken down and removed by various enzymes in the blood. There is also evidence that microglia can degrade and remove beta amyloid to a degree. When in small amounts, beta amyloid is part of a dynamic system in which it is constantly being deposited and also constantly being removed.

Two other facts bear mentioning. First, beta amyloid deposits are associated with the production of a substance called nitric oxide. Second, beta amyloid deposits are sometimes associated with a protein called ubiquitin. I will cover these topics in greater detail later. No one theory seems to satisfy all of the researchers involved in the pursuit of the Alzheimer's mystery. At present, there is not even a satisfactory explanation as to the actual purpose of beta amyloid in a normal, healthy person.

There are two other pieces missing in the puzzle. First, they commonly find plaques during the autopsy of elderly people who did not demonstrate any signs or symptoms of Alzheimer's disease prior to their death. Second, in those patients with definite Alzheimer's there is abundant evidence to demonstrate that neurons were dying in their brains even when there were no beta amyloid plaques nearby. Later, I will discuss these two pieces of the puzzle in detail.

5-2   Cells Produce Some Amyloid

Where does amyloid originate? Research shows that cells in the brain can make it. Neurons may be a key source, but they are not the only source of beta amyloid in the brain. In neurons, the long-stranded amyloid precursor (initial) material is made, and then is quickly moved down the axon to the terminal and synapse. The synapse, where the nerve impulse transmits to the next neuron, is a very busy place. There must be a reason why neurons want to keep a supply of amyloid precursor material near the busiest place of their cell membrane.

Other cells in the brain that make amyloid include astrocytes, oligodendrocytes, microglia, and cells that are part of the capillaries (small blood vessels) in the brain. Neurons make more of the amyloid than the other cells, according to some researchers.

If all cell types in the brain have the capacity to make amyloid precursor material, do cells in other body tissues and organs also possess the ability to make it? Yes, but once again it is something for discussion in greater detail later.

5-3   Blood Platelets Are Storehouses of Beta Amyloid

Does beta amyloid from outside the brain enter into the brain from the circulating blood? The answer is yes.

Circulating blood platelets contain large amounts of beta amyloid, and are a significant source of amyloid deposited in the brain. There is evidence that shows that beta amyloid can cross the blood-brain barrier.

Blood platelets, also known as thrombocytes, contribute to the blood's ability to clot after an injury to tissue.

It is important to remember that beta amyloid is present in the platelets of normal, healthy people who do not have Alzheimer's disease, as well as the platelets of those with the disease. The material inside the platelets is the same. However, some researchers have found that the platelets themselves may be different when comparing those of people with Alzheimer's versus those without the disease. The platelets of Alzheimer's patients demonstrate higher fluidity in their membranes. A later section of this book will address this property of increased platelet membrane fluidity.

A few researchers have known for a long time that the blood carries amyloid. A paper published in 1975 supports this point. Also determined two decades ago was that increased amyloid, a condition referred to as amyloidosis, was associated with various illnesses. Some of the illnesses associated with elevated amyloid levels are rheumatoid arthritis, multiple myeloma, tuberculosis, advanced cancer tumors, leprosy, and certain renal diseases ending in kidney failure. The 1975 research also noticed an association of high amyloid levels in some people over the age of 80.

5-4   Neurofibrillary Tangles: Tau Protein and Glycogen Synthase Kinase

NOTE: Many of the references listed at the end of the book under Chapter 4's heading are also the basis of this section.

Like most cells, the health status of neurons depends upon the microtubule network, among other things. Microtubules are necessary for the movement of things inside cells. They move nutrients in and wastes out. Microtubules are flexible. They assemble when needed and disassemble when they are not needed.

Tau Protein segments (or fibrils) keep the microtubules stable so that movement of things inside of cells may proceed. The altering of tau protein occurs through the addition of extra phosphorus groups to the molecules. This hyperphosphorylation causes tau protein fibrils to bind to each other in pairs instead of to microtubules. The microtubules stop functioning, which leads to cell damage. The tau protein fibrils form paired helical filaments of tau (PHF-tau) after becoming hyperphosphorylated, and they accumulate into neurofibrillary tangles. One of the first signs in brain tissues of Alzheimer's patients is the appearance of neurofibrillary tangles in neurons.

In laboratory experiments, tau protein can be hyperphosphorylated by a number of enzymes. In neurons in the human brain, the enzyme thought most responsible is glycogen synthase kinase.

Why would glycogen synthase kinase do something to cause microtubules to stop working, which leads to neurofibrillary tangle formation and deaths of neurons?

Glycogen synthase kinase is an enzyme associated with glucose metabolism. The brain uses glucose as its primary fuel. There is a need for a constant supply and neurons, unfortunately, do not store much of it. Glucose that can be stored (if there is a relative abundance of it) is stored in the form of glycogen. When many molecules of glucose attach to each other in long branching chains, it is termed glycogen.

The enzyme that promotes this building of glucose molecules into branching chains of glycogen is glycogen synthase. If a cell has abundant glucose supplies, they convert for storage into glycogen through the action of this enzyme (glycogen synthase).

What if a cell, such as a neuron, does not have extra glucose that can be stored as glycogen? There needs to be a way for the cell to stop the actions of glycogen synthase. The enzyme that does this is glycogen synthase kinase.

In review, if a cell has a large supply of glucose molecules, it converts them for storage into glycogen through the actions of glycogen synthase. If a cell has used up its glycogen supplies and must use all new glucose molecules immediately as food, the enzyme, glycogen synthase kinase stops the action of glycogen synthase.

If the cell has abundant food, we say it is "well fed." If it does not have abundant food, it is in a "starved" or "fasting" state. Normally, the use of these terms refers to humans or other animals. Their use also refers to the status of cells, including neurons.

The enzyme working more in "fed" cells is glycogen synthase.

The enzyme working more in "fasting" or "starved" cells is glycogen synthase kinase. These concepts will be covered in greater detail later.

5-5   Plaques Versus Tangles: The Debate

There is a debate among the Alzheimer's disease research community as to what develops first in Alzheimer's patients, amyloid plaques or neurofibrillary tangles.

Some researchers state that amyloid plaque accumulation is the most important event in Alzheimer's disease. An argument for amyloid as the primary factor in Alzheimer's is the finding that in the rare cases of particular families with high numbers of cases of the disease, a particular genetic defect results also in higher amounts of amyloid production. Defects of the presenilin genes are examples.

The disturbing thing about using amyloid plaques as the primary features of Alzheimer's is that neurons in the brains of patients can be dying even when they are not near any plaques.

The opposing view in this debate is that neurons with neurofibrillary tangles as a result of tau protein hyperphosphorylation are the most important on which to focus. The fact that neurons are dying even when they might not be near amyloid plaques supports this. Neurofibrillary tangles occur in neurons that are dying in both situations: next to amyloid or far away from amyloid.

There are also researchers who find both abundant amyloid plaques and abundant neurons with neurofibrillary tangles in the brains of people who had no Alzheimer's symptoms when they died.

In summary, though amyloid plaques and neurofibrillary tangles may be present, the determining factor for the development of symptoms associated with Alzheimer's disease is the loss of neurons in the hippocampus and related structures. The important evidence is 1) neurons are dying in areas throughout the brain, and 2) the brain is shrinking in size in Alzheimer's patients. Later we will see how plaques, tangles, and brain shrinkage are all connected.

5-6   Alzheimer's Genetics: Apo E 4, Presenilin, and Chromosome 21

Many scientists in the field of Alzheimer's research believe that this disease is purely genetic in origin. They feel that, eventually, proof will show that this is so, in spite of an abundance of evidence that shows it is not.

Individuals with Down syndrome are born with three number 21 chromosomes instead of the usual two. The gene responsible for amyloid is located on chromosome 21. Having three chromosomes instead of the usual two represents a 50 percent increase in chromosome 21 material. Therefore, in Down syndrome, amyloid produces at a rate 50 percent greater than normal.

Chromosome 21 can exhibit a gene mutation that in the past they believed played a large role in the cause of Alzheimer's disease. However, research has shown that this genetic mutation defect of the amyloid precursor gene did not play a significant part in the vast majority of people who developed Alzheimer's disease. At most, less than two percent of cases link to the chromosome 21 amyloid gene mutation.

Two other genes called presenilins exhibit possible mutations that may contribute to the development of Alzheimer's disease. Presenilin 1 displays a genetic mutation linked to some people who develop the disease prior to the age of 60. Presenilin 2 displays a genetic mutation linked to Alzheimer's development in a particular family in Germany and to one in Italy.

The location of the gene for apolipoprotein E is on chromosome number 19. Apo E is a lipoprotein that transports cholesterol and amyloid in the brain. It is found in three forms (or alleles): apo E 2, apo E 3, and apo E 4. Research shows that those individuals who inherit the apo E 4 allele seem to have a slightly higher chance of developing the disease compared with those who inherit the apo E 2 or apo E 3 alleles.

Researchers have determined that mutations of the presenilin genes can result in increased production of amyloid (when "favorable conditions" exist). Laboratory experiments show that a deficiency of the presenilin 1 gene results in the slowing down of amyloid production.

The actual percentage of Alzheimer's patients who develop the disease as a possible result of having a presenilin gene mutation is very small.

Presenilin genes exert their effects in the endoplasmic reticulum and Golgi apparatus inside cells, which just happen to be the same places in the cell that make, store, and prepare cholesterol molecules for use.

The majority of Alzheimer's cases cannot be linked directly to presenilin gene mutations, amyloid gene mutations, or to the apo E 4 allele susceptibility. Of those cases possibly linked to one of these genetic factors, the symptoms of the patients and the patterns of brain tissue damage are about the same. This means that in spite of the different chromosomes involved, the final pathways of Alzheimer's disease are just about the same and are common to them all.

Less than 10 percent of people with Alzheimer's have a strong family history of the disease; this means that over 90 percent of all people with the disease have no one else in their family who has Alzheimer's.

Keep in mind that studies of twins reveal that Alzheimer's is not a purely genetic-based disease. Most people with the presenilin gene defects, amyloid gene defects, or apo E 4 allele still do not develop Alzheimer's disease.

Researchers who still believe that Alzheimer's disease is purely genetic in origin continue to look for possible genetic influences. The references for this section list other chromosomes thought to play a role.

All of these genetic studies seem to relate to the situations where the gene defects or mutations cause greater-than-expected amounts of amyloid deposited in plaques, compared to situations without a particular genetic influence or susceptibility. However, <u>in Alzheimer's, neurons that are not near to any amyloid plaques are also dying.</u>

This leads me to agree with those researchers who think that amyloid production is actually a response or reaction to some particular condition present in the brain that is killing neurons. Amyloid fibrils in small amounts do not kill neurons.

There is only one situation in which someone's genetic make-up guarantees the development of Alzheimer's disease. That situation is in people born with Down syndrome. We will discuss the development of Alzheimer's in this group later.

5-7   Normal Aging

Thus far, we have discussed amyloid deposits in the brain as they relate to Alzheimer's disease. However, amyloid deposits are in tissues throughout the body. Amyloid deposits frequently occur in association with various diseases. It is important to keep in mind that amyloid build-up is not something that occurs only in the brain.

If two hallmark signs of Alzheimer's disease are amyloid plaques and neurofibrillary tangles, do older persons considered "normal" (that is, who have normal mental functions with no signs of Alzheimer's disease or any other dementia) ever develop these plaques and tangles in their brains?

The answer is yes. Numerous studies have shown that sometimes plaques and tangles are in the brains of normal, non-demented people in their senior years.

As plaques and tangles accumulate in greater amounts in areas of the cortex on the sides and front of the brain, there is a greater chance that the person will have had Alzheimer's type symptoms of dementia at the time of their death.

The cause of the dementia symptoms is actually the loss of neurons. As more neurons die, the chances of the person having Alzheimer's-type symptoms are increased.

The actual extent of amyloid plaques in the brain does not correspond to dementia symptoms as much as does the extent of neurofibrillary tangles. As previously discussed, neurons may develop neurofibrillary tangles and die, even when there are no amyloid plaques nearby.

Studies of centenarians, people over 100 years old, have shown that their brains may be the same as someone who is only 60 or 70 years old. If the centenarian had extensive plaques, tangles, and lost neurons in the cortex and hippocampus, then it is more likely that he or she would have had symptoms of dementia at the time of death. Fewer plaques, tangles, and lost neurons correlate with the less likelihood of developing dementia symptoms.

5-8   Cerebral Amyloid Angiopathy and HCHWA-D

The previous section described how amyloid might accumulate in the brains of people who are not (or not yet) suffering with the obvious symptoms of Alzheimer's disease. This section will review the two diseases specifically linked to amyloid accumulation, but may or may not be associated with definite Alzheimer's disease.

In the first disease, called cerebral amyloid angiopathy or CAA, amyloid accumulates in the brain and blood vessels. It deposits in the blood vessels so extensively that the blood vessels begin to have points of bleeding or hemorrhages. These occur at normal or even low blood pressures. This is unusual since strokes in the brain of the hemorrhage type usually occur in people with high blood pressure (hypertension). However, brain hemorrhage is the usual cause of death in people with CAA.

As in Alzheimer's disease, people with CAA are typically elderly persons. People with CAA may also experience seizures, a finding seen in people with Alzheimer's. Many researchers believe that CAA is a pre-Alzheimer's condition because of the many similarities between the two, which include symptoms of dementia. Microscopic examinations of brain tissues from people with CAA also exhibit neurofibrillary tangles and areas of demyelination of nerve axons.

There are two other things regarding people with CAA. They sometimes display symptoms of rheumatoid arthritis, and microscopically, the brain tissues show signs of the protein ubiquitin. Rheumatoid arthritis and ubiquitin are topics of discussion later.

The blood-brain barrier shows signs of increased permeability in CAA as well as in Alzheimer's. This may allow a major blood protein called albumin to enter the brain. Albumin carries amyloid in the general blood circulation. (Remember that platelets also carry amyloid.) There are also amyloid receptors in blood vessels in the brain.

A very rare disease, called Hereditary Cerebral Hemorrhage with Amyloidosis-Dutch Type (HCHWA-D), affects a group of individuals who are usually younger than those with CAA. First identified in several Dutch families, the cause of the disease is a true genetic mutation on chromosome 21, the same chromosome that controls amyloid production. Though they are usually younger, people with HCHWA-D are similar to people with CAA in that they experience hemorrhage-type strokes at normal or low blood pressure, and they tend to develop symptoms of dementia. In HCHWA-D, amyloid deposits occur in heavier amounts and accumulate in very large arteries to a greater degree than in CAA.

A final point is that the amyloid material found in Alzheimer's disease, CAA, HCHWA-D, Down Syndrome, and in normal aging is basically the same. In addition, there are other disease and medical conditions accompanied by amyloid accumulations.

Other organs and tissues are involved outside of the brain; hence, the amyloid material may be slightly different compared to the amyloid made by the neurons and astrocytes inside the brain. It is interesting to note that amyloid from outside the brain is deposited inside the brain in the various diseases already discussed. You may ask, do the laboratory tests performed only on brain tissues of those deceased with Alzheimer's show more than one specific kind of amyloid material?

The answer is yes.

5-9   Transporting Amyloid

Amyloid plaques in the brains of Alzheimer's patients, as well as in other people, consist of beta amyloid fibrils aggregated (accumulated) in large amounts. These plaques do not dissolve easily. Amyloid fibrils by themselves are soluble.

Amyloid is transported by various components of blood. Blood platelets carry amyloid. They are critically important in the body's response to bleeding.

Apo E is a transporter of amyloid, especially in the brain. The more typical role of apo E is to transport cholesterol and other lipids. High-density lipoproteins (HDL's) and low-density lipoproteins (LDL'S) can carry amyloid as well.

Another vehicle for transporting amyloid in the bloodstream is albumin, one of the major proteins in blood.

Neurons and other cells in the brain produce amyloid. For large amounts of beta amyloid to aggregate into plaques, there have to be ways for amyloid fibrils to pass through the blood-brain barrier.

Research shows that there are receptors for amyloid in blood capillaries in the brain. This is one way for amyloid to cross the blood capillary walls. As previously discussed, in Alzheimer's, CAA, and HCHWA-D, the amyloid plaques accumulate along the blood vessels in the brain. As amyloid continues to deposit, the integrity of the vessels is affected. They become more permeable and are more likely to hemorrhage.

Normally, albumin is unable to cross the blood-brain barrier. If vessels become more permeable because of amyloid accumulation, then albumin crossing the barrier brings substantially more amyloid fibrils across, leading to continual build-up of plaques.

The picture presented here is one of a cascade downwards as far as the health of the brain is concerned. Once sufficient amounts of amyloid plaques are present, the damaging continual accumulation of amyloid proceeds without stopping.

5-10   The Blood-Brain Barrier in Alzheimer's

There is a debate in the Alzheimer's research community as to whether the blood-brain barrier is abnormal in people with Alzheimer's disease. Many researchers say it is compromised and contributes to the disease process, while a few scientists believe there is no difference between the blood-brain barrier of an Alzheimer's person and that of a healthy, non-demented person.

One way to detect brain tissue damage is if substances were present in brain tissues when normally they would not. Albumin is one of those substances that will not normally cross a healthy blood-brain barrier, but it can cross a damaged, abnormal one.

Amyloid materials accumulate in the brains of Alzheimer's persons in two areas: around the neurons and along blood vessels. Precise experimental and microscopic examinations of blood vessels with amyloid accumulations demonstrate that the blood-brain barrier in these particular vessels is indeed altered.

Amyloid does not accumulate in brains in a concrete, uniform pattern. Many blood vessels in an Alzheimer's patient's brain may not have an appreciable amount of amyloid in association with them. Will blood vessels without amyloid demonstrate an abnormal blood-brain barrier? The answer is no. This has caused some researchers to conclude that there are no blood-brain barrier changes in Alzheimer's patients.

Evidence shows that the degree of damage to the blood-brain barrier relates to the amount of amyloid accumulation associated with a particular blood vessel.

The aging process can alter the blood-brain barrier.

There is research that details specific changes of the barrier associated with aging. The walls of capillaries become thinner, which may result in a decreased ability to compensate for leaks in the blood-brain barrier.

There is also research with laboratory animals that demonstrates that the vessels in the hippocampus may be more susceptible to the changes occurring with the aging process than are those in other areas of the brain.

In conclusion, amyloid deposits alter the blood-brain barrier. This holds true for people whether or not they have Alzheimer's symptoms. In vessels free of amyloid, the barrier functions remain normal, except for the possible effects of aging.

One of the signs of altered barriers in blood vessels is an increased permeability. Blood vessels with significant amyloid deposits are more leaky.

In an experiment, laboratory animals had their blood cholesterol levels raised with medication. The increased cholesterol resulted in decreased permeability of the vessels and of the blood-brain barrier. Cell membrane fluidity decreased, and the vessels became less "leaky." In other words, higher blood cholesterol levels resulted in a stronger blood-brain barrier.

CHAPTER 6
The Conditions That Lead to Most Cases of Alzheimer's

6-1   Weight Loss or Natural Thinness

<u>Note: The information in this section does not apply to those who develop Alzheimer's disease in association with Down Syndrome, brain surgery, or head injury. Body weights of people in those three categories do not play a role in their developing Alzheimer's. This information also does not apply to the two or three percent (or less) of Alzheimer's patients that developed the disease primarily through genetic influences.</u>

Weight loss is not merely a common finding in Alzheimer's disease; it is a universal finding in every Alzheimer's study examining body sizes of people with the disease. There are no studies stating that weight gain is a common finding.

There is one small study of 392 patients (published in 2003) which claims that being overweight is a significant risk factor for later developing Alzheimer's. The study's authors found a "striking relationship" between being overweight at the age 70 and developing Alzheimer's 10 to 18 years later. However, these authors failed to emphasize that the patients were exhibiting weight loss as the years passed by, as evidenced by their decreases in Body Mass Indexes (BMI) listed in the study. My father-in-law would have been someone that these authors would claim as proof of their conclusions. Vance Wolff was overweight to the point of being obese. However, he did not develop Alzheimer's disease until after he lost weight.

In the case of vascular dementia, obesity is most definitely a risk factor, along with high blood pressure and active atherosclerosis. Remember that it often takes an experienced physician to truly differentiate vascular dementia from Alzheimer's disease in a patient.

Many people with Alzheimer's seem to be constantly walking around, thus they call them "wanderers." Is it possible that the weight loss is the result of the person's higher level of physical activity?

The answer is no. Researchers who looked closely at this conclude that people with Alzheimer's do not have higher levels of physical activity when compared to normal, healthy, non-demented people.

Do people with Alzheimer's have higher rates of metabolism, and, therefore, lose weight because their bodies burn calories faster than others do? The answer again is no. The resting metabolic rates of people with Alzheimer's are not different from those of healthy, non-demented people.

In Alzheimer's, the brain exhibits shrinkage. Some researchers have found that the body weights of people measured as BMI (Body Mass Index) are the best indicators of changes in their brains. Low body weight directly correlates with brain shrinkage.

At first glance, one would think that Alzheimer's caregivers are intentionally starving their patients. This is not true, of course. However, it does cast doubt on Alzheimer's-associated weight loss studies based solely on interviews with caregivers. There may be a bias on the caregiver's part in favor of saying that his or her Alzheimer's patient eats the same amount of food as anyone else without the disease. They do not want to give the impression that they are not feeding their patients. This is understandable. However, the fact remains that people with Alzheimer's do have abnormal eating patterns that contribute to continued weight loss.

Also unreliable are studies based on one-time encounters between investigators and Alzheimer's patients. Data from these types of studies always leads one to conclude that Alzheimer's causes weight loss, which is actually the opposite of what is occurring.

This brings us to another of the many debates within the Alzheimer's research community. Does Alzheimer's disease cause a person to lose weight, or is it just a coincidence? Does the weight loss begin before people develop the disease? If that is the case, does the prior weight loss have anything to do with the development of the disease?

<u>Weight loss occurs prior to the development of the disease</u>. In studies in which researchers observed elderly people over several years, discoveries prove this was definitely the case. In our family, Vance Wolff lost weight before the appearance of any memory problems.

In a study of 8,800 women, those who gained weight after menopause did not seem to be developing Alzheimer's disease.

In a study of 8,400 older people admitted to hospitals, they determined that thin people had far more medical complications and death than did people who were overweight. Obesity was a factor only in the people who were 100 percent above their normal weight. This means that older, thin people are at a greater risk for medical complications and death when compared to all other groups, except those who weighed twice their normal weight.

Studies in Catholic nuns from ages 75 to 99 showed that the easiest way to predict possible physical health problems was by monitoring their body weights. Those nuns who began losing weight had far more health problems and deaths than those who did not lose weight.

In studies on people who go on hunger strikes, they found that those who were already thin when the strike began faired much worse than those who were at normal or above-normal weight. This is perhaps an expectation, but what was surprising was the finding that within 60 hours (two and one-half days) of starting the fast, body protein began breaking down and an accelerated weight loss process began in the thin hunger strikers. This means that thin people may start experiencing real tissue damage within three days of improper or insufficient food intake. They did not conduct these studies in older people, who we might predict would be at even greater risk if they were already thin and began to eat poorly (for whatever reason).

There are studies that show that 10 percent (or less) of people with Alzheimer's may go through a phase of overeating and may gain weight as a result. Unfortunately, there is no replacement of the lost neurons. Any weight gain as a result of adequate nutrition will not improve dementia symptoms.

Finally, in a study of 2,000 men and women, ages 50 to 93, researchers found that there is a tendency for people to lose weight as they age. Along with the weight loss over time, they discovered that the blood cholesterol levels tended to decrease as well.

6-2   Altered Taste and Smell

An altered sense of smell is one of the first symptoms seen in patients who later develop Alzheimer's disease. We have already reviewed evidence showing that weight loss is evident in individuals before Alzheimer's disease strikes, with the exception of those with Down's Syndrome, head injury, or brain surgery. Enjoyment of food depends upon aromas and flavors, thus an impaired olfactory system would naturally seem to adversely affect this important aspect of eating. If food does not smell or taste "the way it used to," then a person (over time) may be less inclined to eat enough food to maintain their body weight.

Research has shown that smell identification abilities of people remain stable up into their sixties. Between the ages of 65 to 80, however, half of all people exhibit declining performance of smell. After age 80, almost three-fourths of individuals develop an impairment of their olfactory abilities. These declines in smell and taste performance occur even when there are no obvious medical problems present.

If a person displays symptoms of the initial stages of Alzheimer's disease, which include olfactory problems, then the resulting poor eating patterns may lead to more weight loss and further development of additional Alzheimer's symptoms.

Remember that the olfactory tissues are part of the brain, which means that there are neurons in these tissues. Researchers have shown that these neurons display the same changes seen in the rest of the brain tissues in people with Alzheimer's. There are amyloid plaques, neurofibrillary tangles of tau protein, and dying or dead neurons.

6-3   Weight Loss (and Low Cholesterol) is Common in the Elderly

The intended purpose of this section is to demonstrate that weight loss is common in the elderly population. If a person is losing weight, it must be due to disease or to the lack of adequate food intake. Malnutrition is the lack of adequate food intake, and the most obvious sign of this is weight loss.

Under-nutrition and semi-starvation are appropriate terms that mean eating fewer calories of food than are needed to maintain weight. Starvation would imply an extreme lack of food such that death occurs. Semi-starvation, as used in this book, means eating enough to stay alive, but not enough to maintain weight at a stable level.

There are many reasons for the weight loss commonly seen among the elderly. Some of the more common reasons given for weight loss in the elderly are depression and/or mental health status, interactions of prescribed medications or their side effects, poor dental health, financial status, alcoholism, and various diseases.

There are also many older people placed on dietary restrictions when overweight, but never taken off the restrictions after having achieved an acceptable weight. These people continue to lose weight, due in part to the reluctance of staff members to make recommendations regarding a physician's standing orders.

There are also situations in which the nurses on staff of an institution fail to give the clients enough time to eat their meals. The elderly do many things at a slower pace, including eating.

In home settings, an elderly spouse caregiver may have difficulties ensuring adequate food consumption for both of them, not just the one receiving care.

Another problem may be that the foods eaten by the elderly person losing weight are not nutritious. Various vitamin deficiencies may be present as a result.

A common finding in the elderly is decreasing blood cholesterol levels. These decreased levels accompany the weight loss from which many older folks suffer. One of the Framingham Heart Study research groups concluded from studies that a decline in total blood cholesterol is very common among the elderly, and occurs even in situations where there are no special dietary restrictions or medication interactions.

Of the references listed at the end of the book for this section, many document the common findings of malnutrition and weight loss in the elderly. Other reports record the common findings of decreasing blood cholesterol levels in the elderly. Others detail both weight loss and decreasing cholesterol in the older population.

There are references detailing the findings of higher death rates found in older people whose weight and blood cholesterol are decreasing. Also illustrated is research showing older people, who were at low body weights and then experienced weight gain, had lower death rates compared to those who stayed at the lower body weight.

In conclusion, weight loss from malnutrition (semi-starvation) is common in the elderly. The decreasing blood cholesterol levels that result go hand-in-hand with the weight loss.

6-4   The "Healthy Old" Have "High" Cholesterol Levels

Accompanied by decreasing blood cholesterol levels is the shrinking body size from malnutrition (semi-starvation) prevalent in older populations. Those senior citizens caught in this situation have higher rates of disease (including Alzheimer's) and death. If this is true, then are elderly individuals with adequate body weights and higher cholesterol levels healthier, and do they have lower death rates?

The answer is yes, although this seems to go against everything those in the medical and nutrition worlds have professed over the last forty years.

Published research, that is readily available, supports the fact that older people with higher blood cholesterol levels are healthier and experience lower death rates. It is not a secret.

Cholesterol is one of several factors in heart disease. As will be learned in later sections, it is actually a minor factor for the majority of people. Generally speaking, very high cholesterol levels are a heart disease risk factor only in people up to ages 50 to 60, and always in conjunction with other factors, such as high blood pressure or smoking. After age 60 or so, high blood cholesterol levels have no influence over who will or who won't have a heart attack. This issue will be fully covered in later sections.

One explanation sometimes given for the connection between lower cholesterol levels and increased death rates is that there is presumably some disease present in the subjects that hasn't yet been diagnosed. There are times when this is true. However, it is unscientific to use this as a general dismissal of the evidence linking low cholesterol levels to higher disability and death rates.

If someone is 100 years old or older, he or she is a centenarian. People in their nineties are nonagenarians. Eighty-year olds are octogenarians, etc.

In an Italian study of people ages 50 to 100, of the centenarians judged healthy, all possessed a higher body fat content. This does not mean that they were obese by medical standards. Rather, it means they were not "slim and trim."

In another study, researchers followed 10,000 people ages 35 to 74 for 14 years. Those people over 70 with low cholesterol levels had higher death rates compared with people over 70 with high cholesterol levels.

In a study of 2,500 men ages 25 to 84, very high blood cholesterol levels constituted a risk for coronary artery disease in the younger men. However, the association between high cholesterol and heart disease reached "zero" statistically in the older men.

In a 200-bed nursing home, researchers followed patients for three years. Those people with declining cholesterol values had the highest death rates.

From 1959-1987, a study was conducted with people ages 45 to 92. Those in their 50's and 60's with high cholesterol values suffered from atherosclerosis and heart attacks at higher rates. People ages 70 and older with high cholesterol, however, were healthier and had lower death rates than those with low cholesterol levels.

In the mid-1980's, a study in California followed 1,000 men ages 50 to 89. Those men over age 70 with low cholesterol levels were found to be three times more likely to be suffering from depression, as compared to 70-year-olds with high cholesterol. Depression is often evident in Alzheimer's disease.

In Finland, a study of 700 older men showed how low blood cholesterol levels, low body mass index (thin bodies), and low blood pressure were all associated with mental disability.

In Greece, researchers followed 500 people in a nursing home from 1978 to 1988. Survival of those people reaching age 80 and beyond was dependent upon having higher blood cholesterol levels.

In Connecticut, research documented 997 people for four years. Those aged 70 and older with high cholesterol (over 240 mg/dl) did not have higher rates of coronary artery disease as was expected. Many of these older people had a low HDL number accompanying their higher total blood cholesterol, and they still did not develop heart disease as supposedly expected (according to the "experts").

There exist many published papers based on the Framingham Heart Study, an ongoing study that began over 40 years ago, with people living in Framingham, Massachusetts. Documented and studied in this project were atherosclerosis (and related diseases) and the connections to cholesterol, life style, diet, and various other things.

In a study based on Framingham data, octogenarians judged the healthiest had high LDL numbers and moderately low HDL numbers. According to currently accepted medical standards, the arrangement of high LDL and low HDL numbers is supposed to be a guarantee of heart disease.

In an Italian study, researchers also concentrated on people ages 80 and older. They followed

318 octogenarians and found that those with high blood cholesterol levels had the lowest death rates.

In another study based on Framingham data, 2,800 women ages 56 to 70 were the subjects of an analysis of death rates and blood cholesterol measurements. Researchers discovered that the women in this group with the lowest death rates had cholesterol values between 240 and 280 mg/dl. In women over age 70, those with a blood cholesterol measurement below 240 mg/dl had the highest death rates. The authors concluded that women over 55 should not attempt to lower their cholesterol levels to 200 mg/dl or less, because those women in the study who did ended up with the highest death rates.

In yet another study based on Framingham data, they tracked over 4,000 men and women from 1951 to 1981. In this study, high blood cholesterol levels at or about age 50 linked to higher death rates. After age 50, high blood cholesterol did not link to higher death rates.

In another Framingham study, they followed 5,200 men and women ages 40 to 80 from 1948 to 1980. High blood cholesterol at age 40 was associated with a higher death rate. By age 80, high cholesterol was associated with low death rates. From ages 50 to 70, the authors found no definite relationship between high blood cholesterol and either higher or lower death rates. As a result of this study, the authors concluded that physicians should be very cautious about placing people over age 65 on treatments or medications that would lower blood cholesterol.

In a French study of 92 women in a nursing home whose average age was 82, the lowest death rates occurred in those women with an average blood cholesterol measurement of 7.0 m mol/L, which is the same as 270 mg/dl.

In a Japanese study of 45 centenarians from the Tokyo area, researchers judged those with higher blood cholesterol to be healthier and to have a better mental status.

Japanese people, on average, have the longest life spans in the world. People living on the island of Okinawa have the longest life spans of those in Japan. This means that citizens of Okinawa are a concentrated group of the longest-living people on the planet. In 1994, the ratio of centenarians in Okinawa was one centenarian for every 4,300 people. As a comparison, in the United States, the ratio is approximately one centenarian for every 10,000 people. In this study, one of the common factors shared among centenarians in Okinawa is high blood cholesterol.

In the (year 2000) previous long version of *Alzheimer's Solved*, I wrote a section about the thymus gland. Basically, the medical community thinks only of the thymus' connection to our immune system. But it also has an influence over blood cholesterol levels. In fact, thymus gland extract is "nature's statin", because in certain situations, this substance acts to limit our liver's production of cholesterol. As we age, the thymus shrinks and withers away, so that eventually, there is no further production of thymus extract in the body. This then allows the liver to produce more cholesterol, which raises blood cholesterol levels. And this is how nature provides for humans to have higher cholesterol levels in the senior years. This is more proof that it is both natural and healthier for humans to have higher cholesterol levels in the senior years.

Back before Mevacor and the other first statin drugs were developed, some researchers considered producing thymus gland extract (artificially or from animals) as an alternate treatment for high cholesterol.

In conclusion, from this point on, please remember that it is healthy for folks in their senior years to have "high" cholesterol levels.

6-5   Head Injury, Brain Surgery, Down Syndrome

There are people who have developed Alzheimer's disease in a manner that does not have a direct correlation with low blood cholesterol levels. These individuals may even be overweight and have higher-than-average cholesterol levels. These individuals fall into one of two categories.

The first group includes people who at some time have had a head injury or who have undergone brain surgery. The time span between the injury or surgery and the development of Alzheimer's is usually years, not weeks or months. The mechanism by which the disease develops in people with a history of head injury or brain surgery will be thoroughly explained in a later chapter.

The second group of people developing Alzheimer's disease outside of the scenario of long-term semi-starvation consists of people with Down syndrome. These folks eventually develop Alzheimer's if they live beyond the age of 35. The way these individuals develop the disease is directly related to the cholesterol molecule, but it is not a situation of semi-starvation. You will find a thorough explanation in the chapter covering Down Syndrome and Alzheimer's.

6-6   Aging and Decreased Regeneration Ability

Regeneration means two things. First, it means the ability of cells to reproduce in order to replace those cells that have died or are dying. Second, in cells such as neurons (that do not reproduce), regeneration refers to their ability to repair damage.

The ability of our bodies to regenerate after damage, disease, or normal wear-and-tear, decreases as we get older. The human brain is not an exception to this principle of reduced regeneration capability in older people.

One way researchers have proven this principle is through experiments with superficial skin wounds. In one experiment, healthy people ages 15 to 55 voluntarily subjected themselves to having skin wounds inflicted on their thighs. The older people, though judged healthy in all respects, experienced longer healing times of their wounds as compared to the healing times of the younger people.

There are also experiments at the microscopic level that demonstrate the precise differences in cell performance that leads to reduced healing capacity in older people. While wounds heal in the elderly, the process is slower. Tissue regeneration capability decreases as the age of the person increases.

Researchers cannot do ongoing experiments on the brains of humans that measure response to damage inflicted intentionally. There are experiments, however, using laboratory animals from which we can draw conclusions that may apply to humans.

Neurons do not reproduce. However, they do possess the ability to repair damage to some degree. In experiments with the brains of mice, researchers discovered that old mice exhibit decreased levels of enzymes that protect brain tissue from oxidation damage. This would lead to a greater potential for oxidative damage to brain tissues in older mice as compared to younger mice.

It is reasonable to assume from experiments like this, that the brains of elderly humans are at greater risk for oxidative damage.

CHAPTER 7
Characteristics of Semi-Starvation

(Average readers may wish to skip this somewhat technical chapter.)

7-1   Alzheimer's and the Cortisol Connection

The typical Alzheimer's individual has high levels of cortisol circulating in the blood. It has not been explained why these individuals exhibit high blood cortisol, known as hypercortisolism.

The scientists who believe that Alzheimer's disease revolves around the study of apo E 4 or amyloid accumulation in the brain are unable to explain the high cortisol.

Those who believe that the genes with which you are born are the cause of Alzheimer's have not been able to explain the high cortisol levels.

Researchers who think Alzheimer's is a result of exposure to aluminum, mercury, or some other environmental agent cannot explain the high cortisol levels.

This section will explain why Alzheimer's patients typically exhibit high cortisol levels. In fact, most of the keys to understanding Alzheimer's disease are in this section and the next one.

Cortisol is the primary glucocorticoid hormone. The adrenal glands, located above each kidney, produce the glucocorticoids. Cortisol molecules originate from molecules of cholesterol (I wonder how many health professionals are aware of this fact).

Immediately after the adrenal glands secrete cortisol into the circulating bloodstream, there are three effects. First, cortisol causes cells throughout the body to give up protein. The main cells affected by this are muscle and bone cells. This action of cortisol is protein mobilization.

Second, cortisol forces fat tissue to release fat molecules into the circulation. We refer to this as fat mobilization.

The primary fuel of all cells is glucose, which comes from carbohydrates. Glucose molecules can also be made from proteins and fat molecules in a process called gluconeogenesis. This process is a third action of cortisol, namely, the production of glucose from protein and fat.

Cortisol's effects, therefore, are to immediately increase the amounts of protein, fat and glucose in the bloodstream.

There is a normal rhythm of cortisol production by the adrenal glands. The highest output occurs between 9:00 and 11:00 in the morning. It gradually tapers off during the rest of the day. The lowest amounts of production are in the middle of the night while sleeping.

In addition to the normal daily rhythm of production, the adrenal glands will secrete cortisol as an immediate reaction to stress. Some of the types of stress that may cause this include physical injuries, serious infection, surgery, intense heat or cold, and psychological stress.

The actions of cortisol occur quickly, soon after the adrenal glands produce it in the morning or after a stress stimulus. It quickly deactivates, though its effects last for hours. As our day gets going and we begin moving around in the performance of our daily activities, the cells in our body will have a readily available supply of proteins, fats, and glucose.

Let us now discuss the role of the brain. The adrenal glands release cortisol into the bloodstream after the pituitary gland in the brain secretes a signal in the form of adrenocorticotropic hormone, abbreviated as ACTH. The pituitary gland secretes ACTH in response to a signal from the hypothalamus. This signal is actually a substance called corticotrophin releasing factor, abbreviated CRF. At some point in time, a satisfactory amount of cortisol will be circulating in the blood. Once this level has been reached, the hypothalamus and pituitary stop secreting ACTH and CRF, which then causes the adrenal glands to stop releasing cortisol. This is an example of a feedback control system.

We refer to this entire arrangement as the hypothalamus-pituitary-adrenal axis, or HPA axis. During the proper time in the daily rhythm or in times of stress, the HPA axis sequence occurs.

Both physical and psychological stresses will cause an increase in blood cortisol levels. In the brain, the mechanism of stress-caused increase in cortisol involves the hippocampus. The hippocampus has actual nerve connections to the specific cells in the hypothalamus that secrete CRF, which starts the process of cortisol release by the adrenal glands. This illustrates how the limbic system influences our reactions to stress.

In a normal, healthy person, the cortisol is highest in the morning and lowest in the middle of the night. This daily rhythm is the result of two influences, the timing of meals and the pattern of physical activity.

Researchers at one time reasoned there must be some defect in the HPA axis to account for high cortisol levels typically occurring in Alzheimer's individuals. Careful testing revealed, however, that the HPA axis system in those with Alzheimer's did not differ from the system in normal, non-demented people.

The hippocampus exerts control over the hypothalamus. Some call this control regarding the HPA axis "holding the reins of a wild horse." Damage to the hippocampus can result in loss of control of the hypothalamus. The secretion of excess CRF can occur, resulting in high amounts of cortisol in the blood. Cortisol crosses the blood-brain barrier. Experiments have shown that the hippocampus is very vulnerable to damage by cortisol.

Excessive cortisol damages the hippocampus, which then causes the HPA axis to produce more cortisol. We refer to this concept as the "glucocorticoid cascade hypothesis."

Continued research revealed that in advanced cases of Alzheimer's, this pattern may indeed be occurring, but for the most part, the HPA axis is functioning normally in most people with Alzheimer's. If the hypothalamus, pituitary, and adrenal glands are not actually failing to do their jobs in the regular manner, what causes the high cortisol levels found in individuals with Alzheimer's? Even in the beginning stages of the disease, before discerning a definite diagnosis, high cortisol levels are present.

Some authors believe that the emotional and psychological stresses of today's lifestyles are the reasons for the high cortisol levels that can supposedly lead to Alzheimer's disease. They believe it is important to combat today's high-stress lifestyle. The way to do this, they believe, is by incorporating daily periods of meditation, spiritual relaxation, and consuming various herbal supplements.

These authors are wrong in their opinions. The high cortisol levels in Alzheimer's individuals are not from the stresses of today's high-pressure lifestyles. They are not due to abnormal function of the hypothalamus, pituitary, or adrenal glands. The shrinking atrophy of the hippocampus may distort the HPA axis in advanced Alzheimer's disease, but it does not play a role in the beginnings of the disease.

The cause of the high cortisol levels seen in the typical Alzheimer's person is malnutrition (or the term I prefer, semi-starvation). Pure starvation would result in death in a short amount of time. The reference to slow weight loss over a long period is more accurately known as semi-starvation.

It is unclear as to why researchers have failed to recognize that high cortisol levels in Alzheimer's individuals is due to being in a condition of semi-starvation. The almost universal characteristic of weight loss in Alzheimer's is well known, and most physiology books will state that the lack of food is one of the stresses that causes increased cortisol output.

People conducting research in individuals with anorexia nervosa are aware that high cortisol levels are present during times of active weight loss. If the individuals are able to return to normal weight, the cortisol levels return to the typical daily rhythm of a cortisol peak in the morning and low levels at night. This rhythm is lost during periods of starvation and in Alzheimer's.

The cells in our body store only enough glucose to last 12 to 24 hours. If someone has not eaten enough food to replenish the lost glucose, the cortisol mechanism begins to take over, leaving its normal daily rhythm. The body begins consuming itself (the mobilization of proteins and fats).

Cortisol forces all cells in the body to donate proteins and fats. The body assumes that proper eating in a timely manner will allow for cells to replace the lost proteins and fats during times of rest when the cortisol levels are low. If an individual does not consume the proper amounts of food, then the body will stay in starvation mode. Continuously high cortisol levels will force all cells, including those in the brain, to continually donate proteins and fats that will be used to make glucose molecules.

Perhaps one reason for missing the semi-starvation connection between cortisol and Alzheimer's is due to resumption of proper feeding of the patients, especially if they are in a nursing home facility. The damage already done to their brains is irreversible, but a regimen of nourishing meals can block the production of abnormal cortisol levels. Some Alzheimer's patients can even become overweight. This may be due to damage in the area of the hypothalamus that controls aspects of feeding behavior.

In times of stress, including starvation, the adrenal glands produce epinephrine and norepinephrine, in addition to cortisol. Epinephrine and norepinephrine "speed up" the processes of your body that are used in physical activity. Blood glucose levels rise faster, the heart beats faster, and blood pressure increases. You become "ready-to-go," with a feeling of extra energy. We normally associate these actions of epinephrine and norepinephrine with the "fight-or-flight" syndrome, but they occur in times of semi-starvation, too.

Like cortisol, some researchers will miss the elevated norepinephrine and epinephrine levels in Alzheimer's patients. I believe this is again due to resumption of adequate meals within a proper time frame.

Norepinephrine can be particularly confusing to Alzheimer's scientists. It acts as a hormone in the general circulation after the adrenal glands produce it. The production of norepinephrine also occurs in several areas of the brain, where it acts as a neurotransmitter.

The blood-brain barrier keeps the norepinephrine in the general circulating blood from affecting the specific areas in the brain where neurons make and use it as a neurotransmitter.

The confusing thing is that in patients with Alzheimer's, these specific brain areas exhibit decreased levels of noreinephrine (the neurotransmitter). These Alzheimer's patients, and anyone in a condition of semi-starvation, will usually have increased levels of norepinephrine, the hormone, circulating throughout the body. What effect then does starvation have on norepinephrine in these specific brain areas?

In experiments with laboratory animals, researchers show that after only two days of going without food, the brain levels of norepinephrine decreased.

In Alzheimer's patients' brains, areas where neurons producing norepinephrine are dying will naturally show continued decreased levels of this neurotransmitter.

Cortisol raises the blood levels of cholesterol, too. Just as in the cases of protein and fats, the cholesterol molecules come from the cortisol-caused forced "donation" by cells throughout the body, and not by a type of instantaneous synthesis. We will explore this concept of cortisol causing increased blood cholesterol levels in later sections.

During the night while sleeping, the cells of a well-nourished body make all necessary repairs and store up glucose for the energy requirements of the next day. Cholesterol synthesis occurs at the greatest rate in the middle of the night. It is not a coincidence that cortisol levels in a well-nourished body are the lowest in the middle of the night.

In the morning, all of the cells in your body are in good condition and ready to start the day. However, there is no way of knowing at this point which particular cells will be working hard through the day and which ones will have an easier time. For example, someone working on their feet all day will need more energy (glucose) re-feeding and cell repairs to their leg muscles than someone who sits all day. A person who does more lifting with their arms will then need more upkeep during the day for their arm muscles. Someone who sits and types all day will need more repair and energy refeeding in the cells of their hands and wrists.

The actions of cortisol (the forcing of all cells to "donate" proteins, fats, and cholesterol) will allow those cells that have worked the hardest during the day's activities to repair and replenish themselves to a degree. Again, the time spent sleeping is when the cells can do the best job of this, in a well nourished body.

The secretion of cortisol into the bloodstream causes cells throughout the body to "donate" cholesterol molecules, along with proteins and fats. Cortisol molecules originate from cholesterol molecules, so it is reasonable that cortisol works at the cell membrane to cause these "donations" to occur. As a result of the temporary output of cortisol in a well-nourished body, the blood level of cholesterol increases while the average cell will lose a few cholesterol molecules. Again, nature assumes that the lost cholesterol molecules (and proteins and fats) will replenish during times of rest.

To make cholesterol molecules requires materials, a large amount of energy, and thirty enzymes. Each cell needs hundreds or even thousands of cholesterol molecules. During the day when we are active, however, our bodies decide that it is more important to use these resources for the physical actions we perform while awake, and to delay production of cholesterol molecules until we are asleep. It is not a coincidence that when cortisol levels are high that cholesterol production is low.

The key enzyme in cholesterol synthesis is HMG-CoA reductase. Statins, the drugs that result in lower cholesterol levels, inhibit this enzyme. Your body will lower the amounts of cholesterol molecules made if the cells already have enough of them. This feedback control works in this way; the actual presence of a cholesterol molecule close to the HMG-CoA reductase enzyme will interfere with its action. This stops the process of cholesterol production in that part of the cell. If there are not enough cholesterol molecules, the odds are good that one will not get near to the HMG-CoA reductase enzyme to interfere with it, and production continues until there are enough. Cells will not ordinarily produce too many cholesterol molecules by this mechanism.

Research has shown that cortisol molecules will do the same thing! If a cortisol molecule gets near to the HMG-CoA reductase enzyme, it also will interfere with its actions and stop the production of cholesterol molecules.

In books that show the details of the steps of cholesterol molecule production, you will see three things listed as able to interfere with the HMG-CoA reductase enzyme: 1) adequate cholesterol already present in the cell, perhaps from dietary sources; 2) statin drugs or similar drugs; 3) fasting or starvation.

What the books may not tell you is that fasting or starvation interferes with cholesterol production through the actions of cortisol. Starvation results in higher cortisol levels, which in turn stop production of cholesterol molecules. Remember that poor food intake over a period of as short as two days can result in higher cortisol production.

The reason for this is that the body needs to preserve energy wherever possible during times of relative starvation. Our body assumes that the remedy for any shortfall in cholesterol production will occur during a later time of adequate nutrition. A cell halts production of cholesterol molecules in two situations. These are during the times when adequate cholesterol molecules are already present, and during times of starvation.

In 1986, researchers published a paper about an experiment exposing laboratory animals to glucocorticoids (cortisol is the primary one) for long periods. The hippocampus in each animal's brain suffered damage. However, if the animals received adequate nutrition, the damage minimized.

In 1985, researchers published a paper about an experiment in which laboratory animals received an artificial form of cortisol called prednisolone. After 21 days of this, there were large reductions in the amount of cholesterol in their brains.

7-2   Glucose/Glycogen Metabolism

The cells of our body use glucose molecules as the primary energy source. Breads, potatoes, and any other food classified as a starch or carbohydrate are forms of glucose. Our bodies have the capability of creating glucose molecules from fats and proteins. Making glucose from fats and proteins is gluconeogenesis. If there are not enough carbohydrates, proteins, or fats eaten in the diet, our body will feed upon itself, utilizing continuously high cortisol levels.

The important things to remember are that glucose molecules transport to the cells of the body in the bloodstream, and that once inside of the cells the glucose molecules are stored as glycogen. Glycogen forms in the cells by linking together glucose molecules into long branching chains.

Typically, the cells of our body can store enough glycogen to last from 12 to 24 hours. However, neurons in the brain can store only enough glycogen to last about two minutes! The metabolic rates in the brain are very high. It takes a lot of energy to pump the nerve impulses through the billions of interconnecting neurons.

If the brain's neurons can only store two minutes' worth of glucose in the form of glycogen chains, it seems obvious that a continuous, uninterrupted supply of glucose molecules in the bloodstream is necessary. Neurons in the brain do not get preferential treatment, however, compared with other cells in the body. The only advantage that neurons in the brain have over other cells in the body is that glucose molecules can cross the neuron cell membranes without having to have insulin molecules present.

If there are not enough glucose molecules in the bloodstream, a condition called hypoglycemia exists, or "low blood sugar." An excessively high amount of glucose in the blood is hyperglycemia, or "high blood sugar."

We are discussing this because another one of the hallmark signs in patients with Alzheimer's disease is low brain glucose metabolism when compared to a normal, non-demented subject. The brain of an Alzheimer's patient typically is taking up less actual amounts of glucose.

Some would say that the Alzheimer's brain takes up less glucose because it has atrophied to a smaller size. Researchers have found, however, that this is not the case. The neurons in still-healthy brain areas are taking up less glucose per volume of brain tissue. These measurements are independent of the total amount of brain tissue.

If the total body blood sugar is low (hypoglycemia), then it stands to reason that the brain would get less glucose.

Do Alzheimer's patients exhibit hypoglycemia? The answer is yes, although there are exceptions. If the researchers are performing the tests on Alzheimer's patients who are in an organized and controlled environment, such as a nursing home, then they will probably be well nourished. Even Alzheimer's patients, if they have eaten well during the days before the glucose test, will not turn out to be hypoglycemic. If they test the patient when first diagnosed, and before he/she is under regular professional care, then the chances are good that the patient will test as hypoglycemic.

In situations of lasting hypoglycemia, the brain seems to suffer more damage than other tissues in the body. Researchers have shown that after only three days of little or no food there is a reduction in brain glucose metabolism of anywhere from 24 to 30 percent. If someone were to last for three weeks on little or no food, the drop in brain glucose metabolism exceeds 50 percent, compared to a normal, well-fed person.

Finally, what if the person who is not eating enough happens to have already reached such a degree of thinness that he/she does not have very much body fat left?

There is research that shows that if they deprive cultures containing laboratory animal's brain tissues of their normal amount of glucose, then the starving (but not dead) cells started producing beta amyloid within four days.

In another research laboratory, researchers slowly deprived cultures containing neurons of all glucose. The researchers specifically used neurons from each brain's hippocampus. As they eliminated the glucose supply, there appeared neurofibrillary tangle formations of tau protein. There also were signs of ubiquitin, which I will cover in a later section. The neurons exhibited increased amounts of calcium ions crossing their cell membranes, and they eventually died.

As beta amyloid accumulates in brain tissues, it causes further interference with glucose metabolism. There is experimental evidence using neurons from the brains of laboratory animals that show that amyloid blocks glucose transport into them. In turn, this leads to even less glucose and further degeneration of the neurons.

As amyloid plaques accumulate in association with the brain's blood vessels, transporting glucose from the blood into all of the brain tissues, and not just neurons, are negatively affected.

These last two paragraphs cite research that can explain why the brains of Alzheimer's patients will still show reduced glucose metabolism even if the patients are now being well fed. Once amyloid plaques accumulate in large quantities in the brain, they do not go away.

The typical Alzheimer's patient shows high cortisol output by the adrenal glands, which is outside of the normal daily rhythm.

Evidence exists which demonstrates that occasional exposure of brain tissues, including neurons from the hippocampus, to cortisol does no permanent damage. However, continuous exposure of these brain tissues to cortisol results in decreased glucose metabolism and cell damage.

There have been tests on humans that demonstrate that increasing the glucose levels in blood can enhance memory and thought processes. Some researchers have even achieved improvement of memory in some Alzheimer's patients merely by increasing the blood glucose levels. However, glucose feeding does not constitute a cure. Remember there is no replacement for the dead neurons in the brain. The effect is probably due to an improvement in the function of the remaining neurons.

There are two important terms in discussing glucose/glycogen metabolism. They are "fed" and "fasting." Glucose/glycogen metabolism in tissues relates to these two terms in that the state of the tissue will indicate the phase in which it exists.

If a cell in your body has an adequate amount of glucose, it will be in a "fed" condition. Glucose molecules actively gather into long branching chains for storage, known as glycogen.

In the opposite condition, where there is not enough glucose for the cell, we consider it to be in the "fasting" condition. The cell is not linking glucose molecules together into glycogen chains. Rather, it is breaking the chains down into individual glucose molecules.

Insulin is a hormone produced by the pancreas that does two things: it lets glucose from the blood get across the cell membrane into the interior, and it stimulates glycogen formation (synthesis) for storage of glucose.

Glucagon is another hormone produced by the pancreas. Its main target is the liver, which is rich in glycogen. Glucagon promotes glycogen breakdown, which results in glucose molecules releasing into the bloodstream. Glucagon raises the blood sugar levels in this way.

An individual cell is in either the fed condition or the fasting condition. Either glucose turns into glycogen (fed), or glycogen is being broken down into glucose molecules (fasting). A cell cannot be in both states at the same time.

We as humans are the sum total of all of the cells in our bodies. If we are gaining weight, then we are in the fed condition. If we are losing weight, then we are in the fasting condition.

Depending on what our daily activities happen to be, some cells in our body may be in the fed state and others may be in the fasting state. If someone walks five miles without saying a word, then the leg muscle cells are probably in the fasting state while the muscle cells in the tongue are in the fed state. On the other hand, if one gives an hour-long speech while sitting down, the tongue muscle cells would probably be in the fasting state and the leg muscle cells would be in the fed state.

In each cell, enzymes that are active in the fed condition are different from those that are active in the fasting condition. A cell cannot be in both phases at the same time.

An enzyme will continue to promote reactions until the cell does something to inactivate the particular enzyme. One of the ways that a cell can inactivate (stop) an enzyme is to have another enzyme add phosphorus groups to it.

The enzymes involved with the metabolic processes of glucose/glycogen are universally common to all the cells of the body. They are also involved in controlling cell processes that are not directly involved with glucose/glycogen metabolism.

The key enzyme involved with the linking together of glucose molecules to form glycogen is glycogen synthase.

If the cell senses that the supply of glucose molecules is decreasing and it is burning more than it is bringing in, it switches to the fasting state. The cell must stop the actions of glycogen synthase. It does this by adding phosphorus groups to the glycogen synthase enzymes. The enzyme that does this is glycogen synthase kinase.

Let us summarize. Glycogen synthase is associated with the fed state. Glycogen synthase kinase is associated with the fasting state.

In Alzheimer's brains, the dying neurons display neurofibrillary tangles. These tangles consist of tau protein fibrils that have had phosphorus groups added to them. This hyperphosphorylation causes them to pair up and become twisted. The microtubules, which the tau protein fibrils stabilized, now will no longer perform the movement processes that maintain the neuron, so it eventually dies.

What was the enzyme that caused the extra phosphorus groups to be added to the tau protein fibrils? The answer is glycogen synthase kinase, the same enzyme that becomes active if a cell is in a fasting condition! This tells us that the neurons that are dying in an Alzheimer's patient's brain are starving to death.

The enzyme that removes the phosphorus groups from glycogen synthase enzymes when glucose is abundant again (fed state) is phosphatase 2-A. The real key to a cell's shift from the fasting to the fed state rests with phosphatase 2-A. The natural tendency in a cell is for glycogen synthase kinase to continue adding phosphorus groups to glycogen synthase (and tau protein fibrils, if the fasting state of the cell persists). If glucose molecules become abundant, phosphatase 2-A starts removing the phosphorus groups from the glycogen synthase enzymes, and glycogen formation begins again.

Let us summarize again. If someone is well nourished, there will be abundant glucose molecules in the bloodstream. The pancreas secretes insulin in this situation, which promotes the entry of glucose into the cells and, in addition, promotes the formation of glycogen as a storage form of glucose. Phosphatase 2-A is the enzyme that removes the phosphorus groups from the glycogen synthase enzymes, and glycogen formation proceeds. The cells in this instance are in the fed condition.

If someone is not relatively well nourished and there are beginning to be shortages of glucose molecules, the pancreas secretes glucagon, a hormone that stops further glycogen formation and directs its breakdown into individual glucose molecules. Glucagon prevents phosphatase 2-A from removing the phosphorus groups off glycogen synthase enzymes. The phosphorus groups were added by the enzyme glycogen synthase kinase, which adds them to tau protein fibrils as well if these conditions of fasting persist.

All of the information covered in this section directly connects to cholesterol. To make a molecule of cholesterol requires a lot of energy from glucose "burning", materials (from glucose or sometimes fatty acids), and thirty enzymes. Glucagon, the hormone associated with a fasting condition, inhibits the production of cholesterol molecules at the step involving HMG-CoA reductase.

It has also been determined that insulin, the hormone of the fed condition (when glucose is abundant), increases the production of cholesterol molecules.

7-3   Serotonin, Melatonin, and Chronic Restlessness

Patients with Alzheimer's disease will frequently have changes in their patterns of being awake or asleep. Their medical chart may list insomnia. They will constantly wander around at times that are not appropriate, called a pattern of chronic restlessness.

Researchers have noticed that the levels of two hormones, serotonin and melatonin, are frequently lower in Alzheimer's patients compared to healthy people. Some researchers immediately concluded that the mechanisms of serotonin and melatonin metabolism were not working correctly in Alzheimer's patients. Some said that this might even be a cause of the disease.

More thorough testing revealed, however, that the serotonin and melatonin systems were working as designed in Alzheimer's patients.

Serotonin is not only a hormone. In various places in the brain, it acts as a neurotransmitter. The intestines, as well as the brain in normal healthy people, make high concentrations of serotonin. It produces feelings of calmness, emotional well being, and satiation. Satiation is the state of feeling satisfied after one has eaten a filling meal.

The levels of serotonin produced in the intestines increase after a meal of carbohydrates and fats. Foods high in carbohydrates and fats include potatoes, pastries, cakes, cookies, nachos, breads, donuts, pretzels, etc. Alzheimer's patients sometimes exhibit cravings for carbohydrate and sweet foods.

Serotonin levels increase after eating these carbohydrates and fatty types of foods. Someone with low levels of serotonin indicates that they are not eating enough of these foods. This is another indication of the existence of a state of semi-starvation in Alzheimer's patients. When our bodies make cholesterol molecules, they use glucose and/or fats as the sources of the materials and energy needed in the process.

Melatonin is a hormone made in the pineal gland in the brain. Melatonin is made from serotonin! In humans, melatonin is involved in the regulation of sleep periods. It also has an effect on our emotional mood. The production of melatonin is sensitive to whether it is day or night. There is a definite rhythm, for the enzyme in the pineal gland changing serotonin to melatonin is ten times more active at night than during the day. This is the reason why you feel sleepy at night.

The pineal gland can make its own serotonin for the conversion to melatonin. The gland is also sensitive to circulating levels of serotonin. Increasing the amounts of serotonin will cause increases in the amounts melatonin, regardless of whether it is day or night. This is the reason why you feel sleepy after a large meal.

In experiments, people injected with melatonin began to feel sleepy, regardless of whether it was day or night and regardless whether or not they had eaten.

Laboratory animals that had serotonin injections lost any desires to eat foods containing carbohydrates, even if the animals had not eaten any prior to the injections.

Experiments with laboratory animals show that the pineal gland produces less melatonin when exposed to cortisol and norepinephrine. Remember that in semi-starvation, cortisol and norepinephrine levels are increased. Cortisol and norepinephrine lower the production of melatonin by the pineal gland even at night in laboratory animals with full stomachs. This may be the reason why psychological stresses of various kinds, which boost cortisol and norepinephrine, can cause a sleepless night.

The hypothalamus and hippocampus are sensitive to the amount of serotonin circulating in the blood. This is the link that produces the satiation and feelings of emotional well being that a full stomach can bring. Through the same link, however, high cortisol levels circulating in the blood, produced when it has been a long time since the last meal, produce feelings of hunger and cravings for carbohydrates.

Melatonin also possesses some antioxidant properties.

In some patients with Alzheimer's the serotonin and melatonin levels are not significantly different from normal, non-demented people. You can probably guess the reason for this. If the caregivers of the Alzheimer's patients were successful in getting the patients to eat satisfactorily in the days leading up to the tests, then their serotonin and melatonin levels would be normal.

In patients with significant damage to the hippocampus and other limbic system structures, however, even a filling meal may not prevent the interrupted sleep patterns and restlessness.

7-4   The Inflammation/Cholesterol Relationship

Numerous investigators have determined that in the brains of Alzheimer's patients there are active inflammatory processes taking place. Secondly, scientific evidence seems to show that people who have been taking non-steroidal anti-inflammatory drugs (NSAIDs) over long periods exhibit some degree of protection against Alzheimer's.

Inflammation is basically the protective response of the tissues in our bodies to irritation, insult, or injury. The things that cause the body to mount an inflammatory response include burns from heat or chemicals, cold exposure, bacterial or virus invasions of cells, physical trauma (cuts, scrapes, bruises, etc.), broken bones, and other things.

In the body's system of protection, the inflammatory response must neutralize the agent causing the inflammation and then produce new cell growth to replace the cells damaged and lost.

At the microscopic level, the body responds with special cells, such as macrophages, leukocytes, and extra fibroblasts. Chemical messengers signal that the inflammatory processes have begun.

The steps involved in the actual inflammatory response are very complicated. The processes of inflammation begin when your body senses that things that are supposed to be inside of healthy cells begin appearing outside of cells. Whatever causes cells to open, and let their insides get outside, will start the inflammatory response. Cutting, scraping, crushing, freezing, or burning cell membranes can cause them to open. Chemicals can cause them to burst. Bacteria and viruses or their toxins can cause cells to open. All of these things result in the deaths of the cells, as well as providing the triggers to start the inflammatory process.

What does cholesterol have to do with inflammation? The answer is that in all of these examples, from bacterial infections to significant wounds to various illnesses, there is found a lowering of the blood cholesterol levels. Why do blood cholesterol levels go down in these situations of cells opening up and dying? You would think that the leftover membranes of dead cells would raise blood cholesterol levels.

However, blood cholesterol levels are a measurement of cholesterol molecules on lipoproteins (LDL's and HDL's), not a measurement of free cholesterol molecules that are part of the debris of dead cells.

As the body is quickly trying to generate new cells, it uses the cholesterol in the lipoproteins; LDL's in most of the body and HDL's (such as apo E) in nervous tissues. The result is the lowering of the blood cholesterol values, at least until the healing processes are close to completion.

Accordingly, the manufacturing of new cholesterol molecules speeds up in the inflammatory process. The increasing rates of activity of the key enzyme in the process, HMG-CoA reductase, illustrate this fact.

However, in times of inflammation, if a condition of malnutrition or starvation is present, the manufacturing of new cholesterol molecules does not speed up. In fact, it even slows down.

Experimenters have found that during the inflammatory responses in laboratory animals there was an increase in the amounts of amyloid. There was also a relationship between the amyloid production and the cholesterol production during the inflammation. Discussion of this issue occurs in detail in the next chapter.

We now know that inflammation is associated with a lowering of the blood cholesterol levels. In several experiments, if the blood cholesterol levels were increased in a laboratory animal and the animal is then subjected to an injury or insult, then the inflammatory response is lower in intensity. In other words, boosting blood cholesterol levels qualifies as a real anti-inflammatory treatment. Incidentally, the cholesterol levels in the laboratory animals were increased in some cases by feeding the animals cholesterol, and in others, by using drugs that increased blood cholesterol.

If cells have less access to fresh cholesterol molecules, then they are more likely to have situations where their "insides" can start to leak out. When the body senses that cell "insides" are on the outside, the inflammatory process begins. Therefore, we can logically say that low blood cholesterol levels can be a cause of inflammation even when there are no wounds or infections. What is the most common cause of low blood cholesterol levels? Long-term semi-starvation.

7-5   The Ubiquitin Connection to Alzheimer's

Ubiquitin is a small protein found in the shrinking brains of Alzheimer's patients. It is also in the brains of aging people in areas of damage, even though the people may not be demented. To my knowledge, no medical researchers have explained why they commonly discover ubiquitin in Alzheimer's patients' brains.

The weight loss that results from malnutrition, starvation, semi-starvation, or dieting is due to the body's actions of consuming itself. Cells are broken down and the proteins and fats degraded to produce glucose (gluconeogenesis). The utilization of cholesterol is to replace that which is lost in normal processes, such as renewal of the skin on our bodies. Our bodies have a method of marking the tissues to sacrifice during times of starvation. Ubiquitin is the small protein used to "tag" the cells and proteins that are to be consumed for the good of the body as a whole during times of starvation.

In addition, research shows ubiquitin inhibits the key enzyme in the cholesterol-manufacturing process, HMG-CoA reductase. Couple this with the findings of ubiquitin in the tau proteins of neurofibrillary tangles and you can see why neurons are being consumed during a state of starvation.

Whenever you see a reference to a protein called ubiquitin, the first thing you should think of is the consumption of cell tissue during some type of starvation process.

7-6   The Nitric Oxide Connection to Alzheimer's

First, do not confuse the nitric oxide discussed in this section with nitrous oxide, known as laughing gas.

Several different kinds of cells produce nitric oxide in the body. An enzyme called nitric oxide synthase makes it. The body uses it in a number of different ways, and some areas of the brain use it as a neurotransmitter.

The greatest amount of knowledge concerning nitric oxide relates to its association with blood vessels in periods of physical stress. Nitric oxide molecules are instantly produced in these situations of greater demand for blood flow, and the molecules cause the blood vessels to relax and get larger in diameter. The vessels dilate, and the term used to describe this is vasodilation. When the period of physical stress is over, the demand for blood returns to normal. Nitric oxide production goes down, and the blood vessels "constrict," returning to their normal diameter.

The muscle tissues of the heart need an increased blood supply in situations of greater demand for working skeletal muscles. Nitric oxide molecules will also cause the blood vessels serving heart muscle to dilate in this period of greater physical exertion.

Those people with atherosclerosis will sometimes experience chest pain whenever they suddenly do something strenuous. The pain is from the heart's muscle tissues being unable to receive enough blood flow to meet the suddenly increased need. Many of these people will be able to take a medication that has nitroglycerin as its active ingredient. Nitroglycerin works through this same nitric oxide mechanism to cause the blood vessels serving the heart to dilate. The heart muscle quickly begins receiving more blood, and the chest pain diminishes.

Blood vessels that are afflicted with atherosclerosis have plaques of fat, cholesterol and calcium. Not only does less blood flow through them, but they also are restricted in their ability to relax and dilate when the situation calls for it.

Research has shown that high cholesterol content in blood vessels results in decreased production of nitric oxide. Lower amounts of nitric oxide directly cause the blood vessels to remain in a condition of being unable to relax and dilate.

This relationship of cholesterol and nitric oxide is not limited to blood vessels that are afflicted with the plaques of atherosclerosis. Research has shown that those cells involved with nitric oxide production are sensitive to the amount of cholesterol in their cell membranes in all situations. High cholesterol content in the cell membrane means low nitric oxide production.

The opposite situation also applies. Lower cholesterol content in the cell membrane results in higher nitric oxide production. This results in an increased ability to relax and dilate, which allows more blood to flow. It helps to lower blood pressure.

Research has shown that the blood cholesterol level directly relates to nitric oxide production in an inverse way. Higher blood cholesterol causes lower nitric oxide production. Lower blood cholesterol causes higher nitric oxide production.

Researchers have repeatedly found that in the brains of Alzheimer's patients, there are increased amounts of nitric oxide!

Nitric oxide levels are high in the brains of Alzheimer's patients simply because the cholesterol levels are low. Excess nitric oxide molecules turn into a more harmful type of molecule called peroxynitrite that oxidizes and damages healthy cells. The excess nitric oxide itself can make blood vessels so relaxed that they can actually become weakened. Such blood vessels with low cholesterol content and high nitric oxide levels are at risk for coming apart. We recognize this as a stroke. Brain hemorrhages (strokes) are common in Alzheimer's patients even though they have low blood pressures.

From this point onwards, any references to greater amounts of nitric oxide in the brains of Alzheimer's patients should indicate that conditions of low cholesterol exist.

7-7   The Interleukins and Tumor Necrosis Factor

Cytokines are substances that are involved with the body's response in situations of inflammation. The interleukins and tumor necrosis factor are cytokines, and researchers find them increased in Alzheimer's patients. The word tumor in this term does not actually mean that there is a cancer present. The interleukin cytokines are assigned numbers, and interleukin 6 is the one usually found to be in increased amounts in Alzheimer's patients.

Because they can be elevated in Alzheimer's patients, many researchers view this as further evidence that the disease is a type of inflammation of the brain. The thought is that there may be some kind of defect in these patients' immune systems. Following the patterns discussed in previous sections, the cytokines we are talking about in this section are in actuality part of a normal reaction to the conditions that are present in Alzheimer's patients. These conditions are ones associated with a state of semi-starvation and cholesterol shortage.

Incidentally, the same conditions that produce increases in tumor necrosis factor and the interleukins also lead to increased production of amyloid.

Inflammation is the body's response to a situation where the "insides" of cells are on the outside of them. This tells the body that there is damage to the cell membranes, and the repair and regeneration systems have to go to work. Injury, burns, infection, chemicals, and various stages of semi-starvation leading to a deficiency of cholesterol molecules can cause the damage to the cell membranes. Cytokines like tumor necrosis factor and the interleukins are some of the agents of the body that are responsible for generating the things that are necessary for the repair of existing cell membranes and the "construction" of new ones.

Energy (in the form of glucose) and materials, namely cholesterol molecules and various fatty acids, are the things needed to help repair cell membranes and supply the building blocks for new ones.

Researchers have shown that tumor necrosis factor speeds up the creation of glucose molecules from proteins (gluconeogenesis). Research shows it also stimulates cells to take up existing glucose molecules from the blood and to increase the production of cholesterol, especially in the liver.

If you add tumor necrosis factor to the circulating blood of healthy hamsters, it results in a gradual increase in the blood cholesterol levels. Additional experiments showed that it also raised the blood cholesterol levels of healthy humans, as well.

The interleukins show some of the same properties regarding production of cholesterol. However, the interleukins have as a primary effect the gathering of cholesterol molecules by cells and the incorporation of them into cell membranes. I say this based on research that demonstrated two things. First, the interleukins (and tumor necrosis factor) cause cells to display more LDL-receptors on the surfaces of their membranes. This is the way that cells acquire cholesterol molecules from the blood. Second, adding one of the interleukins by I.V. to the bloodstream of human volunteers lowered the blood cholesterol levels. If cells are instructed to take up more cholesterol, it will lower the blood cholesterol levels temporarily.

In summary, patients with Alzheimer's disease exhibit higher levels of tumor necrosis factor and the interleukins, all of which are cytokines and are part of the body's response to inflammation. These particular cytokines help with the body's mechanism of glucose, cholesterol, and fatty acid production. They also help with the repair of existing cell membranes and the creation of new ones.

7-8   Prolactin and Growth Hormone

Prolactin is a hormone produced by the pituitary gland, which hangs from the brain's base. Though prolactin originates from the pituitary gland in both men and women, it is primarily associated with milk production in women.

Growth hormone, also produced and secreted by the pituitary gland, is very similar to prolactin in its chemical structure. Growth hormone promotes the manufacture of proteins by cells. It also increases the use of body fat for energy production. Growth hormone has a daily pattern of secretion, with the highest amount secreted during sleep, around midnight.

The pituitary gland secretes other hormones, as we learned in earlier sections. Structures in the limbic system, especially the hypothalamus, control the pituitary.

We are discussing prolactin and growth hormone because researchers have found that there are increased levels of these two hormones in the blood of Alzheimer's patients. We, of course, are talking about people over the age of sixty. They are past the normal years of body growth and they are not nursing babies.

Prolactin specifically acts to stimulate cells to increase production of cholesterol molecules. Researchers first discovered this in the study of milk production in nursing mothers. Prolactin is the hormone responsible for breast milk's having cholesterol. All cells having HMG-CoA reductase are under the influence of prolactin to increase cholesterol production if exposed to this hormone. It does not matter whether the person is young or old, male or female.

Growth hormone also stimulates the production of cholesterol, somewhat. It is similar to prolactin in chemical structure. Its main effect is for increasing the ability of cells to take up cholesterol molecules from the blood, along with proteins and fats. After all, for tissue growth or at least maintenance to occur, the cells must bring these things from the blood and into their structures.

Focusing on Alzheimer's, the disease develops primarily in older adults after a period of semi-starvation and weight loss. If prolactin and growth hormone are found to be increased in Alzheimer's patients, then that would mean that normal, non-demented adults should also show increased blood levels of prolactin and growth hormone in times of dieting with significant weight loss.

Research shows this to be true. In adults who are dieting successfully and are experiencing real weight loss, these two hormones are found to be increased in the blood.

In conclusion, Alzheimer's patients frequently have increased levels of prolactin and growth hormone in their blood because their bodies are in a state of semi-starvation.

7-9   Osteoporosis

Osteoporosis is basically a generalized loss of bone structure. The removal of proteins and minerals, mainly calcium, occurs and the bone becomes weaker. Fractures easily occur as a result.

Women who are past menopause seem to develop problems associated with osteoporosis more than men do. Some of the conditions that lead to this disease (besides being an older woman) include deficient consumption of calcium and vitamin D, general malnutrition, and excess cortisol levels in the blood. When you think about it, semi-starvation leads to all of these factors. It is not surprising to learn, therefore, that many Alzheimer's patients simultaneously suffer from osteoporosis.

There is a disorder called Cushing's Disease in which the adrenal glands produce very high levels of glucocorticoids, especially cortisol. The patients will frequently develop osteoporosis. The cortisol forces the bone to "donate" proteins, calcium, and other substances, leaving a very weakened structure. A later chapter will discuss Cushing's Disease in greater detail.

People taking steroid medications (which have the same actions as cortisol, only stronger) can develop osteoporosis.

In conclusion, the findings of osteoporosis in Alzheimer's patients is due to long-term semi-starvation. It is not due to some type of abnormal bone metabolism.

7-10 Cholesterol and Cortisol, Predisone (Steroid) and Cyclosporine Therapies

The adrenal glands produce the natural hormone cortisol from cholesterol molecules. Normally, there is a daily pattern of cortisol production and secretion by the adrenal glands, with the highest amount of cortisol in the bloodstream occurring in the morning. The lowest levels occur during the night, while sleeping. The production occurs outside of this pattern in response to all kinds of mental and physical stresses. Production also takes place during periods of malnutrition and starvation.

Cortisol molecules do not last very long once they are in circulation. Their activity is brief, but their effects last for several hours. The most obvious effect is the raising of blood cholesterol levels. However, this is from the forced "donations" of cells. New molecules of cholesterol are not manufactured to provide this effect. In fact, cortisol stops the manufacture of cholesterol molecules by blocking the key enzyme in the process, HMG-CoA reductase.

Artificial (or synthetic) steroids made by pharmaceutical companies possess the same effects as cortisol, except that the synthetic glucocorticoids are 10 to 100 times more powerful than the body's own cortisol. These synthetic steroids fall under the classification of anti-inflammatory drugs. The most commonly known steroid anti-inflammatory drug is probably prednisone.

How do these synthetic glucocorticoids (like prednisone) stop inflammation? Usually the literature about them states that they reduce inflammation by stabilizing membranes and decreasing the permeability of capillaries (small blood vessels).

It is never stated, however, exactly how the membranes stabilize and the capillaries made less permeable (less prone to leakage). The increase in cholesterol levels brought about by steroids is, in fact, the reason for the stabilization of membranes and the resistance of capillaries to leaking. Synthetic steroids like prednisone are 10 to 100 times more potent than cortisol. This tells me, therefore, that there will be 10 to 100 times more cholesterol molecules available almost instantaneously. As a result, the symptoms of inflammation are under control quickly.

Two of the more prominent effects of cortisol and the powerful synthetic steroids are, first, that blood cholesterol levels are raised quickly through the forcing of cells to "donate" cholesterol molecules (and proteins and fats). Second, the manufacture of new cholesterol molecules is blocked.

It is not possible for someone to have exactly the precise amount of cortisol produced by the adrenals to meet the repair needs of the cells, but in the average healthy person it usually balances out over the long term.

It is not possible for a doctor to prescribe the exact amount of synthetic steroid that is required to deal with some person's inflammatory condition. More steroid dosage than necessary will always be prescribed, because any amount less will leave the patient still suffering from the inflammatory condition.

The published effects of overdosing of steroids can be broken down into two categories. If someone taking steroids is eating adequate or more than adequate amounts of food, then that individual will develop unusual body fat deposit patterns in the face, neck, and upper trunk areas.

The second category of steroid side effects occurs in people who are not eating enough. They can develop muscle, bone and skin changes, and eye cataracts.

People may vary back and forth between periods of adequate eating and periods of poor eating. Therefore, there is usually an overlapping of these symptoms in people taking steroids (like prednisone) for years due to some chronic inflammatory condition.

One side effect of long-term steroid use is atherosclerosis, because of the very high blood cholesterol levels. You will see someone with lupus that ends up suffering a heart attack because of the years of chronic high cholesterol levels caused by steroids.

There is also a major problem in people who have undergone an organ transplant. It is a cruel fate indeed to go through the ordeal of a heart or kidney transplant operation, only to end up suffering a heart attack from atherosclerosis. Unfortunately, transplant patients encounter levels of inflammation that only steroids are able to control.

Cyclosporine is another medicine used to control the inflammation in organ transplant patients. It is technically not a steroid, and research indicates it fights inflammation by influencing lymphocytes. However, cyclosporine also raises blood cholesterol levels, so there is still the risk of atherosclerosis with long-term use.

The "side effects" of high cholesterol levels in steroid patients are actually the real reasons for the beneficial results of these anti-inflammatory drugs.

The same can be said about cyclosporine.

This book is primarily about Alzheimer's disease, an illness in which the brain gradually shrinks in size. Brain tissue normally has almost the highest percentage of cholesterol of any tissue in the body. I have spoken at length of how cortisol forces cells outside of the liver to "donate" cholesterol molecules. In an older person with poor eating patterns, the constantly high cortisol levels that semi-starvation produces will pull cholesterol molecules out of the brain tissue in a slow, gradual manner.

Stress will cause an increase of cortisol production. In experiments subjecting laboratory rats to mental stress (the rats were restrained from moving around), the extra cortisol that they produced caused shrinkage of neurons in their brains.

In other experiments with rats, administering synthetic steroids for 21 days resulted in reductions of brain cholesterol content and overall brain weight.

There were researchers who fed prednisone to pregnant rats for one week before giving birth. The baby rats that were born had significantly less cholesterol in their brains than did those born to untreated mothers.

Researchers in Detroit found that people taking prednisone for as little as three months displayed memory problems. The authors cautioned that their research possibly suggests that steroid anti-inflammatory medicines may not be a good treatment to prevent Alzheimer's disease.

Back in 1978, researchers performed brain-imaging tests on fifteen people who had been taking steroids for long periods. All fifteen were suffering from autoimmune diseases. The oldest was only 40 years old. <u>Every one of the fifteen patients suffered brain shrinkage.</u>

7-11   High Cortisol Levels Will "Mask" Low Cholesterol

Cortisol produced in the excessive amounts that semi-starvation brings about will maintain what appears to be adequate or perhaps even higher-than-normal blood cholesterol levels. These levels will vary, because the person's physical activities during the weight-losing period will vary.

The key to remember is that the person is losing weight. The cholesterol is not newly manufactured, but is taken from existing tissues. Cortisol blocks the manufacture of new cholesterol molecules.

At some point, the weight loss is so extensive that cholesterol levels will begin to decrease in spite of cortisol's actions. Much of the damage has already occurred by this time. Muscle damage, possible osteoporosis, diminished fat storage deposits, and skin changes are some of the recognized effects of long-term malnutrition or semi-starvation.

It is time to add brain shrinkage to the list. In younger people, who have a better capability to repair tissue damage, the brain shrinkage may be reversible if adequate re-feeding begins. In older people, who generally have less of an ability to heal and recover from tissue damage, the atrophy and loss of brain tissue is not reversible. It leads to neuron death and Alzheimer's disease.

Patients with anorexia nervosa are people who are definitely losing weight. Researchers find that high levels of cortisol exist in these people. Other researchers who studied the blood cholesterol levels in anorexia nervosa patients have found that the patients will often exhibit normal or even high cholesterol levels in their blood. The authors of these cholesterol studies offer different opinions as to the reasons for the high cholesterol levels found in anorexia nervosa patients. If they would study the research on cortisol in both anorexia nervosa and starvation, then they would see the reasons for the temporary normal or high cholesterol levels seen in these patients. As a consequence of these high cortisol levels, body tissues are being lost and the patients are losing weight.

7-12   The Ammonia Connection

When proteins are broken down into amino acids, further processing requires removal of the nitrogen (amine) groups from the amino acids. This results in the production of ammonia, of which removal from the body is necessary because it is harmful to cells.

One of the signs of the body consuming itself in the weight-losing process of starvation is an increase in the production of ammonia. Ammonia is not usually one of the things routinely tested for in the industrialized nations, because malnutrition and starvation are not common in these places.

A few researchers have recognized that Alzheimer's patients have higher levels of ammonia, but they did not definitely conclude that the cause was possibly starvation/malnutrition.

The excess ammonia levels found in Alzheimer's patients are due to their being in a state of semi-starvation.

CHAPTER 8
The Primary Cause of Alzheimer 's disease

8-1   Long-Term Shortages of Cholesterol Cause Neuron Damage

The mechanism through which head injury and brain surgery patients develop Alzheimer's will be explained in later sections. The mechanism still involves cholesterol.

For the majority of elderly folks who develop Alzheimer's disease, it is due to simply not eating enough foods in general, but especially not eating enough foods with cholesterol in them. Alzheimer's disease is caused by a chronic state of semi-starvation lasting for many months and often, several years. This is coupled with the decreased healing and regeneration abilities of the tissues of older people.

One phrase that is almost a religious chant among people who write books about human health topics is, "Your body makes all of the cholesterol it needs."

After reviewing thousands of research papers regarding all the aspects of cholesterol metabolism, I have yet to find the research study that proves that the human body makes all of the cholesterol it needs during a lifetime. On the contrary, I have found a mountain of research detailing diseases and conditions that are associated with low levels of cholesterol.

There is only one disease that is associated somewhat with "high" cholesterol levels, and that is atherosclerosis/heart disease. We will discuss this in later chapters.

I will describe the mechanism by which low cholesterol levels over a long period of time in an elderly brain are the cause of Alzheimer's disease.

Cells do not make all of the cholesterol molecules they need in the maintenance of their membranes. The proof for this is the fact that cells display LDL-receptors on their membrane surfaces in order to obtain cholesterol molecules from the bloodstream.

In humans, the liver and intestines make cholesterol molecules and send them into the circulation for use by cells throughout the body (including the brain in adult humans). The human body has evolved in such a way that it depends on getting cholesterol from the diet, though many people do not believe this.

Brain tissue consists of cholesterol, fats, and proteins. The human brain is very large relative to body size, and is the most advanced of all in the animal kingdom. It is a hard-working organ with a high metabolic rate. The high metabolic rate sets the stage for oxidation of cholesterol and other lipid molecules.

Myelin, the insulating coating around neuron branches (axons), is absolutely dependent on adequate cholesterol molecules, just as cell membranes are. It is required in sufficient amounts, or myelin will break down, even if the other lipids and proteins are present in adequate amounts.

It is mandatory for neurons to have adequate amounts of cholesterol in the membranes at their synapses, where they communicate with other neurons.

The absolute pinnacle of animal evolution on this planet is that part of the human brain that performs cognitive functions: memory, thought, learning, perception, emotions, etc. We call this part of the human brain the limbic system, and it has the hippocampus and other structures detailed in previous sections. The structures of the limbic system are the reason why humans survived and became the dominant species.

However, the price for this is that all factors must be perfectly and continuously satisfied in the human brain. Cells must have adequate amounts of non-oxidized cholesterol molecules, an adequate supply of glucose, sufficient oxygen, and a functioning protection system. Wastes and oxidized molecules of cholesterol, fats, etc., must be removed.

The brain is not the first in line to receive cholesterol molecules. Our skin is the first to receive them. The skin performs many tasks, including the retention of body fluids, temperature regulation, and acting as a barrier to bacteria. Retaining body fluids is the most important one. Cholesterol is the "waterproofing" molecule that allows skin to be flexible.

Our skin is totally shed every 39 to 48 days, and that requires many cholesterol molecules. Other organs and tissues also require cholesterol in continuous amounts.

As we age, the systems that maintain cell membranes in a healthy condition do not work as well. Adequate nutrition, therefore, becomes especially important the older we get. Because of this, more cholesterol is needed in our diet as we age.

In conditions of semi-starvation we lose weight. The body is feeding upon itself through a mechanism that utilizes cortisol and other substances. Fats, proteins, and cholesterol are removed from some tissues in semi-starvation in order to satisfy the needs of more important tissues, such as the skin. Cholesterol is removed from the brain and is not replaced as long as the person is in a state of semi-starvation.

If the condition persists over a long time, the brain cholesterol levels become lower and the brain shrinks in size and weight. Cells in blood vessels in the brain, as well as the neurons, astrocytes, etc. are all losing cholesterol molecules that are not replaced in this condition of semi-starvation. The body has one last resort to fall back on in conditions like this, the "temporary cell membrane bandage," also known as amyloid. This topic will be covered in the next section.

Large amounts of amyloid, however, cannot do the job of membrane maintenance. Only cholesterol can fulfill this role. Cell membranes begin to leak, and cell deaths eventually occur. The brain does not replace dead neurons. When enough of them die, symptoms of dementia develop.

The hippocampus and other structures of the limbic system are delicate, hard working, and very susceptible to damage in conditions of insufficient "fresh" cholesterol. The limbic system is what separates humans from other animals. Damage to it, as occurs in Alzheimer's, does not at first result in total body death. What will die are the properties that make us human.

Alzheimer's disease progresses at different rates in different people. Factors include alternating periods of adequate and inadequate nutrition (including cholesterol), genetics (to a very small extent), and things like previous brain injury. Other weight-losing conditions produce similar effects in the brain, as we shall see later.

Some authors believe that brain shrinkage, amyloid accumulation, and neurofibrillary tangles are a normal part of aging, but I disagree. Adequate nutrition, including cholesterol, prevents brain shrinkage and amyloid accumulation. As for those studies that find these things in people who were not demented when they died, I say that it merely shows that different people have different thresholds as to precisely when symptoms of dementia first appear.

If someone's brain is shrinking and amyloid is accumulating, sooner or later dementia will develop unless he or she dies first of some other cause.

In humans, our large brain can serve somewhat as a stored source of cholesterol molecules. During times of food scarcity, the brain can supply cholesterol for the other more vital tissues, such as skin.

When food is plentiful, the brain and body can regenerate the cholesterol and fats that were used up. If starvation were to continue, however, brain damage will occur, <u>especially in older people</u>.

I will now review some of the highlights of the references that provide the basis for my conclusions.

The severity of the dementia symptoms in an Alzheimer's patient is related purely to the numbers and locations of dead neurons. The symptoms are not based specifically on the extent and locations of amyloid plaques.

Amyloid accumulates in the brain in association with the blood vessels. The amyloid in blood vessels causes further damage to neurons by affecting the flow of glucose and other nutrients.

Neurons and other cells have the ability to produce amyloid to a limited degree. The amyloid plaques that build up in Alzheimer's brains are found outside of the neurons. This amyloid comes from platelets and apo E. Amyloid in large accumulations definitely harms neurons, but in small amounts, can be removed by microglia, the scavengers of the brain. It is difficult to break the material down, however. Large amounts of amyloid can simply overwhelm the microglia.

The hippocampus and amygdala, structures in the limbic system, are particularly sensitive to damaging processes. Atrophy (shrinkage) appears here first, even though it is gradually occurring throughout the brain.

A number of investigators have found that the cell membranes of neurons are altered in Alzheimer's brains. They have determined that the alteration is a membrane lipid defect, and guess that the causes include oxidation, amyloid, or something else (shortage of cholesterol!).

In Alzheimer's patients, separate studies found lower levels of cholesterol in cerebrospinal fluid and ventricular fluid (the spaces in the brain are called ventricles).

In studies it was shown that lowering cholesterol levels in an effort to combat heart disease revealed some surprising statistics. The people who were successful at lowering their blood cholesterol levels began to die at increasing rates from other conditions not related to heart disease. There was found to be an inverse relationship. To put it in simple terms: as cholesterol levels decreased, death from non-heart related causes increased.

We have discussed the lowering of cholesterol by a condition of semi-starvation. We will now briefly discuss the lowering of cholesterol by drugs and medications.

Back in 1972, an early drug that lowered cholesterol was shown to interfere with the ability of cells from mice to process oxygen normally. This led to defects in the ability of the cells to produce energy from glucose.

Experiments have been performed which show that intentionally lowering blood cholesterol affects brain function by altering neuron cell membranes.

In rats it was shown that a drug that lowered cholesterol was particularly harmful to neurons from the hippocampus.

In experiments with statins, the new drugs used for lowering cholesterol, applying one of them to human fetal brain cells in cultures led to structural changes and cell death.

In a 1975 study, a group of patients with brain shrinkage were found to have decreased levels of cholesterol in their cerebrospinal fluid compared to people without brain shrinkage.

In a Japanese study, the amount of brain shrinkage increased in proportion to the decrease in blood cholesterol levels. Blood pressures were found to go lower as blood cholesterol decreased. In other words, as blood cholesterol levels decreased, the patients' brains got smaller and their blood pressures went lower.

In a study of children, it was shown that even a moderate degree of malnutrition is harmful to intellectual development.

Malnutrition in the elderly has been linked to impaired cognitive function. Lower blood cholesterol levels were specifically shown to have a negative effect.

In a study of various factors that may have an effect on the development of Alzheimer's disease, one thing that was shown to be common in the medical histories of these patients were periods of malnutrition/clinical starvation.

In a recent Italian study, Alzheimer's patients were shown to have lower blood cholesterol levels than normal, healthy people. They were also shown to have lower blood cholesterol levels than patients with vascular dementia.

A Polish study also found that Alzheimer's patients had lower cholesterol levels compared to healthy, non-demented people.

In a 1988 study done in Finland, blood cholesterol tests were done one time on Alzheimer's patients when they were admitted to a clinic. They were already diagnosed with the disease and the results varied. The authors concluded that blood cholesterol was not a reliable predictor for Alzheimer's disease. Of course, the readers of this book know that if the caregivers were able to successfully get the Alzheimer's patients to eat for the few days before the test, then their cholesterol levels would be normal. The other factor to consider is that high cortisol production can "mask" low cholesterol levels by boosting cholesterol at the expense of cells throughout the body (including the brain).

How is it possible that the low cholesterol connection to Alzheimer's disease has been missed up to this point?

There is a bias against cholesterol in the medical and medical research worlds. This is parallel to the bias against cholesterol in the health and medical agencies of the government, in the health book publishing business, and in many parts of the food processing industry. I understand why this bias exists. It is because heart disease is a major killer of people in the industrialized nations. And most importantly, it is because people have been conditioned to believe that heart disease is caused purely by cholesterol in the foods we eat.

Now in the world of Alzheimer's research, many scientists believe that apo E is the key to the disease. They are aware that apo E is responsible for transporting cholesterol in the brain. Since cholesterol is "bad for you", and "your body makes all the cholesterol it needs", then surely apo E (and apo E 4) might somehow cause Alzheimer's disease by flooding the brain with an excess of cholesterol. Many have tried to show that this is the case, and they all have failed, provided one really analyzes their efforts. Yet, some researchers are still attempting to show this.

As an example, in a study done in 1995 in the state of Washington, researchers stated at the beginning that their purpose was to show that high cholesterol levels were the possible cause of Alzheimer's disease (I am paraphrasing their words). They also tried to tie into this plan the carrier of cholesterol in brain tissues, apo E and its "bad" variant, apo E 4. However, at the end of their work, they were unable to show that high cholesterol levels were the cause of Alzheimer's.

Not being satisfied with this result, the authors of this study stated that the Alzheimer's patients that were used in their research obviously must have had high cholesterol levels in the years before they developed the disease, and that these previous high levels must have been the cause. Since the researchers did not have any real evidence to base this conclusion on, they suggested that longer-term studies would probably show this to be the case. My opinion is that these researchers would have better served their colleagues simply by accepting the results of their work.

Now it definitely is possible that the Alzheimer's patients in this study may have had high cholesterol levels in the years before they showed signs of the disease. But the earlier high cholesterol levels prevented them from developing the disease in those earlier years! The high levels did not cause it.

As a second example of the mistaken idea that Alzheimer's is caused by high cholesterol levels, researchers in a 1998 paper from Arizona decided to invent new guidelines on what constitutes high blood cholesterol.

The title of the paper was "Elevated low-density lipoprotein in Alzheimer's disease correlates with brain abeta (amyloid) levels." In the abstract, the authors state that their work demonstrates "…..for the first time that elevated serum cholesterol, especially in the form of LDL, influences the expression of Alzheimer's disease-related pathology." In other words, these scientists stated that their research showed that high blood cholesterol might cause Alzheimer's.

Now the abstract, which is the opening summarization paragraphs of the paper, did not include any actual measurements of blood cholesterol levels. So I reviewed the entire published paper in order to find the numbers and statistics that these authors used as a basis for their conclusions.

However, let me first reproduce the recommendations of the National Cholesterol Education Program (NCEP), which presents the official guidelines of the U.S. government and the medical world in general. The NCEP defines low total cholesterol as being under 200mg/dl, and that everyone should try to work towards this goal. High total cholesterol is defined as being above 240 mg/dl, and people in this category are said to be at risk for heart disease/atherosclerosis. The NCEP also recommends that low-density lipoprotein, or LDL, be measured. Low LDL is defined as being under 130 mg/dl, and this is a second goal that everyone should try to reach. If your LDL is over 160 mg/dl, then you are judged to be at risk for heart disease/atherosclerosis.

In summary, the universal recommendations for avoiding heart disease are to stay in the low cholesterol ranges, which are judged by the medical community to be under 200 mg/dl for total cholesterol and under 130 mg/dl for LDL cholesterol.

Returning to the Arizona research study, the authors analyzed 64 people diagnosed as having Alzheimer's when they died. Their average age was 81 years. For comparison purposes, the authors selected 36 people judged to not have Alzheimer's when they died. The people in this smaller group were also younger by three years, with an average age of 78 years.

The older group with Alzheimer's had an average total cholesterol measurement of 176 mg/dl. Their average LDL cholesterol was 124 mg/dl. Both of these numbers are definitely in the low ranges according to the government and medical community in general. However, the authors of the 1998 Arizona paper claim that these are high cholesterol levels! This is what I meant when I said the authors invented new guidelines on what constitutes high blood cholesterol levels in order to justify claims that Alzheimer's is caused by high cholesterol.

These authors said these were high levels because those in the smaller (and younger) group that were selected and who did not have Alzheimer's had slightly lower cholesterol levels compared to the larger (and older) group that did have the disease. My response to this data is simply that if these younger people without Alzheimer's had lived another three or four years, they too would be showing signs of the disease.

8-2   The Real Purpose of Amyloid

In this section, and for much of the remainder of this book, I will use the term 'amyloid' instead of the more precise term 'beta amyloid.'

Amyloid plaques are accumulations of amyloid protein found around the neurons and alongside the small blood vessels (capillaries) in the brains of Alzheimer's patients.

It is important to remember, however, that neurons are dying in Alzheimer's brains even in places where there are no amyloid plaques.

As was explained, a shortage of cholesterol over a long period of time is the cause of the processes that eventually lead to the deaths of neurons in Alzheimer's disease. Where does amyloid fit in the overall scheme of things?

I have reviewed thousands of research articles in the effort to find the answers to Alzheimer's disease. Almost every one directly discusses amyloid in some way. Amyloid is also the subject of many articles not connected to Alzheimer's at all. It seems that there are a number of other diseases and conditions where it is not unusual to find amyloid.

No scientist familiar with amyloid has ever published what the definite purpose of the substance is. Many scientists have suggested possible roles for amyloid, but none (to my knowledge) have ever gone beyond offering guesses.

I am not a research scientist, but I am able to state what the real purpose of amyloid happens to be, based on my findings from reviewing the scientific literature.

Amyloid is the body's temporary substitute for cholesterol molecules. Amyloid is to be used as a short-term "bandage" for cell membranes until more cholesterol is provided.

Cholesterol is not only the most important molecule in your body, but it is practically the only one that is common to all of the different types of cell membranes in the organs and tissues. Cholesterol molecules, however, require energy, materials and at least 30 different enzymes in order to manufacturer them. It also takes time to make them, which is very important to keep in mind.

If a cell needs more cholesterol molecules than it can manufacture, it can get them from the circulating blood by displaying LDL-receptor proteins. The cholesterol in the blood comes either from the liver (manufactured or from food) or from cells through the actions of cortisol. However, this too, takes time. There also may simply not be enough cholesterol molecules available.

This is where amyloid enters the picture. Almost all cells (including neurons) have a ready supply of amyloid in the form of a long strand called amyloid precursor protein. It is usually 700 to 800 amino acids in length. If a situation arises where cholesterol molecules are needed but cannot be supplied, the cell "slices" off fragments of amyloid that are from 25 to 42 amino acids in length, and then inserts these amyloid protein fragments into its membrane. Later, presumably when adequate numbers of cholesterol molecules are again available, the amyloid protein "bandages" are removed from the cell membrane.

Amyloid protein fragments are a substitute, and therefore, not as good as cholesterol. If amyloid were equal or even superior to cholesterol, then all cell membranes would consist of amyloid instead of cholesterol. But amyloid will help to protect the cell for at least a short time, provided that the membrane does not contain too much of it.

Neurons, like most cells in the body, can produce some amyloid "bandage" material from an internal supply (the amyloid precursor protein). However, in Alzheimer's disease, the amyloid plaques consist of large accumulations of amyloid that are outside of the brain cells.

The amyloid that accumulated in the Alzheimer's plaques is already circulating through the blood as part of blood platelets, albumin and apo E.

What are the circumstances in which apo E proteins are found to be carrying amyloid protein in the brain? When there are not enough cholesterol molecules available.

Why is amyloid one of the substances found in albumin in circulating blood? It is because albumin provides protein in situations where tissues are trying to repair damage from various causes, and repairing tissues is actually the repair of cell membranes. To repair cell membranes you need the temporary membrane bandage material until enough cholesterol molecules are available, and that material is called amyloid.

Why do blood platelets contain amyloid? When tissues are damaged such that bleeding occurs, blood platelets are responsible for two things: stopping the bleeding by forming a clot, and then beginning the healing process. What is helpful to have when beginning the process of healing tissues, which is actually the healing of thousands or millions of cell membranes? Amyloid, which is nature's temporary substitute when sufficient cholesterol molecules are not yet available.

However, there is no obvious bleeding in Alzheimer's disease, except for those times when a weakened blood vessel breaks. Why would platelets seem to be continuously, yet gradually, releasing amyloid in Alzheimer's disease patients? That question will be answered in a later section of this chapter.

If one analyzes the processes involved in the metabolism of amyloid, it becomes obvious how they are very similar to those involved in the metabolism of cholesterol.

Cells are able to manufacture cholesterol molecules and generate amyloid protein fragments. The difference is that cells require energy, materials, and time to produce cholesterol molecules, while amyloid protein fragments are just sliced off a long strand of amyloid precursor material.

Cells are able to obtain both cholesterol molecules and amyloid material from the circulating blood. They both originate in the liver. A difference is that blood cholesterol used by cells is carried on low-density lipoproteins (LDL's) while the amyloid in blood is usually part of platelets and albumin. Remember that in brains, however, both amyloid and cholesterol can be transported on apo E.

Neurons that are lacking the desired numbers of cholesterol molecules, but are still alive and functioning, will try to protect themselves by inserting amyloid fragments into their membranes. They will eventually die, however, if they are unable to satisfy their cholesterol requirement. Amyloid is not a good substitute for cholesterol over the long term.

Plaques of amyloid around neurons will also eventually kill them. The reason why circulating blood platelets would release their amyloid will be explained in a later section. However, for now, why would the released amyloid accumulate and form the "clumps" that we call amyloid plaques?

The answer is related to the fact that amyloid protein fragments are like cholesterol molecules in that they both possess a surfactant property. This means that they have the ability to "get close" to water molecules. Actually, only a part of them can come into close contact with water, while the other parts act as a barrier to water by repelling it. Though this may seem confusing, the important thing to remember is that this is the reason why amyloid protein fragments will spontaneously clump together when they are in the fluids around brain cells. Unfortunately, the clumps that we call amyloid plaques are harmful to the cells that are adjacent to them.

Why are amyloid plaques particularly abundant alongside the small blood vessels (capillaries) in the brain? Because these vessels are where blood carrying the amyloid (released from platelets) first enters the actual brain space. The concentration of amyloid is highest at this point, so it makes sense that amyloid plaques would form here first. It is also important to remember that the blood vessels themselves are experiencing shortages of cholesterol molecules. They are also incorporating amyloid into their cell membranes, the result of which is a weakening of the blood vessels. Strokes at low or normal blood pressures can be the result of amyloid accumulation in and around blood vessels.

This is a good place to clear up any confusion regarding the transporting of amyloid and cholesterol, especially in relation to the blood-brain barrier.

In a normal, healthy person, cholesterol is transported to the cells throughout the body on low-density lipoproteins (LDL's). Cells that need cholesterol will display LDL-receptor proteins on their cell membrane. A passing LDL will connect with an LDL-receptor and deliver cholesterol to the cell.

LDL's are relatively large and will not cross an intact, healthy blood-brain barrier. This does not really matter, however, because the brain's blood vessels display LDL-receptors just as all cells do. The cholesterol molecules are shuttled across the walls of the blood vessels to then be taken up by a waiting apo E. In the brain, apo E can both pick up and deliver cholesterol molecules.

The end result of this is that in an adult, the levels of cholesterol in the brain ultimately are related to the cholesterol levels in the rest of the body.

Amyloid is transported in the circulating blood in blood platelets and albumin. Amyloid is also transported on apo E. Apo E is the transporter of cholesterol and amyloid in the brain, and is also found in blood throughout the rest of the body.

In a normal, healthy person, albumin does not cross the blood-brain barrier. Albumin will cross the barrier if there is damage to it, as in cases of surgery or severe head injury. Remember that albumin is a large protein that delivers the necessary amino acids (and amyloid) used in the repair processes.

Amyloid from the circulating blood enters the brain in two ways, in most instances. In a normal, healthy person with an intact and healthy blood-brain barrier, amyloid is delivered across the barrier the same way that cholesterol molecules are, by utilizing LDL-receptors.

The second way that amyloid can cross the blood-brain barrier is because of a generalized condition of low blood cholesterol levels. Amyloid released from blood platelets will cross the barrier, because low blood cholesterol levels can affect it as well.

There are two categories of amyloid protein fragments. One category consists of amyloid circulating in the blood as part of platelets, albumin, and apo E. This is that amyloid which crosses the blood-brain barrier and ends up in the amyloid plaques of Alzheimer's disease.

The second category is amyloid made by cells for insertion into their membranes should it become necessary. In neurons, amyloid protein is manufactured and processed in the endoplasmic reticulum and the Golgi apparatus. Remember from an earlier section that cholesterol molecules also are manufactured and processed in the endoplasmic reticulum and the Golgi apparatus.

Amyloid that is no longer useful is excreted from the body in urine. Remember that oxidized cholesterol molecules from the brain are excreted from the body in urine.

Apo E, the transporter of cholesterol molecules in the brain, also carries amyloid. In experiments, amyloid placed in neurons from the hippocampus attract apo E that has cholesterol molecules attached. It can be concluded from this that amyloid plays a role in helping cells to regain needed cholesterol molecules. Amyloid in cell membranes also seems to attract special cells involved with the defense and repair of tissues.

Apo E's carry cholesterol and help neurons in laboratory cultures stay healthy and even thrive. When researchers add aged, mature amyloid to these cultures there is a toxic reaction in the neurons. Adding extra amounts of apo E protected the neurons from the aged, mature amyloid. In other words, the extra cholesterol from apo E provided a protective effect.

Special laboratory mice called "apo E-deficient mice" are genetically altered in such a way as to prevent their brains from having any apo E. This means that the brain cells in these mice must manufacture all the cholesterol molecules themselves. The brain cells cannot count on obtaining cholesterol from the blood. When researchers injure the cells or cause inflammation, the production of amyloid in response to these insults is much greater. In other words, the lack of an extra supply of cholesterol molecules results in greater damage, as evidenced by the increased amyloid generation.

Chemicals that cause oxidation of mice neuron cell membranes in cultures resulted in increased production of amyloid. Neurons physically damaged with fine needles also displayed an increased production of amyloid. In cell cultures where they gradually deprived neurons of blood and its nutrients (including cholesterol), the neurons began to shrink and at the same time produced amyloid protein fragments.

Amyloid inserts into the cell membrane bilayer. If there are small amounts of amyloid present in the membrane, it helps to protect the cell from stresses and insults of various kinds, including oxidation. However, if the cell membrane has a large amount of amyloid protein, gaps (or channels) will develop, allowing harmful agents to enter the cell while beneficial items leak out through these channels. The cell will not survive if the higher amounts of amyloid remain in the membrane.

There is proof that amyloid protein fragments actually bind to cholesterol molecules. This certainly helps since their purpose is to be inserted into the cell membrane bilayer. In fact, amyloid binds to cholesterol better than to any other components of a cell membrane.

Experiments show that they are unable to insert amyloid into a cell membrane bilayer that has a high degree of "lipid packing." In other words, if the cell membrane already contains a large amount of cholesterol, then amyloid protein fragments are not able to enter the membrane!

Some types of amyloid protein fragments have an adhesive "glue-like" segment, parallel with cholesterol sulfate, the "glue" that is present in hair and skin molecules.

Amyloid is thought by some to be an expected thing to find in all people who are getting older. However, people over the age of 70 classified as being very healthy will have the same levels of amyloid circulating in their blood as younger healthy people. In normal, healthy people of any age there is a balance between the accumulation of amyloid and its removal. Amyloid deposits are in a state of dynamic turnover, again, providing the person remains healthy.

Amyloid is difficult to degrade (break down), and its removal is a slow process. In Alzheimer's, the production and accumulation of amyloid gradually overwhelms the removal process. Remember again, however, that neurons are dying even in places where there are no amyloid plaques. They are dying from a long-term shortage of cholesterol.

In neurons that are stressed but still functioning, amyloid is moved down the axons and accumulates at the synapses. This is because the activity of a neuron is highest at its synapse. The synaptic membrane is the most critical part of a neuron's membrane, and cholesterol content is extremely important. This is why the neuron is quick to insert amyloid here if cholesterol molecules are in short supply.

Researchers can often find amyloid in other parts of Alzheimer's patients' bodies. The highest concentrations of circulating amyloid are found in the blood of Alzheimer's patients who were in an advanced state of weight loss and body-wasting. These patients also exhibited low blood cholesterol levels.

Amyloid has been found in organs and tissues throughout the body, including the liver, ovaries, testes, kidney, spleen, pancreas, salivary glands, intestines, skin, skeletal muscle, and heart muscle.

Cells on the edge of tissues that have been subject to a traumatic injury produce amyloid fibrils. This is additional to amyloid that has arrived in platelets and albumin.

Experiments with laboratory animals show that the axons of neurons exhibit amyloid accumulations after a head injury.

Research shows amyloid is associated with cytokines such as tumor necrosis factor and the interleukins. Cytokines are involved with cholesterol metabolism.

Complement is the name given to a protein in blood that acts like an enzyme during various types of inflammatory reactions. Researchers have shown that amyloid protein fragments are produced as one of the responses when complement is activated in an inflammatory reaction.

Researchers have shown that blood amyloid levels increase when the body is involved in a substantial stage of inflammation from some cause. If treatment with an anti-inflammatory medication happens to be effective in calming the body's inflammation, the blood levels of amyloid will go back down to their normal levels.

We witness the same thing in cases of severe bacterial infection accompanied by an increase in blood amyloid levels. If antibiotic treatment turns out to be able to control the infection, then there will be a decrease in blood levels of amyloid.

I was able to find evidence that shows that amyloid levels are increased in <u>untreated</u> cases of a wide variety of illnesses and conditions. These include (but are not limited to) rheumatoid arthritis, multiple myeloma, tuberculosis, and severe bacterial and viral infections. Extensive physical trauma and/or surgery, kidney dialysis (long-term) and advanced malignant cancer cases are also associated with increased amyloid levels.

In a separate series of searches, I found a very interesting common factor shared by the diseases and conditions in the previous list. People with <u>untreated</u> cases of rheumatoid arthritis, multiple myeloma, tuberculosis, severe bacterial or viral infections, and several other conditions almost always have low blood cholesterol levels. In addition, low blood cholesterol levels are associated with extensive physical trauma and/or surgery, kidney dialysis (long-term), and advanced malignant cancer cases.

It is important to remember that there is a definite connection between low cholesterol situations and increases in production of amyloid. Again, this is not something found in any medical journal or textbook of which I am aware.

Some researchers believe that a few cases of Alzheimer's disease were the result of a mutation in the Presenilin gene. However, this mutation does not guarantee that one will develop the disease. There is only the possibility that the chances may be mathematically slightly higher.

Demonstrations indicate that a mutation in the Presenilin gene results in an increase in the production of amyloid by cells at those times when amyloid creation warrants (oxidation stress, injury, etc.). However, what is the normal role for the Presenilin gene in the regular workings of the cell?

It involves the cell's processing of cholesterol molecules!

Scientists found that healthy cells close to invading cancer tumors produce amyloid before the tumor cells cause them to die. In other research, levels of amyloid increased in the blood of patients who were suffering from malignant cancers.

Aggressive, rapidly growing cancer tumor cells require large amounts of cholesterol, and quickly, too.

Rapidly growing tumor cells will take up all available cholesterol molecules from healthy cells that are in close proximity. It is for this reason that researchers have seen amyloid produced by normal cells that are close to tumor cells. The removal of the cholesterol molecules from the healthy cells occurs and they are trying to "bandage" their membranes with amyloid.

8-3   Cholesterol Prevents the Neuron Death Caused by Amyloid

Many researchers believe that atherosclerosis is definitely one of the causes of Alzheimer's disease, because of three reasons.

First, the connection between a history of heart disease/atherosclerosis and Alzheimer's. Secondly, there is the example of experiments using rabbits and high-cholesterol rabbit food (rabbits would never normally eat food containing cholesterol, for they are vegetarian animals).

Researchers fed the rabbits cholesterol until their blood vessels clogged with atherosclerotic deposits. The vessel blockages prevented cells from being nourished, and as they became weak and damaged, they generated amyloid. The authors concluded that this was proof that atherosclerosis (from excess cholesterol) leads to Alzheimer's.

Other scientists refer to these rabbit experiments when writing their own medical articles on Alzheimer's. Readers of this book, however, can recognize the flaw in these conclusions. The condition created in the rabbits was actually a type of vascular dementia, not Alzheimer's disease. In Alzheimer's, amyloid is found in a continuous layer alongside blood vessels. Individual cells may produce some amyloid as they grow weak and die. The most important thing is the fact that in Alzheimer's brains there are neurons dying in areas where there is no amyloid.

In the rabbit experiments, a clogged artery resulted in dead cells just past the point where blood flow was restricted. As they died, some amyloid was produced. Analysis of the process occurring in the rabbits proves that it should not be considered as evidence that atherosclerosis cause Alzheimer's.

What is the third reason why the scientific community believes that the cause of Alzheimer's disease is heart disease/atherosclerosis? It comes back to the medical world's universal bias against cholesterol. Simply put, all cholesterol is bad for you.

The references listed for this section all show that adequate cholesterol prevents the production of amyloid by cells. They also show that cholesterol can protect cells from already-existing amyloid deposits.

Some of the authors of these articles did not seem anxious to accept the results of their experiments. It was obvious to me that they wanted to show that cholesterol causes Alzheimer's damage from amyloid.

There was a research group in Germany that intended to show that the high cholesterol levels we associate with atherosclerosis would be a cause of Alzheimer's disease. Their intention, however, was to show that lower cholesterol levels would prevent the production of amyloid, which was the opposite way to approach the situation compared to the rabbit experiments.

The German scientists used a drug to remove cholesterol molecules from the cell membranes of rat hippocampus neurons. As the neurons were losing cholesterol, they produced amyloid. When the removal of almost 70 percent of the cholesterol molecules occurred, the cells stopped making amyloid. The authors admitted that their drug treatment started to affect the viability of the neurons. In other words, the brain cells were dying. It should come as no surprise, therefore, to learn that amyloid production stopped in the neurons. Remember also that cells only store a limited amount of amyloid.

The cholesterol-lowering drug that halted amyloid production (by killing the neurons) was a statin drug.

8-4   Platelet Membrane Fluidity

Blood platelets (thrombocytes) are the smallest cells in blood. Platelets are not to be confused with red blood cells, which are involved with transporting oxygen.

The function of platelets is to activate the blood-clotting mechanism (coagulation), an important part of the body's injury/repair system. Once formed, a platelet lasts for only about ten days. They are then removed in the spleen.

Platelets are one of the two primary sources of circulating amyloid, the other being albumin. It makes perfect sense for platelets to carry amyloid, because they are the first blood components in the repair/healing process to begin working at the site of an injury. The amyloid protein fragments fulfill the role of "temporary cell membrane bandages" until later in the healing process, when molecules of cholesterol are available and can be incorporated into an organized structure of newly repaired cell membranes.

An injury that produces bleeding will "activate" platelets in that area, and the blood-clotting process starts. The term "platelet activation" simply means that platelets have started the mechanism of coagulation.

Over ten years ago a small number of researchers found that the platelets of Alzheimer's patients displayed increased membrane fluidity. A measurement of increased membrane fluidity means simply that the membranes are more "leaky."

Research has revealed that the total blood cholesterol levels are the most important factor influencing the membranes of platelets. It directly affects the ways that platelets function, too. The following is a summary of the relationship between blood cholesterol levels and blood platelets.

Higher blood cholesterol levels results in low platelet membrane fluidity, greater "stickiness" between platelets, and a quicker tendency to form blood clots. Platelets in blood that has a higher cholesterol content become "activated" more readily.

Lower blood cholesterol levels result in the opposite of everything in the preceding paragraph. Low cholesterol causes increased platelet membrane fluidity, less "stickiness" between platelets, and a tendency for bleeding to last longer before a satisfactory clot forms.

Low blood cholesterol levels are also a danger, with respect to platelets. Low cholesterol content of platelet membranes (increased membrane fluidity) causes them to not be "activated" very quickly. If a clot does not form very quickly, the extended bleeding can obviously become a major problem, possibly life-threatening.

Hemorrhage (uncontrollable bleeding) is one of the causes of death in Alzheimer's patients. A classic heart attack is not, although the patient may have had a history of atherosclerotic heart disease.

Platelets are one of the two major sources of amyloid in the blood, with albumin being the other. Both platelets and albumin have a role to play in the tissue repair process, but I shall concentrate on platelets in this section. Albumin's role (of supplying protein) actually takes place after the clotting process is completed.

At the site of an injury in someone with "satisfactory" or high blood cholesterol levels, the platelets activate and a clot forms. Platelets release amyloid protein fragments, only at the injury site. These blood platelets (if tested) would reveal normal or decreased membrane fluidity (less likely to "leak").

In Alzheimer's patients, the platelets have increased membrane fluidity. They are more likely to "leak" their contents, and that includes amyloid protein fragments. The platelets are circulating in the bloodstream, so it stands to reason that if the platelets are leaking amyloid, it should be accumulating in a continuous manner along the blood vessels. This is precisely what they discover in Alzheimer's blood vessels.

Shortages of cholesterol molecules in the blood circulation, therefore, result in weakened blood vessels that have a continuous "coat" of amyloid. The amyloid comes from "leaking" blood platelets (increased membrane fluidity). The weakened blood vessels are subject to hemorrhaging, and the defective platelets may be unable to form a satisfactory clot in time to stop the bleeding.

Will every Alzheimer's patient exhibit platelets with increased membrane fluidity? The answer is no, and there are two reasons for this.

First, if the patient's caregivers have managed successfully to get the patient to eat adequately, then the blood cholesterol levels would be normal or perhaps even high. Platelets would have normal membranes, especially when you consider that they are replaced every ten days.

Second, Alzheimer's disease may be the result of a head injury and/or brain surgery. Blood cholesterol levels and platelet membrane fluidity are not the critical factors in these cases.

8-5   Cell Cholesterol, Liver Cholesterol and Amyloid

There are three ways by which individual cells provide cholesterol molecules for their membranes. First, they can manufacture them in the endoplasmic reticulum and the Golgi apparatus.

Cells are not able to make all of the cholesterol molecules they need. To satisfy an unmet need for cholesterol molecules, a cell will display LDL-receptors on its membrane surface. This cholesterol in the blood originates in the liver and the intestines.

The third way also involves the use of LDL-receptors, but the cholesterol molecules are from the membranes of other cells throughout the body. The actions of cortisol force all cells to "donate" cholesterol molecules.

In summary, cells provide cholesterol molecules for membranes by making them, getting them from the liver, or getting them from other cells through cortisol's actions.

The liver provides cholesterol molecules in two ways. First, the liver manufactures cholesterol molecules, which requires material, 30 enzymes, and energy. The second way is the easy, shortcut method for providing cholesterol molecules. The liver obtains them from the diet after consuming foods of animal origin.

What if conditions are such that cells cannot make enough cholesterol and the circulating blood does not contain enough, either? In such a situation, the cells will use amyloid to try and temporarily plug the gaps in their membranes. There are two sources of amyloid.

First, a cell contains a limited amount of long strands of amyloid supply material (amyloid precursor protein). By slicing off sections of this supply, the resulting amyloid fibrils can be inserted into the membrane.

The second source of amyloid is within the circulating blood. Platelets have large amounts of amyloid for those times of generalized cholesterol shortages. Albumin also carries some amyloid.

Amyloid can protect cells for a short time, provided that it has not yet accumulated in large amounts. However, amyloid is not the same as cholesterol, which is what cells really need for optimal function.

Amyloid has some type of "irritating" or signaling factor about it that triggers its collection by macrophages (microglia in the brain) at a later time, presumably when adequate cholesterol molecules are again available. What if cholesterol molecules continue to be in short supply? The eventual result for most cells is death.

8-6   The Real Significance of Glycogen Synthase Kinase and Phosphatase 2-A

In its simplest terms, we are dealing with the differences between the "fed" and "fasted" states. Put another way, is the cell adequately nourished, or is it starving?

The enzymes in this section's title govern a range of processes in the cells of our tissues. Glucose/glycogen metabolism and cholesterol synthesis are processes controlled with some of the same enzymes.

When food is plentiful, glycogen synthase and HMG-CoA reductase become active. Glycogen synthase turns glucose molecules into strands of glycogen, the storage form of glucose.

HMG-CoA reductase is more active in this "fed" condition and an increase in the production of cholesterol molecules is the result.

During the periods of the "fasted" state (semi-starvation), the cells of the body need a way of halting enzymes like glycogen synthase and HMG-CoA reductase. Adding phosphorus groups to the enzymes can achieve this. The adding of phosphorous groups is the work of other enzymes called kinases. Examples of these are glycogen synthase kinase and HMG-CoA reductase kinase.

During times of fasting, the body shuts down these and other enzymes associated with the fed or well-nourished state by phosphorylating them.

When food is plentiful again and the cells need enzymes like glycogen synthase and HMG-CoA reductase to start working, it is necessary to remove the phosphorus groups. The removing of phosphorus groups is done by enzymes called phosphatases.

Let us summarize. When food is scarce, glycogen synthase and HMG-CoA reductase are blocked through the addition of phosphorus groups. The enzymes that do this are glycogen synthase kinase and HMG-CoA reductase kinase.

When food is plentiful again, the phosphatases remove the phosphorus groups so that glycogen synthase and HMG-CoA reductase can become active again. One of the enzymes that can remove phosphorus groups is phosphatase 2-A.

An important thing to remember is that the kinases and phosphatases have power over several different processes that occur in cells.

What happens if the "fed" or well-nourished state does not return in a reasonable length of time? In other words, what enzymes are more active in a state of semi-starvation , and what enzymes seem to be inactive?

Logic tells us that the kinases would be more active during a state of fasting or semi-starvation, and the phosphatases would seem to be inactive. It might even appear that there is a shortage of phosphatases.

What happens if the conditions of fasting or semi-starvation continue to occur in such a manner, that they overshadow an occasional period of adequate nutrition (fed state)? Continuous semi-starvation conditions result in weight loss, of course. In a microscope we would see cell shrinkage and cell death as the body is, in effect, consuming itself.

How would our body get cells to "sacrifice" themselves for the good of the rest of the tissues?

The kinases would simply continue to act, and this would result in cell shrinkage and death so that other cells can last (hopefully) through the period of extended semi-starvation. As the kinases continue to act, one of the things that occurs is the hyperphosphorylation of tau proteins. Hyperphosphorylated tau proteins become neurofibrillary tangles. More importantly, since tau protein is supposed to govern the microtubule functions of the cell, the turning of tau proteins into tangles results in the unraveling of the microtubules. If microtubules are not functioning in order to move things around inside of cells, then the cells shrink and die.

What enzyme is most responsible for adding phosphorus groups to tau protein, resulting in the formation of neurofibrillary tangles? Glycogen synthase kinase!

Researchers have found what seems to be a shortage of the enzyme phosphatase 2-A in the brains of Alzheimer's patients. They believe this shortage of phosphatase 2-A is some type of defect. The real reason for the apparent deficiency of phosphatase 2-A is that a continued condition of semi-starvation exists!

With the restoring of adequate nourishment, phosphatase 2-A becomes active again and the kinases discontinue their actions. The phosphorus groups are removed from the tau proteins that are in the neurofibrillary tangles, which cause them to "untangle." The tau proteins then act to reorganize and stabilize microtubules, which restores the cytoskeleton of the cell. HMG-CoA reductase becomes active again, producing cholesterol molecules. The cell resumes the normal functions that are associated with a condition of good health.

Microtubules move things inside the cell. In a previous section, we discussed the evidence that shows the need for an adequate amount of cholesterol in a cell for the tau proteins, microtubules, and other parts of the cytoskeleton to function properly.

Most of the cells in the body are unable to manufacture all of the cholesterol molecules needed for optimum cell function. Cells (especially neurons) need cholesterol from both options. They need to make cholesterol themselves, and they need to gather it from the circulating blood.

What if cells are seemingly receiving adequate nourishment, but cholesterol supplies are blocked?

Scientists genetically breed apo E-deficient mice to not have any apo E, which transports cholesterol molecules in the brain. A lack of apo E means that the neurons in the brains of these mice are unable to obtain cholesterol molecules from the blood, and must rely on only those molecules they make themselves.

These apo E-deficient mice exhibit hyperphosphorylated tau proteins and a disrupted microtubule and cytoskeleton system. These mice also show damaged tissues in the hippocampus and poorer abilities at memorizing tasks, compared to normal mice.

In other experiments, specifically interfering with the production of cholesterol molecules by blocking the activity of HMG-CoA reductase also resulted in the hyperphosphorylation of tau proteins, leading to neurofibrillary tangles and a disrupted microtubule and cytoskeleton system.

Let me close this section by mentioning a rare genetic disease called Niemann-Pick type C disease, discussed in more detail in a later chapter. In this disease, cells are unable to utilize cholesterol molecules obtained from the bloodstream. In Niemann-Pick type C patients, the tau proteins become hyperphosphorylated and form neurofibrillary tangles. A disruption of the microtubule and cytoskeleton systems takes place. Close examinations by researchers revealed that these damaging changes in the brains of Niemann-Pick type C patients are identical to those seen in Alzheimer's brains.

8-7   Calcium Ions and Cholesterol

In Chapter 5, I discussed that large accumulations of amyloid around neurons cause them to die. Individual amyloid protein fragments can be inserted into the membrane temporarily and are even able to protect the cell, to a limited degree. However, large accumulations of amyloid seem to coalesce around neurons and cause damage.

Researchers have found three things occurring when amyloid plaques accumulate around neurons, and all contribute to the deaths of these brain cells.

Dense amyloid plaques damage the neuron's glucose metabolism. In a previous section there are references that show how an impaired cell membrane alters the cell's ability to process glucose for energy production.

Large amyloid plaques will bind to the cell membranes of neurons and pull cholesterol molecules out of the membranes, leading to abnormal glucose metabolism.

Amyloid fits into cell membranes because there is an area on each amyloid protein fragment (or fibril) that specifically adheres to cholesterol molecules. A large, dense accumulation of amyloid in plaques would not only bind to neuron membranes, but would tend to pull cholesterol molecules out of those neuron cell membranes.

Amyloid plaques placed next to neurons in cell cultures caused the hyperphosphorylation of tau proteins. Neurofibrillary tangles then appeared, followed by cell death. Again, dense amyloid plaques pull cholesterol molecules out of neuron cell membranes by forces of adhesion. Previous sections discussed how low cholesterol levels in a cell lead to hyperphosphorylation of tau proteins and neurofibrillary tangles.

The third observation was that dense amyloid plaques cause openings in the neuron cell membranes that are next to the plaques. These openings or gaps in the cell membrane are channels. It is through these channels that excess calcium ions will flow into the cell, and this leads to eventual cell death. The cause of these membrane openings (or channels) is the ability of dense amyloid plaques to pull cholesterol molecules out of the membrane by the power of amyloid's adhesive property towards cholesterol.

Let me remind you again that neurons are dying even in areas where there are no amyloid plaques. However, the presence of these plaques increases the amounts of neurons dying. Either way, cholesterol is involved in the process.

How do excess amounts of calcium ions inside of a cell lead to its death?

Research has shown that excess numbers of calcium ions inside of a cell will lead to the blockage of the actions of HMG-CoA reductase, the key enzyme in the cholesterol production process. Specifically, calcium ions are part of the cell's natural mechanism for "turning off" the actions of HMG-CoA reductase. In fact, each cell maintains a supply of calcium ions inside of an inner membrane to use when it is appropriate to slow down the cholesterol production process. The enzyme that normally does this is HMG-CoA reductase kinase, and it uses calcium ions to add phosphorus groups, which stops the activity of HMG-CoA reductase. If the phosphorous groups are removed, then the manufacturing of cholesterol molecules will start again.

I mentioned that a cell keeps a supply of calcium ions in an inner membrane. This inner membrane consists mainly of cholesterol molecules, just like the cell membrane. There is normally a self-adjusting balance between inner membranes and the cell membrane with regard to cholesterol molecules. If the cell membrane develops gaps from shortages of cholesterol molecules, then similar damage occurs in the inner membranes. The situation you then have is a high level of calcium ions loose and uncontrolled inside of the cell. These ions have come from two sources: outside of the cell and from the interior storage compartments.

The interior calcium ion storage compartments are located in the endoplasmic reticulum of the cell. Remember that this is the initial site of cholesterol metabolism. It is, therefore, logical that the cell would have a supply of calcium ions there for the purpose of halting the process when there are already enough cholesterol molecules to satisfy the needs of the cell.

It is evident that a "vicious cycle" regarding calcium ions and cholesterol can develop, and it can lead to cell death. Channels (or gaps) in a cell membrane allow calcium ions to leak into a cell. Shortages of cholesterol molecules can cause this. The excess of calcium ions now inside of the cell can halt production of new cholesterol molecules by leading to the inactivation of HMG-CoA reductase. The membranes inside of the cell also begin to deteriorate as a result of this, which, among other things, will allow the calcium ions from the interior storage compartment to release. This leads to further blocking of the cholesterol production process. As the cell membranes break down even further from lack of cholesterol molecules, death of the cell approaches.

Researchers in an experiment using cell membrane bilayers from rat brains found that increasing the concentration of cholesterol molecules in the membranes will drastically reduce the numbers of channels.

Another research team performed experiments that produced results that are, basically, the reverse of those in the previous paragraph. In these experiments, researchers utilized a drug that created openings in cell membranes. Calcium ions leaked in and cell damage occurred. Also released were calcium ions from the cells' interior storage compartments. What drug caused this? A cholesterol-lowering statin.

8-8   Altered Taste and Smell (Olfactory Damage)

Alzheimer's patients have been shown by research to have deficits in taste and smell abilities. The olfactory system detects odors and flavors other than the basic salt, sweet, bitter, etc. Not only do the structures of the limbic system intimately connect to the olfactory system, but they evolved from it.

Humans have lost the advanced system of smell identification seen in other higher mammals, but in return we have gained tremendous powers of memory, learning, and thought processes.

Both the limbic system structures and the olfactory structures are among the most active areas of the brain. The more active a brain area is, then the more that area requires a supply of fresh cholesterol molecules (as well as oxygen and glucose). It is for these reasons that olfactory tissues are affected in Alzheimer's patients, along with the limbic system structures.

Researchers have found that amyloid plaques and neurofibrillary tangles are present in the olfactory tissues in the brains of Alzheimer's patients.

Another "vicious cycle" of events can occur that involves the olfactory system. Damage to the olfactory system makes food seem less flavorful. If food seems to not taste very good, then the patient may become even less interested in eating.

All patients with Down syndrome develop Alzheimer's disease. They also exhibit the same type of damage to their olfactory structures. I shall discuss the processes that cause patients with Down syndrome to develop Alzheimer's in a later section. There is a definite connection to cholesterol, but it does not involve a long period of semi-starvation.

8-9   The Primary Cause of Alzheimer's Disease

In the majority of cases, Alzheimer's disease is caused by long-term shortages of cholesterol in an elderly brain. The two exceptions are in the instances of patients with Down syndrome, and people with a history of head injury or brain surgery. Later sections discuss these exceptions.

No researchers have ever performed an experimental study with human subjects that can be used as proof of my conclusion. The reason for this is obvious.

In such an experiment, you would start with one hundred people ages 70 to 72, who are of normal weight and similar health histories. All would have to be free of any signs of dementia. In 50 subjects, you would restrict the amount of food they ate (including cholesterol-heavy foods) so that they would consistently be losing weight as the weeks and months went by. In the other 50 people, you would have to make sure that they were eating enough food so that they would maintain or even gradually show increases in body weight over time.

After several years I am confident that the semi-starvation weight loss group (provided that they have not been overly starved to the point of death) would show the following characteristics as compared to the group that maintained weight, or even gradually gained some weight:

1.   Lower blood cholesterol values
2.   Higher blood cortisol values
3.   Lower blood pressure values
4.   Higher tau protein values in blood and cerebrospinal fluid
5.   More signs of mental abnormalities
6.   Decreased brain glucose metabolism
7.   Brain shrinkage (atrophy)
8.   Higher amyloid values in blood

Such an experiment could not be performed, of course. It is inhuman to intentionally starve a group of 70-year old people for a period of years.

We, therefore, must prove the conclusion by looking at published studies from any field of medicine that would apply.

Almost every study performed on the subject found weight loss in Alzheimer's patients. In those studies that also looked at the histories of patients before they showed signs of Alzheimer's disease, researchers found that weight loss began before the outward signs of the disease were evident.

In a 1996 California study, 300 older people were followed for 20 years. The people who later developed Alzheimer's disease had a period of weight loss before it developed. In those patients who maintained their weight during the 20-year period there were no cases of Alzheimer's.

A 1997 Minnesota study showed that Alzheimer's occurred in those patients who also displayed a 200 percent higher rate of anemia. Though this study did not highlight this aspect, people suffering from malnutrition/semi-starvation are at a much higher risk of becoming anemic.

Some researchers believe that the weight loss is due to a defect of some type that causes the patients who develop Alzheimer's disease to have a higher rate of metabolism. Experiments have shown, however, that Alzheimer's patients generally have the same resting metabolic rates as non-demented people. The obvious conclusion, therefore, is that these people are simply not eating enough food, both before they develop the disease and afterwards.

Some researchers think that if Alzheimer's develops at a younger age in a patient, that it would turn out to be a quicker and more aggressive form of the disease. This, however, is not necessarily true, according to a 1993 study in Germany of 90 Alzheimer's patients. Their disease progressed at varying rates that turned out to be unrelated to the ages at the onset of their Alzheimer's diagnosis. Variations in progression of the disease link to variations in food (and cholesterol) intake.

A common finding in tests of the brains of Alzheimer's patients is a decreased rate of glucose metabolism. Researchers believe this is due to some yet to be explained defect. However, it is simply a result of a state of semi-starvation.

In other studies, glucose utilization decreases in the brains of many people as they become elderly. This leads to damage to the point that neurons die.

A 1989 study showed that fasting in human subjects leads to decreases in brain glucose utilization of as much as 50 percent, compared to a normal, well-nourished brain.

There are a great number of studies showing that the weight loss from successful dieting will lower the blood cholesterol levels in people. After all, that is one of the reasons for people to go on a diet. Successful dieting means that the patient is in a state of semi-starvation.

Remember, though, that during periods of weigh loss, the over-production of cortisol can increase blood cholesterol levels at times.

Both human and animal experiments involving periods of fasting show that the activity of HMG-CoA reductase is reduced. The decreased activity of the HMG-CoA reductase enzyme results in less production of cholesterol molecules.

In a 1995 Framingham study, the researchers found a steady decline in the average cholesterol levels of patients over the decades as they aged. Weight loss in the elderly (as mentioned previously) and the decreasing cholesterol levels are connected.

In a 1995 study, researchers performed detailed studies of the cell membranes from brain tissues of Alzheimer's patients. They found that the membranes were thinner and had 30 percent less cholesterol in them as compared to brain tissues from normal, healthy subjects.

As was already stated, experiments that involve the intentional starvation of elderly people over long periods are just not appropriate. There are, however, many animal-based experiments in the medical literature, and we can draw conclusions from them that apply to Alzheimer's.

In a 1987 experiment, researchers starved adult rats for periods of 12 to 14 hours. The manufacturing of cholesterol molecules stopped during the starvation periods.

In a 1994 experiment, researchers deprived rats of food for five to seven days. They then studied the limbic system structures of the rat brains. The researchers found markedly increased amounts of lipid peroxidation in the tissues (the cholesterol and fat molecules were being oxidized).

In other experiments, long-term starvation in adult rats caused their brain tissue to shrink and neurons in the hippocampus to die. Resuming adequate nutrition in these adult rats did not reverse the damage. The experiments showed that the hippocampus is especially sensitive to starvation periods.

In other experiments, fasting in rats produced damage to neurons in the hypothalamus, including the destruction of microtubules.

In a 1982 experiment, nerve tissues from rabbits were placed in cultures but were deprived of nutrition. Over a period of eight hours, the cells started to shrink, with microtubules disappearing and calcium levels increasing.

In a 1993 experiment, researchers subjected rats to periods of malnutrition for up to 220 days. Neurons from each rat brain's hippocampus showed signs of shrinkage. The amount of neuron shrinkage was in proportion to the duration of malnutrition. As neurons shrink and later die, the result is shrinkage in size of the entire hippocampus.

In a 1991 Italian experiment with rats, researchers wanted to produce results that would support the concept that high-fiber, low-fat diets were beneficial for brain tissues. They fed rats a high-fiber, low-fat food formulation for periods lasting 4 to 32 months. After sacrificing the animals at various times, they found there was less cholesterol in their brain tissues. They also found more "microviscosity," which is another way of saying increased membrane fluidity. The authors of this study concluded that these results should be considered as being beneficial. However, these results actually lead to Alzheimer's disease.

In the examinations of the brains of elderly people who were not demented at the time of death, researchers found amyloid deposits, slight brain shrinkage, and some evidence of neurofibrillary tangles in each hippocampus.

Findings almost identical to those were in the brains of people who displayed the beginning symptoms of Alzheimer's disease. The brains of older, normal people can appear identical to the brains of people with the initial symptoms of Alzheimer's.

In a 1993 study, researchers in Sweden analyzed 300 pairs of twins ages 50 to 86. Researchers found differences in blood cholesterol levels in about one-half of the pairs of twins raised apart from each other. Twins reared together seemed to have similar blood cholesterol levels. This study shows us that even though our genes have some influence over cholesterol levels, the "environment" has an influence, too. The term "environment" refers to a person's diet, lifestyle, and level of physical activity.

An earlier section listed other twin studies. In most of the cases of identical twins, the development of Alzheimer's disease in one twin did not necessarily mean that the other one would. Different "environments" causing different cholesterol levels readily explains this. The twin with the lower cholesterol levels would be at greater risk for developing Alzheimer's disease.

8-10   Antioxidants and Amyloid

An antioxidant is a substance that provides protection against "oxidants." An oxidant is anything that causes oxidation to occur. Our bodies benefit from the energy we obtain from the oxidation of glucose. Unfortunately, oxidation of various components of cells also occurs. Consequently, our bodies must continually wage a war against undesirable oxidation processes.

Oxidation harms cells by disrupting the integrity of cell membranes. When adding extra oxygen atoms to molecules lined up next to each other in a membrane bilayer, the oxygen creates new forces that pull these molecules out of the membrane. This creates gaps (or channels) in the membrane, which then leads to leakage of cell contents and the inward flow of extra calcium ions. Cell damage and death results.

How does an antioxidant actually protect friendly cells from oxidation? Basically, the protection mechanism involves the antioxidant molecule oxidizing in place of the friendly cell molecule. The antioxidant sacrifices itself.

One free radical molecule cannot oxidize more than one friendly molecule. After that, it is neutralized and harmless.

You can now see why our bodies require a continuous supply of antioxidant molecules, for the "bad guys" are always going to be produced.

The most important antioxidant vitamin in the brain is vitamin E, which is carried into the brain on low-density lipoproteins (LDL's) and apo E.

A cholesterol molecule should only have the one oxygen atom on its end if it is to remain as part of a cell membrane bilayer. If oxidants are able to add a second (or third) oxygen atom, the oxidized cholesterol molecule will not fit into the bilayer arrangement. There also will be a very strong attraction to the water-based fluid surrounding the cell.

Researchers have determined in experiments that amyloid plaques can cause the oxidation of nearby neuron cell membranes. This leads to an inward flow of calcium ions, leakage of cell contents, and eventually the death of the cell. Nevertheless, there is never a satisfactory explanation as to how the amyloid actually causes the molecules in the cell membrane to oxidize. Amyloid proteins do not have an active oxygen atom that is ready to jump onto a cholesterol molecule that is in a cell membrane bilayer.

In my opinion, amyloid itself does not do the actual "oxidizing." Instead, the amyloid plaques actively pull cholesterol molecules out of the membrane bilayer. Remember that each amyloid protein fibril has a place that specifically adheres to a cholesterol molecule. A large accumulation of amyloid, therefore, should be able to have a multiplied force of attraction that can pull cholesterol molecules out of membranes. Once out of its membrane bilayer, a cholesterol molecule can be oxidized more easily by any oxygen molecules or free radicals present in the fluid around cells.

The cholesterol (or phospholipid) molecule does not have to be fully out of the membrane before it oxidizes. The amyloid plaque nearby only has to pull the molecule outward enough for the addition of an extra oxygen atom. At this point, the extra oxygen atom provides the final "boost" that forces the cholesterol out, leaving a gap or channel.

Adding a generous amount of vitamin E to a culture containing neurons and amyloid offers the neurons some protection from oxidation. This protection is due to the ability of vitamin E molecules themselves to undergo oxidation. As a result, the oxidants in the area are neutralized. Amyloid plaques will still pull on cholesterol molecules that are in neuron cell membranes, but there will be a decreased amount of them being oxidized. The final "boost" out of the membrane is therefore less likely.

Adding an extra oxygen atom by itself is sufficient to force a cholesterol molecule out of a membrane. It is a stronger force than the "pulling" by an amyloid plaque. This is why amyloid plaques do not seem to cause an instantaneous "meltdown" of all cell membranes that are in close proximity. The process is a slow and gradual one. The mechanism I just explained would account for such a process (amyloid plaque "pulling" and then an oxidation).

A deficiency of vitamin E does not simply cause Alzheimer's disease. But then again, it cannot hurt to make sure you are getting enough of it in your normal diet. The same is true about vitamin C and any other antioxidant vitamins.

However, the best protection against the damaging processes of oxidation is a supply of fresh, unoxidized cholesterol molecules.

8-11   The Golgi Connection to Alzheimer's

The endoplasmic reticulum (ER) manufactures the proteins, cholesterol molecules, and other lipid molecules needed by a cell. The molecules are then shuttled by microtubules to the Golgi apparatus, where they are stored, modified, or moved by microtubules to wherever they are needed by the cell.

When low-density lipoproteins (LDL's) are brought into the cell from the bloodstream, the cholesterol molecules they carry are shuttled to the Golgi apparatus.

If the Golgi apparatus and/or the microtubules transport system are not functioning correctly for whatever reason, cholesterol molecules will not be properly distributed, and the cell will suffer damage.

In brain cells, researchers have shown that apo E delivers cholesterol to the Golgi apparatus. Apo E enters cells in the brain via LDL-receptors.

Oligodendrocytes are responsible for manufacturing the myelin insulating coatings for the axons of neurons. Myelin contains a great amount of cholesterol. The Golgi apparatus of oligodendrocytes are much larger compared to other cells.

The endoplasmic reticulum and Golgi apparatus are also involved in the manufacture and processing of amyloid. The long-chain amyloid supply molecule (amyloid precursor) originates in the ER and then is stored in the Golgi apparatus. When the conditions call for amyloid protein fragments (fibrils) to be available, the slicing of the fragments occurs in the Golgi apparatus.

People with a mutation of the "presenilin gene" have a slightly increased probability of developing Alzheimer's disease. The presenilin gene controls the ways that the presenilin proteins function, and these proteins are involved in the production of amyloid protein fragments. An increased rate of amyloid production occurs (when the conditions warrant it) if the presenilin genes mutate. The presenilin proteins are in the endoplasmic reticulum and Golgi apparatus.

We are now ready to connect the Golgi apparatus to Alzheimer's disease. Researchers in the Netherlands studied the Golgi apparatus of neurons in the brains of Alzheimer's patients.

The neurons were from the hippocampus, hypothalamus, and various limbic structures. These researchers discovered that the Golgi apparatus in Alzheimer's brains were only one-half the size of those from the brains of normal, non-demented people. The suggestion was that this was a sign for possible use in the diagnosis of Alzheimer's brains.

A research team in Pennsylvania found that the Golgi apparatus in the neurons of Alzheimer's brains are much smaller and fragmented, compared to those in the brains of patients who are normal and non-demented.

Neither research team connected the findings to cholesterol. They instead concluded that it related in some way to amyloid.

The smaller and fragmented Golgi apparatus in the neurons of Alzheimer's brains is an obvious sign that there is a shortage of cholesterol molecules.

When confronted with the shortage of cholesterol, the neuron tries to produce amyloid protein fragments, "nature's temporary substitute for cholesterol." It is not a coincidence that this production of amyloid occurs in the Golgi apparatus.

Back in 1980, researchers fed one group of rats a diet very high in cholesterol. The other group of rats was fed the normal rat food that did not have cholesterol.

The rats eating the special diet naturally developed high blood cholesterol levels. When examined, the Golgi apparatus from these high cholesterol rats were larger and contained as much as four times the cholesterol as the Golgi apparatus from normal rats.

If cells that are overloaded with cholesterol contain Golgi apparatus that are larger than normal, then it is reasonable to conclude that a smaller and fragmented Golgi apparatus is a sign of a shortage of cholesterol.

The neurons of Alzheimer's brains, therefore, contain smaller, fragmented Golgi apparatus because there is a shortage of cholesterol molecules.

8-12   The Lysosome Connection to Alzheimer's

Lysosomes are compartments inside of cells that contain hydrogen peroxide or digestive enzymes. The bilayer membrane of a lysosome is similar to the cell's membrane, so naturally it contains cholesterol. Lysosomes provide the cell with a digestive system. Not only can food for the nourishment of the cell be digested, but so too are invading bacteria and friendly cell structures that have been damaged somehow.

In a healthy cell, the membrane of a lysosome prevents its potentially harmful digestive enzymes from contacting vital structures of the cell. Unfortunately, many non-healthy conditions can cause the membrane of a lysosome to break. The subsequent release of the digestive enzymes in such a great quantity is hazardous to the cell, and may lead to its death. If lysosomes containing hydrogen peroxide break open, reaction from oxidation causes damage to the cell. Some researchers believe that the membranes of lysosomes are more susceptible to the stresses of disease or oxidation. The cell membrane may still be intact even though the lysosomes inside are rupturing their membranes and releasing the contents. As the cell's internal structures and fluids digest and oxidize, its future becomes questionable.

Studies of dying or dead neurons have revealed that defects in the membranes of lysosomes may be the initial event in the cascade of damage. A shortage of cholesterol would lead to a defective membrane around a lysosome, causing it to rupture.

CHAPTER 9
Neuron Injury

9-1   Brain Injury, Brain Surgery

Blood platelets and albumin contain great quantities of amyloid. Both are involved in the repair of tissues after injury. As my conclusions proposed, amyloid is nature's temporary cell membrane repair material.

1. Are amyloid deposits found in the brains of people who have suffered a head/brain injury?

2. Do people with a history of head/brain injury develop Alzheimer's disease at a higher rate than those who do not have a history of head/brain injury?

The answer to both is yes.

Many different research teams have found that a head injury increases one's chances of developing Alzheimer's disease. I found only one study (from the Netherlands) that did not conclude a relationship.

I have chosen to include a history of surgery on the brain as a risk factor, especially in the cases where a large surgical area is involved.

The primary factor would be whether the injury, or surgery, had occurred in or close to the hippocampus and other limbic system structures.

The length of time between the injury and development of the disease also varies. This is determined by both the location and the size of the injury.

Large accumulations of amyloid are difficult if not impossible to remove by the body's scavenger system of macrophages and microglia. We know that amyloid plaques can slowly damage neurons that are in close proximity. These two aspects may be the reason why there may be a long period of time between the date of injury and the first symptoms of Alzheimer's disease.

Are there deposits of amyloid in tissues elsewhere in the body as a result of injury? The answer is yes, as we learned in an earlier session. In other parts of the body, however, new cells will replace any damaged and lost cells close to the amyloid deposits. Unfortunately, neurons in the brain do not produce.

9-2   Boxing and Alzheimer's, Parkinson's Diseases

The goal in a boxing match is to score a knockout over an opponent by repeatedly beating an opponent's head with one's fist. A knockout is actually a concussion severe enough to cause a loss of consciousness.

When a punch lands on the head, brain tissues squeeze against the inner rigid walls of the skull in two places. First, the brain tissue under the place where the fist lands compresses as it quickly forces the head backwards. Second, it affects tissues on the opposite side of where the blow struck as the head movement stops because of the fighter's neck and back muscles, which react to resist the movement of the head.

Every blow to the head results in bruising and the rupture of tiny blood vessels that provide nourishment to the neurons in the brain. Bleeding and swelling occur immediately, with the severity of the punch determining the extent.

If a boxer's career is a long one, the cumulative brain damage can ultimately be substantial. This damage can occur in all areas of the brain, with the result being a variation of symptoms that afflict retired boxers.

One of the most famous boxers of all time, Muhammad Ali, is now suffering from Parkinson's disease. Parkinson's symptoms of muscle rigidity, tremor at rest, loss of reflexes, etc., are due to the gradual loss of neurons in the brain that control various muscle groups. These neurons are in the substantia nigra, a part of the mid-brain.

Many researchers now believe Parkinson's disease closely relates to Alzheimer's disease. We will discuss Parkinson's in detail in a later section.

A more familiar affliction that is suffered by ex-boxers is dementia pugilistica, or punch-drunk. A punch-drunk boxer exhibits mental confusion, slowness and loss of memory. The symptoms get worse as the boxer ages, even if he is no longer fighting.

Research shows that at autopsy, the brains of ex-boxers who became punch-drunk before they died are similar to Alzheimer's brains. The ex-boxer's brain tissues display amyloid plaques, neurofibrillary tangles and loss of neurons. This also provides further support for my conclusion that amyloid is nature's membrane repair material.

The symptoms of a punch-drunk boxer will more closely resemble classic Alzheimer's disease if the damage is in or near to the hippocampus and other limbic structures.

The fair thing to do would be to provide those young people interested in boxing careers with the medical information explaining the damage a boxer is likely to suffer.

CHAPTER 10
Vance Wolff's Other Medical Ailments

10-1   Low Cholesterol Symptoms: Keys to Other Diseases

During the long period of time that Vance Wolff was losing weight and keeping his blood cholesterol levels low, he exhibited signs and symptoms of several other conditions and diseases. After determining that his Alzheimer's disease was caused by low cholesterol levels over a long period of time, I decided to investigate these other signs and symptoms.

I was able to find a tremendous amount of evidence linking cholesterol to Vance's other conditions. Just as in the search for the cause of Alzheimer's disease, I was never able to find a clear statement in the published studies that said, "Rheumatoid arthritis can be caused by low cholesterol levels" or "Some types of epilepsy can be caused by low cholesterol levels."

It can take many months or years of low cholesterol levels before the signs and symptoms of Alzheimer's disease appear in an elderly patient. Some of the following conditions, however, may develop over shorter periods.

Some of the other symptoms that Vance Wolff experienced at various times during the years that Alzheimer's disease was stealing his mind include the following: headaches, low blood pressure (hypotension), seizures, cataracts, muscle aches and weakness, irregular heartbeats (arrhythmias), skin eruptions and arthritis-like joint pains.

10-2   Low Cholesterol and Headache

While Vance was losing weight, and successfully maintaining the weight loss, he was also taking one of the first statin drugs that lower cholesterol levels. The diet he religiously followed was a low-fat, low-cholesterol plan.

One thing we noticed at the time was that he seemed to be plagued with frequent headaches. In my research of Alzheimer's disease, I chose to not pursue a specific connection between cholesterol and headaches. This is because a symptom of headache can be associated with so many different conditions.

Another interesting thing is that one of the old home remedies for treating the headache associated with an alcohol hangover involves the drinking of some kind of raw egg mixture. As you know, eggs are a major source of cholesterol.

As mentioned before, Vance was taking one of the statin drugs that lower cholesterol levels. One of the most common side-effects of these cholesterol-lowering drugs is headache.

There is some research linking NSAIDs to a reduced incidence of Alzheimer's. NSAIDs have an effect on cholesterol metabolism, and this will be discussed later.

10-3   Alzheimer's and Low Blood Pressure (Hypotension)

After Vance successfully lost weight and lowered his blood cholesterol levels, he began to occasionally experience dizziness when rising out of bed or a chair. Sometimes he fainted for a few moments.

We learned that Vance was now suffering from extremely low blood pressure, or hypotension. This is the opposite of high blood pressure (hypertension). Blood at low pressure may be unable to reach the brain against the force of gravity when the person is rising upwards. Dizziness or a fainting spell can result from the brain's blood deprivation, even if it is only for a few seconds.

Is low blood pressure a common finding in patient's with Alzheimer's disease? The answer is yes. Some Alzheimer's patients may have had high blood pressure in the past, just as some may have had heart attacks from atherosclerosis. Nevertheless, before and during the development of Alzheimer's disease, low blood pressure is the rule and not the exception.

Those who have a history of brain injury or surgery are one exception to the rule. Blood cholesterol levels, or blood pressure, do not necessarily play a major role in the development of Alzheimer's in those cases.

Some investigators have analyzed the history of high blood pressure and its relation to Alzheimer's. Back in 1989, researchers followed a group of elderly women with hypertension for several years. Researchers noticed that the only women in this group who developed Alzheimer's disease were those who experienced a decrease in blood pressure measurement over time. They were also the ones who lost weight.

Other researchers have noticed the trend that older people with consistent hypertension seem to be more likely to develop vascular dementia. Is it possible for someone with definite Alzheimer's to have hypertension? Yes. In addition to the exception to head injury or surgery, those Alzheimer's patients who have manage to gain weight after developing the disease may show higher blood pressures, and higher cholesterol levels, too.

Some researchers who are aware of the hypotension in Alzheimer's patients believe it is due to an alteration in the ways that the brain influences blood pressure regulation. But the brain's nervous control mechanism over blood pressure does not account for the other things we see in the blood vessels of Alzheimer's patients.

Arteries have a thin layer of muscle in their walls, while veins do not. These muscles play an important role in the ability of arteries to constrict and relax, depending on the physical conditions that are present. During periods of physical exertion, the heart beats stronger and faster. The muscle layers act to maintain the integrity of the arteries while they enlarge, which provides more blood flow in a safe manner.

Cholesterol molecules are vital for muscle cells and non-muscle cell tissues that make up the walls of the arteries.

Arteries that have been subjected to a long-term shortage of cholesterol would be associated with three signs or symptoms: amyloid deposits, low blood pressure (because of weaker strength), and hemorrhaging at low blood pressures.

A syndrome that fits these characteristics is cerebral amyloid angiopathy. These patients suffer brain hemorrhages (strokes) even though they have low or normal blood pressure. At autopsy, amyloid deposits and other Alzheimer's-type cell damage is visible. In my opinion, cerebral amyloid angiopathy is a condition that leads to Alzheimer's disease.

I have made it a point of stressing that the hemorrhages occur at low or normal pressures. This is because most in the medical community assume that anyone who suffers a brain hemorrhage must have had hypertension. This may be true for those under the age of sixty, but it turns out to be a false assumption when it comes to the elderly.

Researchers have found that people in their seventies and beyond with low blood pressure have a greater chance of dying from a stroke than people with high blood pressure. In fact, people aged eighty-five to one hundred who are active and healthy, seem to have blood pressures in the upper ranges.

When researchers include cholesterol levels, the age barriers begin to be less of an influence. In a 1997 analysis of the "Seven Countries Study," men dying of stroke in their sixties were shown to have low blood cholesterol, as well as low blood pressure

In an earlier section, we learned that the elderly people who are healthy and active seem to have higher cholesterol levels. We can now say that they also have higher blood pressures. We are not talking about those people who have what is termed as malignant hypertension, which means very high blood pressures almost all of the time. Statistics in the studies that are referenced at the end of the book will provide some average blood pressure values for the "healthy old." As an example, in a 1993 Italian study of people over the age of seventy-five, the lowest death rate was seen in eighty-year olds with blood pressures equal to or more than 160/95.

Expanding on the connection between blood cholesterol levels and blood pressure, excessively high blood cholesterol levels are positively associated with excessively high blood pressures, for the most part. Lowering blood cholesterol in these patients produces decreases in blood pressures.

What about people who have blood pressures in the normal ranges? Can Lowering blood cholesterol levels alone push the blood pressure measurements into the range that is below normal?

Yes. In experiments with people placed on vegetarian diets there was a trend for blood pressure readings to drop below normal levels. When people resumed their regular non-vegetarian diet, the blood pressures went back up to the normal range

The most effective way to lower cholesterol levels is by starvation. This also lowers the blood pressure. A lowering of blood pressure is shown after fasting for periods as brief as 48 hours.

One group of people who always develop Alzheimer's disease are patients born with Down syndrome (trisomy 21). Do people with Down syndrome have lower-than-normal blood pressures? The answer is yes.

There was a Japanese study published in 1987 that connected cholesterol and blood pressure. The authors of this study found that as blood cholesterol levels decreased, blood pressures also decreased. An additional finding was that the amount of brain shrinkage increased proportionately. In other words, as cholesterol and blood pressures went down, their brains got smaller. These patients were on the path to developing Alzheimer's, even though the authors of the study were totally unaware of it.

10-4   Low Cholesterol, Nitric Oxide and Blood Vessel Fragility

During times of high physical stress, the arteries must relax and get larger while still maintaining their structural integrity. We call this vasodilation. In fact, this will occur before the physical activity begins. If the brain senses that high physical activity is about to start, it sends "messenger molecules" (acetylcholine) to the cells in the arteries. This tells the cells to release nitric oxide molecules, which in turn causes the arteries to relax and enlarge.

In an earlier section, we learned that high amounts of cholesterol prevent the production of nitric oxide molecules. There is a direct inverse relationship between the two. In summary, high cholesterol leads to lower nitric oxide production. More importantly (for our purposes), low cholesterol leads to higher levels of nitric oxide.

Very high levels of cholesterol, therefore, cause decreased nitric oxide production and decreased vasodilation of the arteries. Over many years, atherosclerotic lesions can form in the arteries. The common term for this is "hardening of the arteries."

In experiments, scientists kept pieces of arteries in high-cholesterol cultures and low-cholesterol cultures. When they added the same amount of acetylcholine to each, the arteries in the low-cholesterol culture dilated more.

In human experiments, two groups of people without atherosclerosis were given equal amounts of acetylcholine. One group had high blood cholesterol levels; the other had normal or low results. The low or normal group displayed increased dilation.

People taking the cholesterol-lowering statin drugs have shown increased vasodilation.

Experiments have shown that high levels of nitric oxide will disrupt the membranes of cells. Calcium ions then get inside the cells in an unbalanced manner and cell damage or death results.

As previously discussed, people with low cholesterol levels can experience more hemorrhages (strokes). Their arteries are literally falling apart. A shortage of cholesterol molecules combined with the increased nitric oxide levels is the cause of this. My term for it is increased "blood vessel fragility."

In summary, very high blood cholesterol levels lead to decreased nitric oxide and decreased vasodilation. Low blood cholesterol levels lead to increased nitric oxide, increased vasodilation, and possibly to increased blood vessel fragility, or "softening of the arteries."

What would be a visible sign of increased blood vessel fragility? If a thin elderly person seems to bruise very easily and it takes a long time for the bruises to heal, then there is a very good chance that the person has had low blood cholesterol levels for a period of time. Vance Wolff was an example of this. As his weight decreased and his blood cholesterol levels went down, he seemed to show greater amounts of bruising on his arms and legs.

We discussed in an earlier section that there are higher nitric oxide levels in the brains of Alzheimer's patients. However, I am the only who states that low cholesterol levels are the cause.

Researchers have shown in experiments that when they add amyloid "clumps" to cell cultures, it causes the cells to release nitric oxide. I believe this is because amyloid deposits will pull cholesterol molecules out of the cell membranes. The decreased cholesterol content causes the release of nitric oxide.

10-5   Low Cholesterol and Seizures

Vance Wolff suffered seizures classified as falling somewhere between absence (petit mal) and tonic-clonic (grand mal) seizures.

Epileptic seizures are common in Alzheimer's patients. In fact, the highest rate of new adult cases of epilepsy occurs in the population that is over sixty-five years old.

As in Alzheimer's, the medical community does not know what causes epilepsy. Let us look at some other interesting findings about epilepsy patients that resemble aspects of Alzheimer's disease.

Most cases of epilepsy originate in the cortex of the temporal lobes of the brain (temporal lobe epilepsy). The structures of the limbic and olfactory systems are in the temporal lobe.

Do some long-term epilepsy patients exhibit brain shrinkage?

Do some epilepsy patients exhibit decreased brain glucose metabolism?

Do researcher's (who bother to look for it) find amyloid in the brains of epileptics?

The answer to the previous three questions is yes. In fact, in experiments not actually connected to epilepsy, Alzheimer's researchers found something very interesting about the drugs that are used to treat epileptics. They added these medications, called anticonvulsants, to cell cultures that contained hippocampus neurons and amyloid deposits. The anticonvulsants protected the neurons from damage by amyloid. The authors did not know why they worked, but later in this section, you will learn about the relationship between anticonvulsant drugs and cholesterol.

After a seizure, epileptic patients typically exhibit increased blood levels of cortisol, growth hormone, and prolactin. In experiments with laboratory animals, increases of tumor necrosis factor and interleukin-6 followed the seizures. These hormones and cytokines are the body's way of increasing cholesterol in the blood and cell membranes. They work to cover both the short-term and the long-term needs for cholesterol.

Patients with Down syndrome will always develop Alzheimer's disease if they live long enough. They also develop epilepsy at a high rate. In fact, almost half of all Down syndrome patients experience seizures if they reach the age of fifty.

Epilepsy patients can exhibit irregular heartbeats (arrhythmias) that can be fatal. Alzheimer's patients and heart arrhythmias are discussed later. For now, however, I want to point out a few aspects of epilepsy and arrhythmias.

A very large nerve connects to the heart (and other structures in the body) and influences the patterns of heartbeats. It is the vagus nerve. The vagus nerve's brain connections are in the structures of the limbic system, so you can see why an epileptic seizure or simply an alteration in limbic activity could cause a heart arrhythmia.

Not only do proper doses of anticonvulsant drugs control seizures, but they also seem to prevent arrhythmias. We will learn later that there is a relationship between cholesterol and the anticonvulsant drugs.

Another similarity between Alzheimer's and epilepsy patients is that both exhibit disruptions in the myelin insulation layers that cover nerve fibers.

Let us analyze the real connections regarding cholesterol and epilepsy. Epilepsy is a disruption of the brain's electrical functions. In a seizure, an uncontrolled electric discharge emanates from the nerve cells of the cerebral cortex. This occurs primarily in the temporal lobe, the location of the limbic structures. During an attack, millions of neurons discharge (fire) at the same time, causing a seizure. As stated earlier, the medical community does not know what causes epilepsy. The following is my opinion of what occurs in the brains of some epilepsy patients.

A signal impulse travels down the nerve fibers as a wave. This wave is the temporary shift of sodium and potassium ions across the fiber's membrane. Fibers with myelin transmit the signal impulses quickly and efficiently, because the myelin prevents the ions from escaping permanently into the surrounding tissues.

The overall structure of the brain consists of millions of neurons and their fibers, all bundled up right next to each other. What would happen if the myelin coatings that insulate and separate the nerve fibers were somehow made to be defective?

As impulse signals travel down the nerve fibers with defective myelin, sodium and potassium ions would be more likely to leak into surrounding tissue. In the brain, however, the surrounding tissues are other nerve fibers! These other nerve fibers, which are going to other brain or body areas, would naturally have defective myelin, also. The ions from the first fibers would penetrate the second ones and cause additional, unplanned signal impulses. A cascade of uncontrolled signal impulses and neuron firings is the result. This is my conclusion as to what occurs in the brain during a seizure.

In other words, a deficiency of cholesterol molecules causes myelin to be thin and defective, and this leads to crossed connections between nerve fibers. The electrical term for this is "short-circuiting." Imagine bundles of wires that have numerous gaps in their plastic insulating coverings. The short-circuits that result when electricity tries to flow through them are in principle an electrical "seizure."

In discussing the drugs that help prevent seizures in epileptic patients, the most common ones are phenytoin (Dilantin), phenobarbital and carbamazepine (Tegretol). If you refer to the Physician's Desk Reference or a similar source, you will see that there is not a clear explanation given as to precisely how these drugs work to prevent seizures. There is also no mention of cholesterol.

How do phenytoin, phenobarbital and carbamazepine help control seizures in epilepsy patients? By raising the total blood cholesterol levels! The manufacturers and doctors who are aware of this property of these drugs may think that it is just an annoying "side effect," but it is the true reason behind their effectiveness.

You may be thinking that if these anticonvulsant drugs raise blood cholesterol levels, then the patient taking them would gradually be at greater risk of developing atherosclerosis. Long-term epileptic patients would be having fewer seizures but more classic heart attacks.

Researchers have looked at this aspect of the anticonvulsant drugs. The researchers found that total blood cholesterol levels increase, but it is due to a rise in high-density lipoprotein (HDL). They found that anticonvulsant drugs do not significantly increase low-density lipoprotein (LDL). As you are aware, atherosclerosis and heart attacks link primarily to high levels of LDL's. Increases in HDL's seem to help prevent atherosclerosis and heart attacks, as long as there are not huge increases in LDL's at the same time. Therefore, if the increase in total blood cholesterol is due purely to increases in HDL's, then the epilepsy patients can take these anticonvulsant drugs and not be overly concerned about heart attacks.

You may again be thinking that something does not sound right in this process. LDL's carry cholesterol molecules to the tissues, while HDL's carry them away from tissues and back to the liver. Therefore, how can increases in only the HDL portion result in more cholesterol in the brain to prevent seizures?

For the answer, remember that cholesterol molecules in the brain are transported on apo E, not on LDL's. Apo E is an HDL in the majority of people!

Neurologists and other doctors who treat epilepsy patients should not really be surprised by my conclusions. This is because of the methods used by epilepsy researchers to cause seizures in laboratory animals. Seizures gradually start occurring after exposing the animals' brains to chemicals that block the manufacture of cholesterol molecules. Some of the chemicals that do this are U-18666A and A Y-0044.

Researchers can also cause seizures by inserting cobalt rods into the brains of laboratory animals. The cobalt rods reduce the cholesterol levels in their brains..

A third way to cause seizures in animals is by injecting kainic acid (kainite) into their systems. Kainic acid removes cholesterol molecules from cell membranes.

Alcohol acts as a solvent on cell membranes and cholesterol in particular. Someone who drinks a large amount of alcohol in a short period is at high risk of suffering a seizure. There is one more situation where we find the development of seizures, and it does not involve alcohol, colbalt rods, kainic acid, or chemicals that block the manufacture of cholesterol molecules. Febrile seizures result from a high fever.

There is a cholesterol connection to febrile seizures, which are more common in children. The health status of both cell membranes and the myelin insulating coatings around the nerve fibers depends on a proper amount of cholesterol molecules and a proper, organized arrangement around them. Normal human body temperature is 98.6 degrees F. The internal temperature, which is what we are most concerned with, is normally 99.6 degrees F. As temperature increases, however, the arrangement of cholesterol and other membrane molecules become less organized.

Research shows that the cholesterol in cell membranes is in a healthy "gel" state at around 98.6 to 100.4 degrees F. At 107 degrees F, and above, the healthy "gel" condition changes to an unhealthy "fluid" condition. In other words, the cell membranes and myelin "melt" at and above this temperature. Cells in cultures at this temperature and above will die.

In humans, fever is an internal temperature (rectal) at or over 100.8 degrees F. The closer your temperature gets to that 107 figure, the more disorganized and the fluid-like your cell membranes and myelin will become. Eventually, the myelin coatings will no longer provide adequate insulation between nerve fibers, and a seizure will occur.

Experiments have also shown that increasing the cholesterol content of cell membranes will provide greater protection against increases in temperature.

Studies have shown that illnesses will frequently result in lower blood cholesterol levels, especially if a prolonged fever is present. We can now see why a high fever can cause a seizure. Why are children especially susceptible to febrile seizures? It is because the temperature in a child during an illness that produces fever can go up higher and faster than in an adult. In a child's body, dehydration from water loss occurs faster, and this can cause the upward spike in body temperature that can result in a seizure.

Doctors sometimes use Valium-type drugs to control a seizure that is in progress. However, if doctors administer Valium or another diazepam continuously, it not only becomes useless, but it actually increases the chances for more seizures to occur.

Once again, drug information sources will say that it is unknown as to why diazepam controls seizures in the short-term, but increases the chances for seizures with long-term use. The answer is that diazepam possesses two separate properties.

First, diazepam (Valium) acts in the limbic system, providing a calming effect that can control a seizure that is occurring. This effect has nothing to do with cholesterol.

Secondly, long-term use of diazepam results in a decrease of cholesterol levels! This is the reason why a patient may actually be more likely to have a seizure after taking the medication for a greater length of time, especially if withdrawn quickly.

In a 1979 study of the clinical chemistry of epilepsy patients, researchers discovered that blood cholesterol levels tended to be low, especially just before a seizure! I also found a scientific paper published in 1949 by C. L. Anderson that showed where researchers in 1927 recognized that epileptic seizures were associated with low blood cholesterol levels. My personal conclusion regarding epileptic seizures and low cholesterol levels were, therefore, not new at all. Others recognized it over 70 years ago!

In a 1983 experiment with rats, researchers found that there were increased amounts of cholesterol deposited in their brains after a seizure. I already discussed the findings in humans of increased cortisol, growth hormone, prolactin, etc., after seizures, all of which lead to increased levels of cholesterol available for brain tissues.

All of these findings lead me to conclude that a seizure may be the body's method of quickly correcting dangerously low levels of cholesterol in the brain. The seizure does two things: it immobilizes the victim so that a mandatory rest period begins, and then increases cholesterol through the actions of cortisol, growth hormone, prolactin, etc.

In a later chapter, we will discuss seizures and other problems that occur in people who have been on kidney dialysis for a long period. During a dialysis session, the patient receives a medication called heparin. We shall discuss this in detail later, but for now, what you need to know is that heparin pulls cholesterol molecules out of blood and tissues. In a 1999 article, scientists in Britain found that seizures resulted from the injection of heparin into the hippocampus areas in the brains of laboratory rats. The true cause of the seizures in these rats was the action of heparin in drawing cholesterol out of the brain tissues.

10-6   Cholesterol and the Eye

Vance Wolff developed cataracts in both eyes after he successfully lowered his weight and blood cholesterol levels through diet, exercise, and statin drug therapy. His ophthalmologist performed successful lens surgery on his eyes. During this time, he was experiencing some memory problems, but he had not yet received a definite diagnosis of having probable Alzheimer's disease. It was because of this history that I decided to investigate any possible connection between the eyes and cholesterol. It seems that everything about the eye revolves around cholesterol molecules.

The eye should be considered as an integral part of the brain. Like the brain, the important parts of the eye must last a lifetime. There are no eye diagrams in this book. The reader is encouraged to examine eye diagrams from another source.

The cornea is the outermost layer of the eye. Both it and the lens are structures with protein fibers that reinforce and maintain their overall shape and organization. This is necessary for proper transmission of light. A very important component of each is a proper amount of cholesterol molecules. In fact, the lens contains the highest concentration of cholesterol molecules of any tissue in the body!

The high amount of cholesterol molecules in the lens is necessary for maintaining the proper degree of separation between the protein fibers. Remember that cholesterol molecules allow a tissue to be flexible. The lens must certainly be flexible, because its job involves constant changes in shape for the focusing of light images on the retina.

Unfortunately, the high cholesterol content of the lens means that there is a high susceptibility to oxidation by the sun's rays, X-rays, smoke and other pollutants in the air, etc. The oxidizing molecules that naturally occur in the body can also damage the lens.

Vitamins C and E are important antioxidants, but the most effective substance for protecting against oxidation damage is a continuous supply of fresh, non-oxidized cholesterol molecules.

A cataract is an opacity in the lens that is caused by the coagulation and denaturing of proteins in the lens. The word opacity is a derivative of opaque, which means the blocking of the light. "Coagulated and denatured proteins" means that the proteins are tangled and clumped together. The cholesterol molecules in the lens serve to keep these proteins separated from each other, especially while the lens changes its shape in the image-focusing movements that are constantly occurring.

Where do the parts of the eye get their cholesterol molecules? The answer is the one given earlier for the brain. In the initial growth period of the eye's structures, cholesterol molecules are made locally in the eye. At some point after growth is complete, however, the general blood circulation provides cholesterol molecules for tissue maintenance. In other words, the cholesterol status in the blood of an adult determines the cholesterol status of the structures in the eye.

The lens has the greatest concentration of cholesterol molecules of any tissue in the body, yet there are no blood vessels in it. Without a constant supply of fresh cholesterol molecules, the proteins would coagulate and clump forming a cataract. The back of the lens meets the vitreous humor, the gel that fills up most of the eyeball. It has no blood vessels floating through it. It receives nourishment from blood vessels at its edge. Apo E has been found by researchers to be present in the retina. Apo E is responsible for transporting cholesterol molecules into the vitreous humor, for use in supplying the back of the lens as well as the retina. Research shows that the cells in the retina are not able to make all of the cholesterol molecules that it needs. The circulating blood must make up the difference.

Between the front of the lens and the back or inside surface of the cornea is the space filled by the aqueous humor. The aqueous humor fluid is in constant circulation, carrying nutrients in, and carrying wastes and oxidized cholesterol molecules away. Aqueous humor fluid is very similar to blood plasma. It is not red, because it contains no red blood cells. The fluid bathes the front surface of the lens and the inside surface of the cornea, then flows out into a vein and into the venous blood of the general circulation.

Before eye growth is complete, cells in the ciliary processes make almost all of the cholesterol molecules needed for the aqueous humor fluid. After development is complete, the cells in the ciliary processes stop making them. The cholesterol content in the aqueous humor fluid of an adult eye mirrors that of the blood. The tiny capillaries in the ciliary processes screen out the red blood cells, but leave in other necessary nutrients, including cholesterol molecules. If the cholesterol level of the blood is low, then the cholesterol level of the aqueous humor fluid will also be low.

It is possible to have very high cholesterol levels and still get cataracts, because atheromatous plaque material can clog the tiny capillaries in the ciliary processes. A NIDDM can develop a cataract this way. Fresh cholesterol does not adequately replenish the aqueous humor fluid, and the cataract formation occurs as a result.

In a state of semi-starvation, cortisol levels rise. Cortisol forces all tissues with which it comes in contact to "donate" cholesterol molecules to the general circulation. Cortisol can reach the lens from the general circulation via the aqueous humor fluid and the vitreous humor gel fluid.

Corticosteroid medications like Prednisone may be one hundred times stronger than our body's cortisol in forcing membranes to give up cholesterol molecules. It is for this reason, that long-term steroid patients are at increased risk of developing cataracts.

The lens and cornea do not have blood vessels, yet we have shown how the delivery of cholesterol molecules to them may occur.

But what of the outer surface of the cornea, which faces the environment, with all of its airborne pollutants, dust, gases and toxins? How does the outer corneal surface get fresh cholesterol molecules? The answer is in the blink of an eye!

The lacrimal glands produce tear fluid, known as lacrimal fluid. There is one gland above each eye. We are familiar with the salty taste of tears. What most people do not know is that human tear fluid contains a high level of cholesterol. We normally blink our eyes thousands of times each day, and each blink washes the eye with fresh tear fluid containing a supply of cholesterol molecules.

Let me review some of the situations that can lead to the development of cataracts, all which leave the lens lacking in sufficient amounts of fresh cholesterol.

Long-term semi-starvation can result in cataracts.

Corticosteroid therapy for some types of inflammatory illness can lead to cataracts. On a related issue, they treat some eye conditions with corticosteroid eye drops. In the short term, they may help, but extended use of them may cause eye problems later.

Someone with excessively high blood cholesterol levels and atherosclerosis may develop cataracts if the tiny capillaries in the ciliary process clog.

Free radical metabolism produces hydrogen peroxide. An excessive amount of hydrogen peroxide in your system can affect the lens and cataracts can develop. We will explore this in more detail in the chapter on Down syndrome. Patients with Down syndrome develop cataracts at a high rate.

Are the companies making statin drugs for lowering cholesterol aware of the connection to cataracts? The answer is yes.

Experiments using other drugs that block the making of cholesterol molecules such as AY9944 and U-18666A, also resulted in the development of cataracts in laboratory animals.

And a 1990 study in England revealed that a strict vegetarian diet was a significant factor for the development of cataracts.

The lens, retina, and cornea require adequate levels of cholesterol. As stated earlier, amyloid is nature's temporary substitute when cholesterol is in short supply.

Can we find amyloid in these parts of the eye? The answer is yes.

In a 1995 Japanese study, in cases of injured corneas, they found amyloid involved. An incidental finding was that there were increased numbers of cataracts in the patients who exhibited amyloid in their corneas.

In a 1996 study of patients with wounded corneas, every patient's tear fluid had amyloid protein!

In a 1996 paper published by researchers at the National Institutes of Health in Bethesda, Maryland, they show amyloid protein found in lenses with cataracts. In animal experiments, adding hydrogen peroxide to lenses produced both amyloid protein accumulations and cataracts!

10-7 Low Cholesterol and Muscle Problems

Vance Wolff developed muscle weakness problems after successfully losing weight and lowering his blood cholesterol using diet, exercise, and statin drugs.

Over the past thirty years, we have seen a disease called inclusion body myositis increasingly in the elderly. The patient experiences progressive muscle weakness. Laboratory testing reveals that the muscles affected exhibit amyloid protein accumulations, tau proteins, ubiquitin, and spaces between cells where muscle tissue has been lost. If you replace the word "muscle" with "brain", it would sound just like a description of an Alzheimer's patient.

Is there scientific evidence that lower cholesterol levels will cause muscle problems? The answer is yes. In fact, for thirty years they have known of the link between muscle disease and the various drugs used to lower cholesterol. The name given to this is CLAM, which stands for "cholesterol-lowering agent myopathy." Almost all drugs used for lowering levels of cholesterol link to cases of CLAM. The patients with it experience muscle weakness and cramps. Statin drugs are the latest medications to be associated with muscle problems.

Low cholesterol levels caused platelet membranes to have increased fluidity. This means that the membranes became weak and leaky. In a 1991 paper, the researchers explained that statin drugs added to muscle cell membranes cause an increase in membrane fluidity. The only way to get the muscle membranes back to a healthy condition was by adding cholesterol.

10-8 Low Cholesterol and Heart Muscle

Another problem that Vance encountered after losing weight and lowering his blood cholesterol levels was an irregular heartbeat, or arrhythmia. The specific arrhythmia diagnosis for Vance was atrial fibrillation. It is due to a disruption in the way that electric signals flow through the heart muscle. The upper heart chambers (atria) quiver and twitch instead of beating uniformly. Blood does not pump very effectively in atrial fibrillation, which leads to problems.

Vance's doctors implanted a heart pacemaker in his chest to control the atrial fibrillation and help with his low blood pressure. This occurred after appropriate medication treatments had failed. Vance's pacemaker performed well.

During this episode Vance was experiencing memory problems, but he had not yet been definitely diagnosed with probable Alzheimer's disease.

In looking back over this history, I decided to see if arrhythmias such as atrial fibrillation were common in other Alzheimer's patients. I also wondered if there was a connection between atrial fibrillation and low cholesterol levels and amyloid accumulations. As you may have guessed, atrial fibrillation is associated with all three: low cholesterol levels, Alzheimer's disease, and amyloid accumulation in heart muscle.

Most of the references for this section's conclusions did not have a direct connection to Alzheimer's disease. The basis for one paper that is concerned with the disease was information gathered in the Rotterdam Study. In this 1997 paper, the researchers found that there was a high prevalence of atrial fibrillation in patients with Alzheimer's disease. There was a very low association rate between atrial fibrillation and vascular dementia. If you will recall, vascular dementia links to atherosclerosis and high cholesterol levels. One can presume from this, that there is a link between low cholesterol levels and atrial fibrillation and Alzheimer's.

The hardest working group of muscles in the body is the heart. There are times when cholesterol may be in short supply, and amyloid protein would be used to "fill the gaps" in heart muscle.

The electrical signals that tell muscle cells in the heart to contract must flow through the cell membranes. If there is a significant amount of amyloid material present in the muscle, then a disruption in the electrical conduction pattern can occur. This is how amyloid can lead to an arrhythmia like atrial fibrillation.

Testing (while the patient is alive) may not detect the presence of amyloid in heart muscle. Echocardiograms do not detect heart muscle amyloid. Most of the time, the discovery of amyloid is by accident, during some type of surgical procedure on the heart or during an autopsy after a patient has died.

A pacemaker will help in correcting an arrhythmia like atrial fibrillation that is due to amyloid accumulation. If there is a large amount of amyloid material, however, a fatal condition called restrictive cardiomyopathy can develop. The only treatment option is a heart transplant operation.

In a 1991 Swedish paper, twelve patients aged eight-two to ninety-two were found at autopsy to have amyloid in their heart muscle, even though their doctors had no knowledge of its presence before they died. Nine had atrial fibrillation arrhythmias in the last years of their lives.

A paper published in 1978 was about the autopsy findings of twenty-three people who died after reaching the age of one hundred. They found in eight centenarians amyloid in their heart muscle.

In a 1996 Mayo Clinic study, they examined eighteen patients with definite amyloid in their heart muscle for any arrhythmias. Eleven had atrial fibrillation.

In a 1996 Japanese study, they found a greatly increased risk of brain hemorrhage in people with low cholesterol levels. Also shown in these patients with low cholesterol was a very high rate of atrial fibrillation.

Finally, researchers examined 5,200 people over the age of sixty-five and determined the rates of atrial fibrillation in this population. The authors of this 1997 study found that one of the factors associated with the people of this group who had atrial fibrillation was low blood cholesterol.

10-9   Low Cholesterol and Joint Inflammation

After Vance lost weight and lowered his blood cholesterol, he began experiencing pain in the major joints in his body. Both shoulders, both hips, and both knees were involved. Although never subjected to the full testing process for it, he seemed to fulfill many of the criteria for a diagnosis of rheumatoid arthritis.

Rheumatoid arthritis is a chronic destructive disease of the joints. It is an autoimmune disease. For some unknown reason, the body is attacking the joints. Processes of constant inflammation occur, although periods of remission also occur. (We are _not_ talking about osteoarthritis in this section.)

Joints are the places in the body where bones come together. Cartilage, which is a gray, fibrous tissue that feels like hard rubber, covers the ends of bones. Fatty acids, phospholipids, proteins, glycerides, and cholesterol molecules make up cartilage.

Cartilage acts as a cushion between bones, so it must be flexible. It is 80 percent water. Under a microscope, cartilage is like millions of tiny water balloons, and this is what provides the cushion effect. Cholesterol molecules are necessary to keep the "water balloons" from leaking.

There are no blood vessels in cartilage. Synovial fluid, which bathes the joints, contains cholesterol along with other materials to both lubricate and nourish the joints.

If the cholesterol content of the cartilage decreases, cells start leaking and inflammation processes appear. The way to halt the chronic inflammation of rheumatoid arthritis is to increase the cholesterol content of joint cartilage. If the process in rheumatoid arthritis continues, cartilage is lost. This eventually allows bone to rub against bone, which is extremely destructive.

Twins studies show that genetics play a very small role in rheumatoid arthritis.

There are numerous studies going back to at least 1977, which show that people with active rheumatoid arthritis have low levels of blood cholesterol. Children with active juvenile rheumatoid arthritis also have low cholesterol.

Japanese researchers in 1987 and 1989 published papers about experiments using laboratory rats specially bred to develop arthritis easily. The rats had arthritic episodes whenever their blood cholesterol levels were low. These researchers also found that they could prevent the arthritis attacks in the rats simply by feeding them a food that had a high cholesterol content.

Deposits of amyloid protein are in the joints of rheumatoid arthritis patients, including children with the juvenile form of the disease.

Some research shows that patients with rheumatoid arthritis over a long period have cerebral atrophy (brain shrinkage), which may be the result of steroid therapy.

A research group documented the finding that most patients with rheumatoid arthritis exhibit weight loss.

Also associated with active rheumatoid arthritis are nitric oxide, ubiquitin, interleukins, prolactin, and tumor necrosis factor. They all link in some way to low cholesterol levels.

Some studies have shown that there are rheumatoid arthritis patients with adrenal glands that do not produce enough cortisol. This could cause the low cholesterol levels in some of these patients.

Patients with joint injuries will sometimes have cortisone injected into the afflicted joint. The patient seems to show improvement in the short term. Additional injections, however, will accelerate damage to the joint. Cortisone acts like cortisol except that it may be up to one hundred times stronger. This forces the "donation" of so much cholesterol that damage will occur later.

There are three classes of medicines used in the treatment of rheumatoid arthritis. The first are the corticosteroids, which bring fast relief, but have many side effects.

Second are the nonsteroidal anti-inflammatory drugs, which are the major choices for treating these patients. They work gradually to bring relief. These NSAIDs have, as a major side effect, problems of intestinal bleeding. They raise cholesterol levels gradually, and this may be the real reason for relief of symptoms.

The third treatment option is a slow therapy that involves the use of gold in various forms. Is there a cholesterol connection to gold? Yes, and we will explore it in another section later.

There have been researchers who have noted some type of connection between Alzheimer's disease and rheumatoid arthritis, but it seems confusing. Current research shows that people who have had rheumatoid arthritis for a long time seem to have less of a chance of developing Alzheimer's disease.

Many researchers have noted that the modern NSAIDs somehow protect against the development of Alzheimer's, and conclude that it is specifically due to the raising of cholesterol levels, as you will see in the section on NSAIDs.

Eskimos that follow their traditional diet have very low rates of rheumatoid arthritis. I maintain it is due to the high cholesterol content of their traditional animal-based diet.

The Pima Indians of the southwestern United States have the highest rates of non-insulin dependent diabetes mellitus (NIDDM) of any small group. They exhibit obesity and high cholesterol levels. Up until thirty years ago, they did not have a high rate of diabetes. Researchers believe the problem began when the Pima Indians started eating a non-traditional diet that was high in starches, fat and cholesterol, coupled with a new sedentary lifestyle.

Other researchers have noted that over the past thirty years the rate of rheumatoid arthritis in the Pima Indians has been steadily decreasing, and I believe it is because the Pima Indians now have higher blood cholesterol levels.

The current higher blood cholesterol levels of the Pimas should also make them less susceptible nowadays to Alzheimer's disease. Perhaps researchers will do a study and see if the Pimas now have lower rates of Alzheimer's.

10-10 Low Cholesterol and Skin Eruptions

After Vance successfully lowered his weight and blood cholesterol levels using diet, exercise, and a statin drug, he began to exhibit skin eruptions that were strange to us. We were informed that he might have psoriasis.

The skin of a psoriasis patient has red patches covered with gray or silver scales. The scales flake off continuously. Frequently, these psoriasis patches are on the elbows, knees, and buttocks.

Most dermatologists believe psoriasis may be some type of autoimmune disease, which means that the body is attacking itself. However, I believe that at least some forms of psoriasis are caused by shortages of cholesterol molecules.

The elbows, knees, and buttocks are areas where the skin must remain flexible. Skin from these areas rubs off at a higher rate. An overall shortage of cholesterol molecules would affect these areas first, and in psoriasis, it frequently does.

Our skin is a barrier that prevents loss of fluid (water) from the body. It also stops bacteria and viruses from entering; and, if fluid loss is not prevented it can lead to death.

Skin is tough, waterproof, and flexible. It consists of proteins, cholesterol molecules, cholesterol sulfate molecules, free fatty acids, and ceramides. Keratin is the primary protein.

Keratinocytes make up 95 percent of skin tissue.

Fibroblasts bind and support the skin tissue layers to the body.

We lose skin cells continuously; this is a natural process. It takes from 39 to 48 days from the time the skin cells first produce to when they shed. This is called epidermal turnover time.

In psoriasis patients, however, the cells in the active patches have a much faster epidermal turnover time. It may be five to eight times faster. We say it is hyperproliferative. The red patches with gray scales flaking off are signs of skin that is growing much faster than normal.

In some cases there are genetic influences in psoriasis. However, speeding up the growth cycle of the keratinocytes alone did not produce the characteristic psoriasis skin lesions. Some other factor must be involved.

That triggering factor is a shortage of cholesterol molecules. Researchers have found that many psoriasis patients with active skin lesions exhibited low blood cholesterol levels. They also have low blood vitamin D levels.

Skin cells can make cholesterol molecules, but they also obtain them from the general blood circulation, because keratinocytes and fibroblasts display LDL-receptors.

The amounts of cholesterol molecules present determine the overall status of the stratum corneum. If the ratios of cholesterol molecules are not in balance with the fatty acids and ceramides, then the rate of cell growth increases drastically, becoming hyperproliferative. The barrier to water will remain intact as a result.

This is the basis of at least some cases of psoriasis. To compensate for a shortage of cholesterol molecules, the skin cells begin reproducing at much higher rates. The resulting skin is rigid, deformed, and continuously flaking off, but at least the water barrier remains intact.

In an experiment, scientists damaged the skin of laboratory animals using trauma and harsh chemicals. During the repair process, there was an increase in the activity of HMG-CoA reductase, a display of more LDL-receptors, and there was an increase in the numbers of apo E. All three things result in increased cholesterol for skin repair, but two involve obtaining cholesterol from the blood in general circulation.

As we age, our skin cells have a reduced capacity to make cholesterol molecules. An experiment revealed that a mixture of cholesterol, ceramides, essential fatty acids, and nonessential fatty acids quickly helped restore aged skin that was intentionally damaged. It also helped younger skin repair itself faster. The most important ingredient was cholesterol. Skin repaired itself even faster when the cholesterol portion was increased.

Scientific papers have been published that show where psoriasis developed in patients taking statin drugs for lowering cholesterol. Experiments with animals showed that applying statin drugs topically to the skin would deplete the stratum corneum of cholesterol. The skin begins to hyperproliferate and starts scaling. The water barrier remained intact.

In a 1996 experiment, researchers had people take statin drugs. They then specifically looked for skin changes. Hyperproliferation began to appear, but the researchers showed that there was no increased water loss through the skin.

In a 1991 experiment, repeated topical applications of statin drugs again to skin of animals caused it to hyperproliferate at first. Eventually the barrier property was lost. Fluid began to seep out of the skin.

In experiments with mice, fasting (semi-starvation) in the animals caused a significant decrease in cholesterol production in skin (as it does in all tissues).

Researchers have found amyloid in the skin of psoriasis patients. In addition, they also found amyloid in people with psoriatic arthritis, which is a type of rheumatoid arthritis that can accompany psoriasis of the skin. These patients with psoriatic arthritis also exhibit low blood cholesterol levels.

In a study, scientists discovered amyloid in the skin of 72 percent of the Alzheimer's patients tested. The skin of 90 percent of Down syndrome patients had amyloid. Only 37 percent of normal, healthy people had skin with amyloid.

Eskimos that still follow their traditional diet, based totally on animals, do not get psoriasis. Eskimos do not develop psoriasis because in eating animals they consume large quantities of cholesterol and vitamin D.

Three types of medications help psoriasis patients: corticosteroids, cyclosporine, and acitretin. All three have the side effect of raising cholesterol levels.

Corticosteroids provide an instant increase in blood cholesterol levels, but have serious side effects with long-term use. Topical steroids provide relief to the skin patches, but repeated use can lead to even more skin eruptions.

Organ transplant cases use cyclosporine to control rejection processes, and it raises cholesterol levels.

The last three psoriasis treatments we will discuss are therapies using ultraviolet light, vitamin D, and methotrexate.

Using a special medical light to shine ultraviolet light on the skin of psoriasis patients results in three different findings. In some patients, it helps cure their skin lesions. In others, it damages the skin even further. In a third group, it causes skin cancer.

The newest way to treat psoriasis is with the use of vitamin D, either in a skin ointment or swallowed as medicine. We are specifically discussing vitamin D-3, which is the active form of vitamin D, known also as calcitriol.

Calcitriol is necessary for your intestines to be able to absorb calcium from the food you eat. Calcium is necessary for bones, teeth, muscle, nerves, and almost everything else in your body.

Psoriasis is the result of skin cells that are growing much too fast. We have discussed the fact that a deficiency of cholesterol causes the skin cells to multiply faster in order to maintain the barrier. Researchers discovered, over ten years ago, that calcitriol slows the rate of skin cell production. It works at the level of the DNA in the nucleus. It has this controlling effect whether it is a topical application or taken internally and transported through the bloodstream to the cells.

Where does calcitriol, the active form of vitamin D, come from? The ultraviolet rays of the sun turn cholesterol molecules in the skin into the vitamin by splitting open one of the four rings in the molecule. After the cholesterol molecule splits, enzymes in your liver and kidneys turn it into a calcitriol molecule.

There are two overlapping mechanisms by which low cholesterol levels lead to the hyperproliferation of skin cells. In one case, it is the lack of calcitriol molecules due to a deficiency of cholesterol molecules. In the other case, there may be enough cholesterol, but not enough sunlight exposure to turn them into calcitriol.

In the northern latitudes where Eskimos live, the darkness of winter lasts for months. How do they satisfy their requirements for calcitriol if there is no sunlight for long periods? By eating the livers and other organs of fish and animals, they ingest oils, which are rich in vitamin D.

Calcitriol, the active form of vitamin D, allows your body to absorb calcium from your food and prevents skin cells from multiplying too fast. A satisfactory amount of calcitriol, therefore, plays a vital role in preventing rickets, osteoporosis, and psoriasis.

The ultraviolet rays of the sun turn cholesterol molecules into vitamin D, which then becomes calcitriol. The energy of ultraviolet rays, which can damage tissue, are neutralized in this process.

We can now explain why the use of ultraviolet light therapy in psoriasis patients can bring about the three different results I spoke of earlier in this section.

In the patients who see a healing of their psoriasis lesions, it must be due to their having an adequate amount of cholesterol in their skin. These patients could have gotten better on their own if they had just spent more time in natural sunlight.

In the second situation, where ultraviolet light therapy made the lesions worse, the patient must have had a shortage of cholesterol molecules in their skin. The energy of the ultraviolet rays caused tissue damage. Normally, neutralization of the ultraviolet energy occurs in the process of creating vitamin D/ calcitriol from cholesterol molecules.

In the third situation, the combination of ultraviolet tissue damage and cell hyperproliferation from a cholesterol shortage progressed to the point of becoming skin cancer. Will adding calcitriol halt the skin cancer once it is established? We will discuss that in the next section.

Researchers in a 1995 study placed keratinocytes in cell cultures. They added a statin drug, which caused the cholesterol content in the cultures to decrease. Ultraviolet light caused more damage to these cultures than to an untreated one that still had a normal amount of cholesterol. The researchers then simply added pure cholesterol to a culture with decreased cholesterol from statin drug treatment. This protected the cells from ultraviolet damage. Finally, the researchers added LDL cholesterol to a low-cholesterol culture, which also protected against ultraviolet damage. It is obvious that the amount of cholesterol in our skin is very important.

Calcitriol prevents cells from multiplying too fast by influencing the DNA. It works whether delivered into the bloodstream or simply applied topically.

In addition, a psoriasis medication that affects the rate of cell multiplication by influencing the DNA is methotrexate. Its normal usage is in the treatment of various types of cancers. It is a powerful drug with dangerous side effects. Consequently, only very serious cases of psoriasis, for which no other therapy currently in use has been effective, utilize methotrexate.

Both calcitriol and methotrexate are effective in preventing skin cells in psoriasis patients from multiplying at excessively high rates. Both accomplish this by influencing the DNA in the cells. Methotrexate is a drug used in cancer treatments. Cancer cells by definition are cells that are multiplying at excessively high rates. I wondered if the molecules are similar in structure, considering the fact that their actions are similar.

If methotrexate can control the overproduction of skin cells in psoriasis, could calcitriol control the overproduction of tumor cells in cancers?

Before my father died of colon cancer, his treatment included chemotherapy. I have never heard of any cancer treatments that used vitamin D or calcitriol. I wondered if any medical researchers had investigated this concept. The answers I found relating to vitamin D and cancer are in the next section.

10-11 Your Body's Natural Cancer Fighter

I hoped to find at least a few scientific papers detailing a possible connection between vitamin D/calcitriol and cancer. I was surprised to see that there are hundreds of published papers on this subject. There are over sixty references for this section listed at the end of the book. There are hundreds more that I could have listed.

Does vitamin D/calcitriol fight cancers in your body? The answer is yes.

Are researchers able to prove, through experiments, that vitamin D/calcitriol stops the growth of cancer cells in laboratory cultures? Yes.

For convenience, we shall just use the term vitamin D in the remainder of this section. Incidentally, vitamin D is also considered by some to be a hormone.

Many researchers have recognized that cancer is associated with low blood cholesterol. However, there is no clear answer as to which comes first. Does a cancer tumor that has already developed then draw great amounts of cholesterol out of the blood for its own tumor growth? Alternatively, does low cholesterol lead to cancer by some undiscovered mechanism?

We are actually discussing a possible mechanism right now. Low cholesterol, resulting from diet and lifestyle, leads to low vitamin D levels. The low levels of vitamin D might lead to cancers. Have any researchers analyzed a possible relationship between cancers and vitamin D levels in blood? Because our bodies use sunlight to make vitamin D, a better question to ask would be about cancers and exposure to sunlight. Do people with more exposure to sunlight have decreased numbers of cancers? Do people with less exposure to sunlight develop cancers at higher rates?

The answer to both of these questions is yes, when speaking of the following cancers: breast, colon, prostate, and ovarian.

Though severe sunburn increases the risk for skin cancer, research shows that regular exposure to sunlight actually prevents skin cancer. The chances for skin cancer and other cancers to develop in patients will actually increase if they begin avoiding the sun. This even holds true for malignant melanoma, according to a study of men in the U.S. Navy. This study concluded that the vitamin D from regular sun exposure blocks the growth of malignant melanoma cells and leads to lower rates of the disease.

We should emphasize that we are talking about regular sun exposure and not regular sunburning.

Cortisol, made from cholesterol, has specific actions on cells. Cortisol forces cells to donate molecules of cholesterol. Its actions do not last very long in the body.

Now we learn that vitamin D/calcitriol, also made from cholesterol, influences the rates of growth of cells in tissues. Its actions do not last very long in the body.

If one eats too much vitamin D, there is a chance that an excessively high amount of calcium may be absorbed. Blood with a high amount of calcium can lead to constipation and loss of appetite. Blood with an extremely high amount of calcium leads to a condition called hypercalcemia. Mental confusion and muscle weakness are some of the signs of hypercalcemia. Over a long period, kidney stones may develop.

There is research for the development of drugs that act like vitamin D towards cancers, but will not increase calcium absorption. These drugs are vitamin D analogues.

What types of cancers are affected by vitamin D or the synthetic vitamin D analogues? Breast cancer, colon cancer, and prostate cancer.

Some of the other cancers that have been found to be susceptible to control by vitamin D or its analogues are: ovarian, endometrial, brain, liver, squamous cell, lung, pancreatic, and malignant melanoma, which was mentioned earlier.

I have never heard of cancer patients receiving vitamin D or calcitriol as part of their chemotherapy. I find this to be amazing when you stop and consider all of the research currently available on this subject.

The only risks in receiving high doses of vitamin D or calcitriol are constipation, some dizzy spells, or perhaps muscle weakness. These are a small price to pay if it means saving your life in a battle against cancer.

Methotrexate is a powerful drug used in the treatment of cancers. Since both methotrexate and calcitriol control the rates of cell growth in psoriasis by influencing the DNA, I wondered if their molecules were similar in any way. If you examine the drawing for this section at the end of the book, you will see that each molecule has three rings that are in a similar position towards each other. There are some nitrogen atoms in place of carbons, but nitrogen and carbon are next to each other in the periodic table. Only one atomic number separates them.

CHAPTER 11
Down Syndrome

Normally we have 23 pairs of chromosomes that provide the plans for what we are made of and how we look. In Down syndrome, there is a third chromosome on number 21. It is for this reason that we also refer to the condition as Trisomy 21. There are various body characteristics common to all Down syndrome patients.

The most significant feature of Down syndrome is mental retardation. This syndrome also occurs as a mosaic, which means that the patient can have a mixture of Trisomy 21 and normal cells. The degrees of mental retardation and physical features of Down syndrome mosaics will vary from patient to patient. In some cases, it may be difficult to positively diagnose Down syndrome without a genetic test.

In an earlier chapter we discussed the fact that people with non-insulin dependent diabetes mellitus almost never get Alzheimer's disease. Patients with NIDDM have much higher blood cholesterol levels in most instances, and this protects them from developing Alzheimer's. Unfortunately, the high cholesterol levels, along with other factors, cause NIDDMs to experience higher rates of heart disease/atherosclerosis.

In other words, I searched for and found a group with low rates of Alzheimer's disease. If I were able to find a category of people with high rates of developing Alzheimer's disease, then they should also have low rates of classic heart disease/ atherosclerosis. I found the group of people for whom I was searching.

All people with Down syndrome have Alzheimer's-type damage in their brains, and those that survive past the ages of thirty-five to forty will eventually develop the full clinical signs and symptoms of Alzheimer's disease. This is a cruel fate for those already having to deal with the mental retardation and body features of this condition.

To my knowledge, no one has satisfactorily explained why all Down syndrome adults eventually develop Alzheimer's disease. You will know the mechanism behind it by the time you finish reading this chapter. It definitely does involve cholesterol.

All Down syndrome patients are on the path to eventually develop Alzheimer's. They show the signs and symptoms of the disease: amyloid plaques, neurofibrillary tangles, cerebral atrophy (brain shrinkage), damage to the hippocampus and other limbic system structures, cerebral amyloid angiopathy with small strokes, olfactory deficits, low blood pressure, cataracts (even in children with Down syndrome), increased platelet membrane fluidity, epilepsy, myelin defects, defects in brain glucose metabolism, ubiquitin, interleukins, prolactin, and tumor necrosis factor.

Down syndrome patients develop Alzheimer's disease regardless of whether or not they possess an apo E 4.

<u>The brain of a Down syndrome baby at birth is essentially normal</u>. The Down syndrome

brain at birth is not a mentally retarded brain. However, the processes of brain tissue changes and the depositing of amyloid begin around the time of birth. After three to five months, the size of the brain has already started to shrink compared to a normal infant of the same age. The axons and dendrites of the neurons exhibit damage by the end of the first year of life. The child is on the path to developing Alzheimer's disease.

The observation that very young children with Down syndrome seem to almost be able to learn things as well as other young children illustrates this situation. However, as they get older, learning becomes increasingly difficult.

If a shortage of cholesterol causes Alzheimer's, and Down syndrome patients always develop Alzheimer's if they live long enough, then logic tells us they must almost never develop classic heart disease or atherosclerosis. Is this true?

The answer is yes. Atherosclerosis/ classic heart disease does not affect Down syndrome patients.

Some readers are aware that Down syndrome patients may be born with a heart defect, but it has nothing to do with conventional heart disease. They may be overweight and have a chubby appearance. Their blood can be high in triglycerides, but it is not high in cholesterol. On the other hand, Down syndrome patients are not in a condition of long-term semi-starvation. What is the link between a thin 80-year-old man with Alzheimer's and a chubby, 50-year-old Down syndrome patient with Alzheimer's?

The answer is that they both develop Alzheimer's disease as a result of a shortage of cholesterol molecules in their brain tissues. They reached this condition, however, in two very different ways.

The thin, 80-year-old followed the path that has already been detailed in this book. The disease followed a long period of semi-starvation.

In Down syndrome there is no shortfall in eating, though some of these patients may have some defects in the ways their intestines absorb food. Instead, a constant chemical process occurs that causes the removal of cholesterol molecules from all of the tissues of the body, including the brain. The genetic defect itself, namely the extra number 21 chromosome, programs this constant removal of cholesterol from tissues.

Before continuing, let me point out something for those readers who plan to look up the references for this chapter. The article by Murdoch, J.C. in a July 1977 issue of the British Medical Journal is available in abstract form by computer on Medline. Unfortunately, the Medline version of the abstract has an incorrect word that is critical to the overall meaning of the sentence in which it appears. The word "with" should actually read "without." Please refer to the actual journal article itself.

The following explanation details why Down syndrome patients always develop Alzheimer's disease and do not develop atherosclerosis/ classic heart disease.

The term "free radical" refers to an oxygen molecule with an extra electron. We call this the superoxide free radical, and it is the molecule most responsible for aging the tissues in our bodies. Superoxide oxidizes beneficial molecules, which over a long time weakens our systems and organs. Antioxidants are supposed to help protect us from superoxide and other harmful free radicals produced every day in our bodies as part of the normal processes that are always occurring.

The body neutralizes superoxide with a two-step process that uses two different enzymes. The first one is copper zinc superoxide dismutase, and it converts the superoxide radical into hydrogen peroxide. Hydrogen peroxide can be harmful to friendly tissues if not controlled, so the second enzyme, called glutathione peroxidase, converts the hydrogen peroxide to water, which is harmless.

The first enzyme, copper zinc superoxide dismutase, forms in our tissues according to genes on chromosome 21. The second enzyme, glutathione peroxidase, forms according to genes on a different chromosome.

Down syndrome patients have an extra chromosome 21, which means that their tissues produce fifty percent more copper zinc superoxide dismutase than normal. This occurs right from the time of birth, which means that fifty percent more superoxide free radicals are converted to hydrogen peroxide molecules, compared to someone without Down syndrome. The enzyme glutathione peroxidase does show some increased activity in converting the dangerous hydrogen peroxide to water, but there is not enough of the enzyme in our tissues to equal the fifty percent increases in copper zinc superoxide dismutase. As a result of this genetically programmed inequality, excess hydrogen peroxide is continually produced in the tissues of Down syndrome patients from the time they are born.

Hydrogen peroxide is a very powerful oxidizing agent, especially towards cholesterol molecules. <u>Hydrogen peroxide can literally explode cholesterol molecules out of cell membranes</u>. The first discovery of this occurred over thirty years.

The power of hydrogen peroxide to remove cholesterol from tissues in large amounts is illustrated by its ability in experimental tissue cultures to strip away the atheroma plaques that clog arteries in heart disease.

Amyloid is nature's substitute for cholesterol molecules. The genes that control the production of amyloid protein are also on chromosome 21; therefore, Down syndrome patients have 50 percent more amyloid generated compared to someone without the syndrome.

The combination of excess production of hydrogen peroxide, which strips cholesterol molecules out of tissues, and excess amyloid production, guarantees that eventually the Down syndrome patient will develop Alzheimer's disease. All of the other conditions, from cataracts to epilepsy, will develop in due course.

CHAPTER 12
Genetic and Metabolic Defects of Cholesterol Metabolism

(Average readers may wish to skip this somewhat technical chapter.)

12-1   Genetic Cholesterol Synthesis Defects

Making cholesterol molecules requires carbon building blocks, energy and many enzymes to create each one. A genetic defect anywhere in the process will have profound effects in the brain of a developing infant.

This section has two references about very rare conditions of cholesterol metabolism. In each, the shortage of cholesterol leads to brain atrophy (shrinkage). You are aware that this is one of the primary signs in Alzheimer's disease, though current medical opinion does not connect it to cholesterol.

In the remaining sections of this chapter, we will discuss several genetic conditions and one that is acquired that result in defects of cholesterol creation or the usage and transporting of it.

You will notice the similarities between these and various conditions and Alzheimer's, such as brain atrophy, cataracts, and so on.

12-2   Cerebrotendinous Xanthomatosis

Cerebrotendinous Xanthomatosis, which we shall refer to as C-X, is also known as VanBogaert's disease. C-X is a rare, purely genetic disease in which there is a defect of cholesterol metabolism. Produced and deposited throughout the body as clumps, or xanthomas, are large amounts of the substance "cholestanol." Xanthomas are in muscle tendons, the nervous system and the blood. Patients can survive into their adult years.

The genetic defect in C-X that causes increases in the production of cholestanol is also responsible for the low blood cholesterol levels seen in the disease. C-X patients commonly possess the following signs and symptoms: cerebral atrophy (brain shrinkage), dementia, cataracts, epileptic seizures, loss of myelin and parkinsonism.

All of these are also associated with Alzheimer's disease.

C-X patients suffer from a type of atherosclerosis, but it is from the deposits of cholestanol, not cholesterol.

Because a genetic defect in cholesterol metabolism causes C-X, one research group thought that treatment with a statin drug would be helpful. A C-X patient, who had low cholesterol levels to begin with, received one of the statin drugs. This patient's blood cholesterol levels decreased even more as a result, and the patient showed no improvement in disease symptoms.

12-3   Smith-Lemli-Opitz Syndrome

Smith-Lemli-Opitz Syndrome is a purely genetic disorder that we shall refer to in this section as SLOS. In SLOS, a defect exists in the enzyme controlling the last step in the production of a cholesterol molecule. Because of this, there exists a severe shortage of cholesterol molecules before the time of birth.

Those born with SLOS exhibit the following signs and symptoms: cerebral atrophy (brain shrinkage), cataracts, epileptic seizures, reduced myelin in the brain and other parts of the nervous system, mental retardation and skin eruptions which I characterize as juvenile psoriasis.

Patients born with SLOS can survive up to at least the age of thirty if they follow a special diet.

Researchers created SLOS in laboratory rats by exposing developing fetal rats still inside the womb to chemicals that blocked the production of cholesterol molecules. The researchers then added a serum rich in cholesterol to the rat embryo, which restored normal development of the fetal rats.

Researchers began feeding cholesterol to children born with SLOS. They consumed a mixture of pure cholesterol of egg yolks and soybean oil.

All children with SLOS who ate a cholesterol mixture exhibited benefits from it. Their brains grew in size, even though the researchers thought that cholesterol from the diet did not cross the blood brain barrier.

This is very important. Earlier in this book we discussed how glucose in the brain itself produces cholesterol for the brain during the early growth years. These experiments with SLOS children prove that the human brain is capable of using cholesterol from the diet for its growth and development.

We have already detailed in the earlier sections how the adult brain depends on cholesterol from the general blood circulation.

In addition to increased brain growth and development in the SLOS children, feeding cholesterol resulted in increased language development and increased motor abilities. There also was an improvement in their overall body growth.

12-4   Mevalonic Aciduria

Mevalonic Aciduria, which we shall refer to as MA, is a very rare genetic disorder in which there is a deficiency of another enzyme in the cholesterol production process. In this disorder, the enzyme is mevalonate kinase. As a result, the shortage of cholesterol molecules causes signs and symptoms in MA patients that you are familiar with: brain atrophy (shrinkage), cataracts, mental retardation, and muscle and skin problems.

12-5   Niemann-Pick Type C Disease

Niemann-Pick Type C Disease, which we shall refer to as NPC, is a genetic disorder that is different from the ones previously discussed. Cholesterol molecules are produced in normal amounts. However, the cells are unable to move the cholesterol molecules around in order for their use. The reason for this is unknown.

NPC is a cholesterol storage disorder because of this inability of cells to move it around. As a result, cholesterol accumulates in massive amounts, especially in the Golgi complex. Cholesterol molecules are present but not used, so the cells react as if there were shortages of cholesterol. Some of the signs and symptoms present in NPC patients are: dementia, seizures, mental retardation, ubiquitin, arthritis and skin problems.

I found no references that said cerebral atrophy (brain shrinkage) was a symptom of NPC. This should not be surprising, because there is not a shortage of cholesterol in the disease. The problem is that the cells are unable to use it.

Researchers studying NPC have found that the brains of these patients have neurons that contain neurofibrillary tangles identical to the tangles found in the brains of Alzheimer's patients.

The researchers did not find amyloid plaques in the brains of the NPC patients. This surprised the researchers, because all of the other signs and symptoms of NPC are almost identical to those of patients with Alzheimer's disease.

Readers of this book, however, know why amyloid is not present in NPC patients. It is because there are large quantities of cholesterol molecules present, especially in the Golgi complex. You will remember from an earlier section that amyloid is generated in the Golgi complex of neurons. This occurs only when the Golgi complexes are experiencing a shortage of cholesterol molecules. There is no such shortage in NPC.

12-6   Metabolic Defect: Fetal Alcohol Syndrome

Fetal alcohol syndrome is present in the babies of mothers who were heavy drinkers of alcohol while pregnant. Children born with fetal alcohol syndrome, which we shall refer to as FAS, exhibit mental retardation, small brain and head size, a characteristic arrangement of the eyes and nose, and heart defects. For pregnant women, there is no safe amount of alcohol consumption. However, in general, greater degrees of birth defects occur in women who were heavy drinkers compared to light drinkers.

The actual mechanism by which alcohol consumption by pregnant women leads to FAS babies is unknown. Here are my conclusions.

In a growing fetus, the brain manufactures cholesterol molecules. The material used by the fetus to make brain cholesterol molecules is glucose. The glucose molecules come from the blood of the mother.

Drinking alcohol just happens to be one of the most common causes of low blood sugar, or hypoglycemia.

Consumption of alcohol lowers blood glucose. In a pregnant woman, therefore, drinking alcohol reduces the amount of glucose available to the developing baby. A shortage of glucose molecules leads to decreased production of cholesterol molecules, especially in the brain. This is the mechanism by which drinking alcohol while pregnant can lead to fetal alcohol syndrome.

My advice for women is to avoid drinking alcoholic drinks entirely while pregnant. If a woman is unable to give up drinking while pregnant, then it is vital for her to eat plenty of starches, to help maintain an adequate blood glucose level.

CHAPTER 13
Alzheimer's Symptoms in Other Illnesses

13-1   Other Illnesses with Brain Shrinkage, Etc.

The purpose of this chapter is to show you that other diseases and conditions exhibit the signs and symptoms of Alzheimer's disease. The one thing that is common to all is a loss of brain tissue, which appears as atrophy.

Younger people have a better ability to regain normal brain size if a situation of good health or better nutrition returns. Older people have less ability to do this.

As we age, we have less ability to bounce back from injury or illness. In most cases, researchers have not been looking for connections between these illnesses and conditions and Alzheimer's disease. A more accurate statement would be that no one has searched for the low cholesterol connection to Alzheimer's disease, and no one has appreciated the significance of cholesterol levels in the illnesses and conditions discussed in this chapter.

As an example, look at semi-starvation in children. Lack of proper amounts of food leads to shortages of cholesterol as well as proteins and other substances. The parts of the body decrease in size as the processes of starvation take their toll. The human brain is also subject to shrinkage during starvation.

Kwashiorkor and protein energy malnutrition are two conditions seen in children who are subject to long periods of semi-starvation. Brain shrinkage is evident in both conditions, and its severity directly relates to the duration of the semi-starvation period.

If provided with the proper amount of nutritional feeding, the brain shrinkage in these children is reversible. This illustrates that younger children can bounce back from a condition of brain shrinkage.

13-2   Anorexia Nervosa

Anorexia nervosa is caused by long periods of semi-starvation. One is classified as having anorexia nervosa if voluntary starvation has reached a point where body weight is 15 to 25 percent below the acceptable standard. Almost 95 percent of anorexia nervosa patients are female. There are complex psychological reasons behind this disorder.

Multiple changes occur in the bodies of anorexics, including the loss of monthly menstrual periods. As their bodies become thinner, we should be able to find similarities between the changes occurring in this disorder and those that we see in Alzheimer's.

The first question to ask is if there are amyloid plaques and neurofibrillary tangles in the brains of patients who have had anorexia nervosa for a long period of time. We cannot answer this question at this time for several reasons. First, we must find these plaques and tangles during special examinations of brain tissue after the patient has died. The goal of treatment, of course, is to prevent anorexics from dying in the first place.

About ten percent of anorexics will die because of this disorder. If they perform an autopsy in a case, it is highly unlikely they would test brain tissue for plaques and tangles. This is because no one up to this point has ever thought that there is a connection between anorexia nervosa and Alzheimer's disease.

Almost all of the other signs and symptoms of Alzheimer's disease are present in patients with anorexia nervosa. Brain shrinkage occurs in anorexia nervosa patients. If treatment is successful and the patient regains weight, then the brain may return to its original size. However, there is also data that shows that it may not. If the anorexia patient should die, I believe that at autopsy, the patient's brain should show the presence of amyloid and neurofibrillary tangles, *but only if the pathologist happened to check for these two things.*

Most of the following signs and symptoms in anorexics that are common to Alzheimer's disease will disappear if the patient resumes eating and returns to a normal weight. Younger people have a greater chance of recovering compared to older patients.

The list includes epileptic seizures, muscle damage, low glucose metabolism in the brain, memory and learning problems, skin eruptions, low blood pressure, elevated growth hormone, elevated tumor necrosis factor, elevated interleukins, elevated prolactin, decreased serotonin and edema.

Anorexics have high levels of cortisol and norepinephrine, which gives the feeling of having more energy than ever. It allows some female athletes to keep going, even though their bodies are wasting away. However, at some point, their bodies will collapse.

Patients with anorexia nervosa may seem to sometimes have normal or even elevated blood cholesterol levels. The cortisol can temporarily mask what is actually a condition of cholesterol deficiency.

Just as in Alzheimer's, some researchers believe that the high cortisol levels are a result of stress or a defect in the HPA axis. The real reason, of course, is that high cortisol levels are the normal response of the body to a condition of starvation.

These patients can die from a heart problem, but it is not a classic heart attack.

They instead may develop a fatal heart arrhythmia, or irregular heartbeat. This is another symptom shared with Alzheimer's patients. The heart muscle of an anorexic becomes thin and weak. At autopsy, I believe that it would show the presence of amyloid in the muscle, but only if the pathologist checked for it.

13-3   Long-Term Kidney Dialysis: Warnings About Heparin

Dialysis means the use of a device to artificially filter the blood in a patient whose kidneys have failed. There are two types of dialysis.

In hemodialysis, the patient's blood is removed from the body and pumped through a filtering device. The treatment takes three to five hours, several times a week.

In peritoneal dialysis, a special solution is pumped into the abdomen where it removes waste, urea and salts from the blood. The solution is then flushed out. Several techniques can accomplish this, but the most common is continuous ambulatory peritoneal dialysis, or CAPD.

We are talking about patients who have been on dialysis for a long time. In many cases, patients just beginning dialysis must do so because of atherosclerosis and high blood pressure, combined with obesity. High blood cholesterol levels and heart attacks are common in these people.

However, as the months and years pass, these same people on dialysis can lose weight to the point of appearing almost anorexic. Their blood cholesterol levels decrease. They are now in the stages of developing Alzheimer's disease, though their doctors may not recognize the association.

Malnutrition and weight loss are common in both types of dialysis. The process itself results in increased production of cortisol by the adrenal glands, probably because of a type of metabolic acidosis, according to researchers. Body tissues degrade and wasting of muscles occurs at a high rate.

The increased levels of cortisol will make the blood temporarily appear to have normal or even high amounts of cholesterol in it. This is masking an actual condition of a shortage of cholesterol. Eventually, the blood cholesterol levels fall.

Researchers have found that blood cholesterol levels are the most reliable indicators for determining whether a long-term dialysis patient is close to dying. As cholesterol levels fall, so too fall the chances of survival. Long-term survivors on dialysis are those who maintain normal or elevated blood cholesterol levels.

Does cerebral atrophy (brain shrinkage) occur in dialysis patients? The answer is yes. Some researchers have even noticed the connection between the falling cholesterol levels and the degree of brain shrinkage. Others have found a direct correlation between the length of time on dialysis and the amount of brain shrinkage. Still others have associated it with the malnutrition and weight loss of long-term dialysis.

There was a study of children on dialysis who were aged eighteen or under. Brain shrinkage had already occurred in 59 percent of these children.

A universal finding in long-term dialysis patients is amyloid accumulation throughout the body. Researchers believe there is a connection between amyloid and the arthritis symptoms and carpal tunnel syndrome frequently seen in these patients.

These patients exhibit arrhythmias (irregular heartbeats). Pathologists discover that many long-term patients at autopsy have amyloid in their heart muscle.

These patients have malnutrition and weight loss, falling cholesterol levels, amyloid accumulation and brain shrinkage. Do they develop dementia?

The answer is yes. In fact, at least 80 percent or more of long-term dialysis patients develop dementia, according to a 1995 study. Before the firm diagnosis of dementia occurs, these patients exhibit memory and learning problems.

Documentation shows the following signs and symptoms, that we know are associated with Alzheimer's disease, occur in long-term dialysis patients. The list includes cataracts, epileptic seizures, nitric oxide, ubiquitin, tumor necrosis factor and the interleukins. Cerebral hemorrhage (stroke) at low or normal blood pressure occurs at a high rate in these patients as their body weight and cholesterol levels decrease. These are hemorrhages not associated with the heparin used during dialysis.

A number of years ago researchers noticed that aluminum was accumulating in the brains of these patients. They developed a condition called dialysis dementia. This condition led some people to believe that aluminum caused Alzheimer's disease.

The types of solutions used in the dialysis procedures were the cause of the accumulation of aluminum in brain tissues. When they modified the solutions, the aluminum stopped accumulating in the brains of the patients.

Careful research discovered the particular damage caused by the aluminum to be different from the damage associated with Alzheimer's disease. People on long-term dialysis with the proper solutions were still becoming demented. Current researchers may not be classifying it as Alzheimer's disease, but it is.

The use of heparin is to prevent the blood from clotting during the dialysis procedure. Physicians must make a judgment as to how much heparin is necessary. Too much heparin may cause a serious hemorrhage. An insufficient amount may lead to clotting of the blood.

Heparin has an additional effect in the body, in that it aggressively lowers cholesterol levels. Heparin is so effective at lowering cholesterol levels that they use it in a special therapy called HELP, which stands for Heparin-mediated Extracoporeal LDL Precipitation. HELP is a treatment for people born with a genetic disease called familial hypercholesterolemia. These people have blood cholesterol levels of 500 to 700 mg/dl or more, and they all develop atherosclerosis and suffer heart attacks at a young age. They also use this drug therapy in transplant cases, where the drugs used for controlling rejection have caused high cholesterol levels.

We now have the complete picture as to the reasons why long-term dialysis patients develop a dementia that I say is Alzheimer's disease. The parts of the picture are malnutrition and weight loss, cortisol production, and heparin. The low cholesterol levels that result will eventually lead to Alzheimer's.

In a 1999 article, researchers in Britain found that they could cause seizures to develop in laboratory rats. How did they do it? By injecting heparin into the hippocampus areas of the rats' brains.

13-4   Long-Term Alcoholism

One of the basic chemical properties of cholesterol is that alcohols can dissolve it. Alcohols act as a solvent upon membranes. They increase the fluidity of a membrane. Another term that means the same thing is disorder; alcohols disorder the membrane. Alcohols act on the cholesterol and other lipids in membranes in a manner that alters their structure in a negative manner.

Ethyl alcohol, or ethanol, is the alcohol found in the beer, wine, whiskey, and other alcoholic drinks.

Alcoholism is the continuous dependence on excessive amounts of alcohol. It is associated with a pattern of unacceptable behaviors. Alcoholics become physically and mentally addicted.

Consuming alcoholic drinks at first may cause a person to act in an excited and uninhibited manner. Eventually, however, the alcohol acts as a sedative. Continuous drinking in a short amount of time may cause the person to fall asleep. Before that point is reached, the person develops slurred speech, slow reaction times, and uncoordinated muscle movements.

How does alcohol actually cause these effects? There is no definite answer. Most references in the medical literature state that alcohol acts as a depressant on the central nervous system and that it causes sedation. I could find no actual biochemical or physiological explanations that explained exactly how alcohol causes these effects.

The following are my conclusions.

One of the chemical characteristics of cholesterol is that it can be dissolved by alcohols, including ethanol. After consuming an alcoholic drink, exposure to the alcohol occurs quickly in tissues throughout the body.

Cholesterol makes up a large part of the brain. Alcohol in blood acts as a solvent on the cholesterol in cell membranes, synapses, and myelin layers.

Eventually, removal from the bloodstream occurs. Until that happens, however, the bilayer cell membranes are in a state of relative disorder and exhibit higher membrane fluidity. The myelin coverings around nerve fibers become thinner.

As alcohol acts on cholesterol molecules in neuron cell membranes, synapses, and myelin, we should expect to see that the speed of nerve impulses would be slower. This slowing of nerve impulses is the primary cause of the slurred speech, uncoordinated muscle movements, and slower reaction time. An epileptic-like seizure may occur.

Let us now discuss alcoholics and Alzheimer's disease. A common finding in both types of patients is brain atrophy (shrinkage). Some researchers think that this is proof that alcoholism can definitely cause Alzheimer's. Others, however, state that even though alcoholics exhibit brain shrinkage and suffer memory losses, they may not have large numbers of neurons dying in the hippocampus and other limbic areas. It is for this reason that they do not believe that alcoholism definitely causes Alzheimer's.

In regards to brain atrophy, the brain may reverse back to normal size if the patient stops drinking, but there is also the chance that it may not. Brain shrinkage occurs in the earliest stages of alcoholism, even before detection of any liver damage.

Alcoholics have memory and learning problems, what we call Korsakoff syndrome. Researchers have found similarities between Alzheimer's patients and those alcoholics with Korsakoff syndrome.

High cortisol levels occur while an alcoholic is actively drinking. Other signs and symptoms include dementia, skeletal muscle damage, parkinsonism, loss of myelin, epileptic seizures, neuron loss in limbic structures, amyloid plaques, neurofibrillary tangles, arrhythmias (irregular heartbeats), and high levels of tumor necrosis factor and interleukins. In rats fed ethanol, feeding cholesterol prevented the increase in tumor necrosis factor and other cytokines.

Heart muscle damage in alcoholics occurs gradually. Amyloid protein accumulates in the process (though references may call it glycoprotein). The muscle damage leads to arrhythmias, though alcohol can affect the rhythm of a heart even in someone who is not an alcoholic.

Does alcoholism directly cause Alzheimer's disease? We must consider the nutritional status of the patient. Malnutrition is common among these patients. A diagnosis of anorexia nervosa may even occur.

In experiments with rats, researchers showed that providing an adequate amount of food leads to an increase in the percentage of cholesterol in neuron membranes and myelin. This occurred at the same time they were feeding the rats alcohol. The researchers concluded that the brains of the rats increased the cholesterol as a protective measure against the alcohol.

This did not occur in rats that were deprived of adequate food while consuming alcohol. These rats exhibited decreasing amounts of cholesterol in neuron membranes and myelin. They found them to have increased membrane fluidity and they developed problems in tasks that involved memory and learning.

Does alcoholism directly cause Alzheimer's disease? The answer depends on three factors. The first one is the age of the patient, because older people have a decreased ability to heal and bounce back after tissue damage.

The second factor is the length of time that the patient has been drinking excessively. Longer exposure to alcohol will obviously result in a greater degree of brain atrophy and tissue damage.

The third factor is the nutritional status of the patient. A well-nourished alcoholic will be more resistant to permanent damage to tissues.

13-5   Cushing's Disease

Cushing's disease is a metabolic disorder resulting from a continuous high level of cortisol in the bloodstream. The adrenal glands, which are on the kidneys, produce cortisol in response to signals received from the pituitary gland in the brain. A tumor of the pituitary gland leads to Cushing's disease because the adrenal glands receive a continuous signal to produce cortisol.

In some cases, there is no tumor of the pituitary gland. The high cortisol levels are due instead to an excessive amount of adrenal gland tissue.

Some of the signs and symptoms of Cushing's disease are unusual accumulations of fat and fluid in the face and upper body, muscle damage, skin changes, osteoporosis, and high blood cholesterol levels. The high blood cholesterol levels are not the result of increased production of cholesterol molecules. Remember that cortisol blocks the synthesis of cholesterol. Cortisol forces all of the cells of the body to donate cholesterol molecules, and this action raises the levels in the blood.

Do the high cortisol levels in Cushing's disease cause brain atrophy? The answer is yes. The hippocampus is especially vulnerable.

Cushing's disease patients who have brain atrophy usually have memory and learning problems. Successful treatment of these patients can result in a reversal of the brain to normal size. The learning and memory problems may disappear in such cases.

Keep in mind that in Cushing's disease the cortisol levels are higher than in Alzheimer's disease. The muscle wasting, osteoporosis, and skin changes occur quickly. The high blood cholesterol levels which result can lead to atherosclerosis and classic heart disease, especially if the patient is continuing to eat an adequate amount of food.

Prednisone and the other synthetic forms of cortisol may be up to one hundred times more powerful than natural cortisol, and they may last longer in your body, too. As a result, people receiving these synthetic steroids will develop the same signs and symptoms as do patients with

Cushing's disease. People taking steroids will develop fat and fluid accumulations in their face and upper body. They will also suffer from muscle weakness and damage, skin damage, and osteoporosis. These changes are all the result of cells throughout the body continuously giving up cholesterol molecules, proteins and other lipids.

Are patients that take synthetic steroids at risk of developing brain shrinkage? The answer is yes. In a paper published in 1985, researchers placed rats on prednisolone, which is a synthetic steroid. It also possesses much more strength than natural cortisol. After twenty-one days the brains in the rats were smaller and had lost cholesterol.

13-6   HIV/AIDS, Kaposi's Sarcoma

Human immunodeficiency virus, or HIV, is the virus that causes AIDS, which stands for acquired immune deficiency syndrome. The AIDS virus eventually destroys the body's protective immune system. The patient then dies after severe infections of disease agents that are not normally harmful to healthy people.

From one-fourth to one-third of all AIDS patients develop dementia. I was already aware that advancing weight loss and malnutrition are common findings in AIDS. With these thoughts in mind, I investigated the disease from the aspect of cholesterol.

Researchers have analyzed the brains of AIDS patients who were demented when they died. These brains exhibited atrophy (shrinkage) and areas where neurons had died. However, the AIDS virus found to be present in these brains was in a random pattern. The areas of shrinkage and dead neurons might or might not have AIDS viruses. Something other than the direct presence of AIDS viruses must account for the brain changes and dementia.

The evidence of weight loss and malnutrition, brain shrinkage, and neurons dying in areas where no viruses were present, led me to search for an answer to the following question regarding cholesterol. As the disease processes of AIDS progress, do the blood cholesterol levels of the patients decrease?

The answer is yes. In fact, it is a universal finding in AIDS patients. Some researchers even consider the decreasing blood cholesterol levels as markers that indicate the status of the patients. As the levels go down, so do their chances for survival.

The decreasing cholesterol levels that are part of the disease cause the dementia that develops in AIDS patients. The dementia does not specifically relate to the presence of any AIDS viruses in the brains of the victims. The progressive weight loss and malnutrition are the cause of the decreasing blood cholesterol levels.

One additional factor plays a part in the decreasing cholesterol levels. The AIDS virus has RNA covered with an unusual type of coating, in that it has cholesterol molecules arranged in a lipid bilayer.

This factor may play a role in the decreasing cholesterol levels. As more viruses reproduce, they use more of the cholesterol molecules in the body, which deprives normal body tissues, including the brain, of these necessary molecules.

It is true that the brains of AIDS patients may be the sites of fungal and bacterial infections labeled as opportunistic. They occur as a direct result of the decreased immunity present in the disease. However, these brain infections occur also in AIDS patients who are not demented. The dementia may develop regardless of the presence or absence of high numbers of virus particles in the brain, and regardless of the presence or absence of other opportunistic infections. The cholesterol levels are the only criteria that matter in the dementia of AIDS.

Memory and learning problems are associated with the brain atrophy in these patients. This is also present in many children infected with HIV.

Adults and children with AIDS have high cortisol levels.

Cholesterol levels continue to decrease, as the condition of a patient gets worse (even though cortisol may sustain the levels temporarily). Some researchers have found that feeding the patient food that is high in fat and cholesterol seems to improve their appearance and health status.

Drugs which attack the AIDS virus directly can be made more effective by covering them with cholesterol. This virus needs cholesterol molecules, and it will take them from any source.

Knowing that statin drugs block the production of cholesterol, researchers added one to an AIDS culture. They found that the statin halted growth of the virus as long as there was not a significant amount of cholesterol already present in the culture.

In a 1987 paper, researchers in New Jersey were working with a chemical mixture that pulled cholesterol molecules out of the membranes of cells. This mixture, called AL 721, was able to kill the AIDS virus simply by this action on its cholesterol coating.

The virus survives best in body fluids containing a significant amount of cholesterol, such as blood, lymph, semen, and vaginal fluid. Normal body perspiration is a fluid that does not contain a significant amount of cholesterol. This is the reason why a carrier cannot transmit the AIDS virus simply by perspiring onto another person.

One of the reasons for the failure of the immune system to attack the AIDS virus, as other invaders are attacked, is due to the cholesterol coating of the virus. The body does not recognize cholesterol molecules as being an enemy of the body, so why should the immune system regard a virus covered with them as a threat?

AIDS patients have amyloid proteins in many areas of their bodies to varying degrees. Researchers have found amyloid plaques, tau protein, and neurofibrillary tangles in AIDS brains that appear to be identical in pattern to those in Alzheimer's brains, but no one ever considers cholesterol as a factor in either AIDS or Alzheimer's.

There is a loss of myelin in the brains of these patients, and they frequently develop epileptic seizure attacks.

There are elevated levels of ubiquitin, interleukins, tumor necrosis factor, prolactin, and growth hormone.

Increased levels of nitric oxide are present, even in children with AIDS.

There are decreased levels of serotonin

There is damage to the hippocampus and other limbic structures.

An altered sense of smell is frequently present.

Low blood pressure (hypotension) is another characteristic. These patients suffer a high rate of cerebral hemorrhage, or stroke, even though they have low blood pressure.

Muscle damage occurs throughout the body, including muscle tissues that do not have large numbers of virus particles.

Arrhythmias (irregular heartbeats) and heart muscle damage are common. Many children and adults with AIDS die as a result of arrhythmias.

Cataracts are common in AIDS patients, although documentation of this does not frequently occur. Many people are aware of the virus infections that involve the retinas of patients, but this is not due to low cholesterol. Shortages of cholesterol definitely cause the cataracts.

Rheumatoid arthritis is common in AIDS patients.

Psoriasis is common, and those AIDS patients with advanced psoriasis are usually very close to dying.

Adding vitamin D to an AIDS culture stops the virus from multiplying.

Kaposi's sarcoma is a cancer that occurs in 15 to 30 percent of all AIDS patients. The tumors consist of cells that are similar to the cells of normal blood vessels, and occur in the skin and throughout the body. Is cholesterol connected to Kaposi's sarcoma? Yes.

In a 1987 paper, researchers analyzed the medical signs and symptoms of thirty-one AIDS patients who had developed Kaposi's sarcoma. <u>Every patient had low blood cholesterol levels</u>.

In another paper also published in 1987, cancer researchers noted that weight loss and malnutrition were common in the AIDS patients who developed Kaposi's sarcoma. Patients not infected with the AIDS virus but who were victims of other cancers would sometimes develop Kaposi's sarcoma. This occurred only after their primary cancers had caused significant weight loss and left them in a condition of malnutrition.

In a 1988 paper, researchers in Germany revealed that Kaposi's sarcoma cells kept in cultures actively took up cholesterol, but that after doing so the cells had less of a tendency to be malignant. In other words, Kaposi's sarcoma tumor cells were more dangerous when there was a shortage of cholesterol.

Patients with advanced psoriasis will sometimes develop Kaposi's sarcoma.

The German researchers also determined that the AIDS virus itself does not directly cause Kaposi's sarcoma.

In a 1993 paper, researchers in California determined that drugs capable of killing tumor cells in Kaposi's sarcoma can be made up to 38 times more effective simply by covering them in a capsule coating that contained cholesterol.

When damage occurs to skin, the new tissue that fills the wound is imperfect and may be lacking all of the necessary components of normal tissue, including cholesterol. Blood vessels must grow rapidly into the area if the tissue is to eventually turn into normal skin. It is my opinion that Kaposi's sarcoma cells will develop in this environment. A sufficient amount of cholesterol already present in tissue will keep the tumor cells from growing further.

In other words, the blood vessel tumor cells of Kaposi's sarcoma are similar in nature to the rapidly growing but imperfect skin cells found in psoriasis. Both develop in conditions of low cholesterol, and controlling both should be possible by providing satisfactory amounts of cholesterol.

13-7   Kainate: "Instant Alzheimer's" in the Laboratory

What follows is a summary of the work performed by various research groups from around the world that utilized kainate, also known as kainic acid.

Applying kainate to rat brain tissue produced the following results, all of which can be considered to be characteristics of Alzheimer's disease.

Kainate directly caused the rapid and violent oxidation of large amounts of cholesterol and other lipid molecules in the cell membranes of neurons.

Myelin is lost after injection of kainate. Axons pack together because of the loss of myelin. Some axons and dendrites degenerate, leading to the death of neurons.

Seizures occurred, the hippocampus was quickly damaged, the blood-brain barrier was altered, and amyloid was produced when kainate was applied to rats' brains.

The brains of older rats were far more susceptible to damage from kainate than were those of young rats.

In conclusion, this evidence demonstrates that kainate creates a type of Alzheimer's disease in the brains of rats.

13-8   Proposed Alzheimer's Terms

I have identified some diseases and conditions that can lead to the development of changes in the brain that are similar to those seen in Alzheimer's disease. Some new terms should be adopted that will identify the connections between these diseases or conditions and Alzheimer's.

The terms are as follows:
1. Anorexia-associated Alzheimer's
2. Dialysis-associated Alzheimer's
3. Alcohol-associated Alzheimer's
4. Cushing's-associated Alzheimer's
5. AIDS-associated Alzheimer's

An alternate method may be to say that we see "Alzheimerism" in AIDS, or "Alzheimerism" in dialysis, and so on.

There are other situations in which "Alzheimerism" develops, such as in long-term cancer patients where there is extensive weight loss and body wasting.

CHAPTER 14
Autoimmunity, Inflammation, and Cholesterol

(Average readers may wish to skip this somewhat technical chapter.)

14-1   Alzheimer's as an Autoimmune Disease

Many researchers believe that the processes occurring in the brains of Alzheimer's patients are the same as those found in people suffering from various autoimmune diseases, in which the body seems to be attacking itself. There is a constant inflammatory response, also called an autoimmune response, though there is no obvious cause for the reaction.

No one can explain exactly why your body's immune system would mount an inflammatory response against itself. Attempts to explain the processes are just descriptions of the various steps seen in normal inflammation that are then linked to the particular body tissue that is involved.

Diseases thought to be autoimmune in nature include rheumatoid arthritis and psoriasis. We have discussed these in previous chapters. There are at least two reasons behind the belief by some that Alzheimer's is an autoimmune disease. The first is that there is a constant activation of inflammatory processes despite no obvious cause. The second is medical evidence appearing to show a slightly reduced rate of Alzheimer's disease among people taking anti-inflammatory medications over long periods.

14-2   Autoimmune and Rheumatic Disorders

Autoimmune diseases are characterized by the apparent alteration of the function of the immune system of the body. No one has ever actually explained why these diseases occur. Again, definitions given for these diseases are just descriptions of what seems to be happening using the terms of inflammation processes.

Rheumatic disorders are those autoimmune diseases associated with connective tissues of the body. Vasculitis pertains to inflammation of blood vessels, which also contain connective tissue.

In addition, there are overlap syndromes, which are combinations of rheumatic disorders. An example of this is psoriatic arthritis, which is a condition where the patient simultaneously has skin and joint problems.

The inflammatory or immune response that characterizes autoimmune and rheumatic diseases is never associated with outside viruses, bacteria, or physical injury.

Previous sections of this book discussed the things that do seem to be in common with autoimmune and rheumatic diseases. They include interleukins, tumor necrosis factor, prolactin, ubiquitin, and several others. These factors are also common in patients with Alzheimer's disease and Down syndrome. Why would your body attack itself? The answer is that in actuality it does not, though rheumatologists and immunologists will not agree with this. The body mounts an inflammatory response whenever it detects things normally found inside of cells as being in the body fluids outside of cells. When does this occur? It happens when damage occurs to cell membranes, which then results in the leakage of cell contents. What are the causes of cell membrane damage?

Infections from viruses and bacteria, very high or very low body temperatures, physical injuries and burns, and shortages of cholesterol cause this damage.

Most autoimmune diseases and rheumatic disorders are actually a continuing response by the body to cell membranes that are simply falling apart. The body is continually sensing that the "insides" of cells are on the outside. There is a constant effort in progress to repair cell membranes. Medical professionals interpret this constant effort as being an autoimmune response.

What is the one class of medications that are helpful in almost every autoimmune disease? The answer is steroids, such as prednisone. How do steroids, which actually are a more powerful synthetic version of cortisol, bring about the relief of symptoms in patients with autoimmune disease? The answer always given is that steroids stabilize the membranes of various parts of cells thought to play a role in inflammation. How do steroids actually stabilize the membranes of cells? Supposedly, no one knows.

For the true answer to this question, we need only to discuss one of the major side effects of steroids, which is the raising of blood cholesterol levels. As stated in a previous section, this is not an annoying side-effect of steroid therapy; it is, in fact, the actual reason behind the relief of symptoms that are brought about by using them. The increased amounts of available cholesterol molecules can be used for the repair of cell membranes. The leakage of cell contents then stops. This results in a decrease in the signs of inflammation.

14-3   Freund's Adjuvant

An antigen is any protein that stimulates the body's immune system to produce an antibody. When scientists want to study the interaction of antigens and antibodies, they use a mixture called Freund's adjuvant. This is an emulsion made by adding water to a special type of oil. They then add various kinds of bacteria or viruses to act as antigens.

For example, to study the antibodies produced by an infection of tuberculosis, they add the germ that produces this disease to some Freund's adjuvant. They then inject this combination into a laboratory animal, which produces an inflammatory response that includes antibodies specific to tuberculosis.

How does Freund's adjuvant actually cause this reaction to occur? In papers published in 1987 and 1989, scientists used adjuvant to produce arthritis in laboratory rats. After injecting adjuvant, the cholesterol levels decreased in the rats. It was then that arthritis and inflammation developed. During the active inflammatory process, the cholesterol levels in the rats increased back to and even beyond the levels that existed before the injections. The arthritis inflammation subsided.

In addition, they discovered that by feeding the rats cholesterol before they injected adjuvant, the researchers prevented the arthritis and inflammation.

The most important molecule of myelin is cholesterol. In multiple sclerosis, patches of myelin flake off nerves in the brain and spinal cord. In a 1985 paper, scientists created the animal version of multiple sclerosis in rabbits by adding Freund's adjuvant to their spinal cords. Cholesterol decreased, leading to the damage of myelin.

Freund's adjuvant also reduces the myelin of nerves outside of the central nervous system, so it produces a condition called peripheral neuropathy in laboratory animals.

The primary use of Freund's adjuvant is to produce the antibody response to an antigen in experiments. It does this by specifically lowering the cholesterol content of membranes. Cell contents then leak out, which in turn activates the body defense system. Thus, this produces an inflammatory response.

This inflammatory response occurs regardless of the presence or absence of an antigen. If there is an antigen, then the body produces antibodies against it. If there is no antigen, scientists would label the reaction as a type of autoimmune disease process.

Freund's adjuvant produces inflammation by removing cholesterol from cell membranes. The temporary substitute for cholesterol in cell membranes is amyloid. Therefore, Freund's adjuvant should be associated with some degree of amyloid accumulation, since it removes cholesterol from cell membranes. Is there any evidence in the scientific literature that associates amyloid with Freund's adjuvant?

Yes. In fact, scientists who study amyloid diseases have used Freund's adjuvant for over thirty years as a way to produce amyloid accumulation in laboratory animals!

14-4   Proposed New Definitions

The conventional definitions for autoimmune disorders state that the immune system has caused the body to attack itself.

Two things trigger an immune or inflammatory response. The first one is based on the recognition that components normally found inside of cells are found in the body fluids outside of cells. Cell membranes are leaking for one reason or another.

The other trigger is the presence of an antigen. This is also the basics of an allergic reaction, especially when the response is far greater than would be expected.

The first situation is the one with which we are primarily concerned. The things that cause membranes to leak or break open completely are infections of viruses or bacteria, temperatures that are either too hot or too cold, physical injury, chemicals or solvents, and a shortage of cholesterol molecules.

The diseases classified as autoimmune fall into the last category. The basis for all is a shortage of cholesterol molecules in relation to various cell types, such as fibroblasts, keratinocytes, synovial lining cells, neurons, etc.

Inflammation can now be defined simply as those processes used in the repair of existing cell membranes or the creation of new ones. The most important molecule for this task is the cholesterol molecule.

Suppression of the immune response or the inflammatory response may now be termed as "satisfying" the immune or inflammatory response. The drugs that suppress the immune system are, in fact, satisfying it. The key to their benefits are that they in one way or another increase the availability of cholesterol. The immune or inflammatory response subsides only after it has been "satisfied."

On a related matter, one might ask why the body would initiate processes that possibly use antibodies if the real cause of cell membrane leakage is simply a shortage of cholesterol molecules, as I propose is the case with autoimmune diseases. The answer lies in the fact that in the beginning, the body does not yet know what has caused the damage to cell membranes. I believe that the body assumes, until proven otherwise, that the cause of the damage might be viruses, bacteria, and so on.

14-5   NSAIDs, Cholesterol and Alzheimer's

NSAID is the abbreviation for non-steroidal anti-inflammatory drug. In other words, an NSAID is a drug that controls inflammation even though it is not a steroid.

The side effect of steroids is the quick increase of cholesterol levels. This is, in fact, the real beneficial aspect of their use in satisfying inflammation.

How do NSAIDs satisfy inflammation? Before we answer that, we need to discuss the reason for including NSAIDs in a book about Alzheimer's disease.

There have been studies showing that patients taking NSAIDs for a long period appear to develop Alzheimer's disease at a slightly lower rate. In other words, sustained use of NSAIDs seems to protect a patient against Alzheimer's.

Most of the patients in these studies were taking NSAIDs as treatment for rheumatoid arthritis. Many years ago (and before the use of NSAIDs became routine), patients with rheumatoid arthritis developed Alzheimer's at a higher rate. It is only in the last two or three decades that the protective property of NSAIDs against Alzheimer's in these patients became evident.

Some examples of NSAIDs are ibuprofen and indomethacin. One of the unfortunate side effects of NSAIDs is bleeding from the stomach or intestines with continued use over a long period of time.

How do NSAIDs satisfy (or control) inflammation? How is it that people taking NSAIDs for a long time seem to have a lower risk developing Alzheimer's disease?

The answer to both questions is the same. NSAIDs raise cholesterol levels.

Aspirin and other NSAIDs promote bleeding with a property that works against clotting. This property is separate from the raising of cholesterol levels.

Cortisol and steroids raise cholesterol quickly, by forcing all cells to donate molecules of cholesterol. NSAIDs, on the other hand, raise cholesterol levels by speeding up the manufacture of molecules, not by taking them away from tissue throughout the body. How do NSAIDs speed up the production of cholesterol?

There are actually at least three processes involving NSAIDs that play a part in the raising of cholesterol levels. The first is the ability of NSAIDs to increase the production of cholesterol molecules regardless of whether inflammation or cell damage is present. The NSAIDs increase the incorporation of pyruvate into the process of manufacturing cholesterol molecules.

Prostaglandins block the release of cholesterol from lipoproteins that come from the liver.

NSAIDs inhibit the creation of prostaglandins throughout the body, so the cumulative effect is an increase of lipoproteins carrying cholesterol from the liver.

The third process that is occurring relates to the fact that prostaglandins themselves block the creation of cholesterol molecules. NSAIDs block the production of prostaglandins not only at the injury site, but also throughout the body. This then serves to increase the amount of cholesterol produced.

Prostaglandins are so effective in lowering cholesterol that some researchers have created synthetic versions of them called analogues. Theoretically, they could use these prostaglandin analogues as a treatment to control atherosclerosis by the lowering of blood cholesterol levels.

Some researchers have warned that doctors who prescribe NSAIDs need to be aware that cholesterol levels will rise, and that this property might increase the risk for the development of atherosclerosis.

Researchers have found that increasing the amount of cholesterol molecules can cause a reduction in the production of prostaglandins.

You will remember that conditions of low cholesterol result in increased membrane fluidity (more leakage) and increased nitric oxide. Researchers have found that NSAIDs act to decrease membrane fluidity and lower the levels of nitric oxide.

The reason for discussing NSAIDs was the evidence that their use seemed to offer protection against Alzheimer's. Two of the hallmark signs of this disease are amyloid plaques and neurofibrillary tangles. One NSAID, indomethacin, has been shown to reduce the production of amyloid in special cell cultures that stimulate inflammation.

In a trial that lasted six months, Alzheimer's patients given an NSAID saw their mental status stay the same or decrease only 1 percent. The Alzheimer's patients who took a placebo, however, experienced a decrease in their mental status of 8 percent. This provided evidence that NSAIDs will not cure Alzheimer's, but they might offer protection against the advancement of the disease, and perhaps its initial development.

14-6   Malnutrition and Immune Problems

The purpose of this section is to point out two important aspects of nutrition. The first is the fact that malnutrition (or semi-starvation) quickly harms the immune system of the body. People who are poorly nourished are more susceptible to disease processes that damage tissue. The body is less able to repair itself, and this obviously centers on the repair of cell membranes and the utilization of cholesterol molecules.

The second point is that the elderly will frequently display problems in their immune system. This correctly links to their nutrition status. The elderly are particularly sensitive to disease processes if they are malnourished. We are already aware that weight loss and malnutrition are common in this population.

14-7   Gold and Cholesterol

Some of the oldest and most effective drugs in the treatment of rheumatoid arthritis are gold compounds. They are also effective in treating psoriatic arthritis.

In an earlier chapter, you learned that some cases of rheumatoid arthritis are the result of shortages of cholesterol molecules. The beneficial effects of steroids and NSAIDs in these patients are due to their influence on cholesterol metabolism.

In the treatment of patients with rheumatoid arthritis, gold has two beneficial effects: 1) gold compounds decrease joint inflammation, and 2) they retard cartilage and bone destruction. Gold compounds do not cure rheumatoid arthritis.

The companies that make the gold compounds state that the mechanism of action is unknown

There are gold compounds taken orally and ones for injection only. They do not produce immediate results. It may take two or three months for benefits to appear.

How does gold help patients with rheumatoid arthritis? It is due to the fact that gold and cholesterol adhere to each other, especially if the cholesterol is part of a lipoprotein such as LDL or HDL. The presence of gold in the blood and tissues apparently keeps the body from losing cholesterol easily. Gold that accumulates in and around joints increases the availability of cholesterol, which lowers inflammation.

Do rheumatologists and the drug companies that make the gold compounds know that gold and cholesterol adhere to each other? Probably not.

Therefore, who does know about it? It is those researchers who use gold to label or mark lipoprotein particles in their experiments.

By labeling LDL particles with gold, it is possible to see how they cross a human placenta or are taken up by skin fibroblasts. There is even a technique for measuring the amount of LDL in whole blood by labeling it with gold.

There are some side effects to gold therapy but the side effects are rarely dangerous. In 1995, there was a study in Finland of patients who died because of their rheumatoid arthritis medications. Out of forty-seven deaths, thirty were due to NSAIDs, eleven due to steroids, and six to other medications. No deaths were due to gold. This was in spite of the widespread use of injectable gold in Finland.

Amyloid is the temporary substitute for cholesterol. In experiments in 1986, scientists created cultures of cells that could force the production of amyloid by using a special substance that created inflammation. The scientists found that they could prevent the production of amyloid by adding gold compounds to the cultures.

I conclude that gold compounds can be beneficial for patients with rheumatoid arthritis simply because cholesterol adheres to gold.

CHAPTER 15
Cholesterol and Other Conditions

15-1   Parkinson's Disease and Cholesterol

This disease is a slow and progressive disorder in which the neurons in the brain that control voluntary muscle movements gradually die. These motor neurons are located in the substantia nigra and other parts of the brain stem.

The deaths of increasing numbers of these motor neurons lead to the development of the symptoms which are characteristics of Parkinson's disease. These are slow movements, rigid muscles, unstable posture, and slow shaking or tremor while at rest. However, many Parkinson's patients do not exhibit shaking or tremor.

The neurotransmitter chemical used by motor neurons is dopamine. The treatment for patients with Parkinson's disease involves increasing the amounts of dopamine available for the neurons that are still alive. The drug used for this is levodopa, which crosses the blood-brain barrier and converts into dopamine.

People of all ages can develop Parkinson's disease, but it is more common in those over the age of sixty.

Dementia that some consider identical to Alzheimer's disease will develop in a high percentage of patients with Parkinson's disease. It is also true that signs of Parkinson's disease can develop in Alzheimer's patients.

Other findings in this disease that are similar to Alzheimer's include learning and memory problems before the dementia develops.

Weight loss and malnutrition are common in many Parkinson's patients, just as in Alzheimer's disease.

Olfactory (sense of smell) problems are almost universal in the disease, as are problems with chewing and swallowing, so continued weight loss occurs.

Cerebral atrophy (brain shrinkage) occurs in Parkinson's disease, just as in Alzheimer's. Even the children who develop Parkinson's exhibit this.

Found in Parkinson's brains at autopsy are amyloid plaques and neurofibrillary tangles. The hippocampus and other limbic structures are frequently involved. I should also point out that the substantia nigra shows damage in patients with Alzheimer's disease, though it is not widely known.

Industrial toxins, pesticides, and other environmental suspects do not cause Parkinson's disease, although some drugs and chemicals can cause similar symptoms.

Studies with twins reveal that most cases are not due to a genetic cause. However, there is a small percentage of people who are more susceptible to developing the disease.

Previous brain injury or surgery increases the risk for Parkinson's disease.

Parkinson's patients exhibit elevated levels of cortisol, growth hormone, and prolactin, just as in Alzheimer's.

There are also increases in nitric oxide, ubiquitin, interleukins, and tumor necrosis factor in Parkinson's patients. Low blood pressure and osteoporosis are common. The brains of these patients exhibit reduced glucose metabolism.

Researchers found that the substantia nigra in the brains of Parkinson's patients contain up to ten times the amount of oxidized cholesterol molecules compared to normal brains. The cause is shortage of fresh, unoxidized cholesterol molecules.

The conclusion that all of this evidence leads to is that in many cases, Parkinson's disease and Alzheimer's disease are probably two versions of the same processes. The difference is a simple one based on chance and genetic variability. In Alzheimer's, the neurons most susceptible to cholesterol shortages are those in the limbic system that are involved with memory, thought, and learning. In Parkinson's disease, the motor neurons in the substantia nigra, involved with voluntary muscle controls, just happen to suffer damage first. We also see combinations of the two diseases.

Just as in Alzheimer's, patients carrying the apo E 4 gene may develop Parkinson's at an earlier age compared to others developing the disease.

In summary, the probable cause of many cases of Parkinson's disease is a long period of cholesterol shortages due to insufficient nutrition, or semi-starvation. It is simply by chance that Parkinson's develops before Alzheimer's. It is important to remember that Parkinson's patients can develop Alzheimer's and vice versa. Remember also that a previous head injury or brain surgery can lead to the disease, perhaps years or decades later. Cholesterol levels may or may not be a factor in such cases.

Parkinson's patients and Alzheimer's patients share almost all of the same laboratory findings, such as brain shrinkage, amyloid, olfactory deficits, and so on. One thing they do not share, however, is the presence of epileptic seizures. Though common in Alzheimer's patients, Parkinson's patients never have epileptic seizures. What is the reason for this?

A 1977 paper provided the reason why Parkinson's and epileptic seizures are exclusive of each other. It is because they both involve the same nerve pathways and circuits in the brain.

Voluntary movements of body parts involve complex feedback mechanisms where some muscles contract while others relax simultaneously. This system is abnormally affected in both Parkinson's and epileptic seizures of the grand mal or tonic-clonic type. The same neuron circuits leading to body muscles are not able to express a classic epileptic seizure if damaged by Parkinson's disease.

In a final way of connecting a lack of cholesterol to Parkinson's, people born with the genetic disease cerebrotendinous xanthomatosis may display the signs and symptoms of Parkinson's disease. Cerebrotendinous xanthomatosis is due to a defect of cholesterol metabolism.

15-2   Vasculitis

Vasculitis is the term used to describe an inflammation of blood vessels. This can affect any arteries or veins. Vasculitis is usually one of the first signs of a rheumatic disease, such as lupus or rheumatoid arthritis.

Researchers have described the condition of some arteries in the brains of Alzheimer's patients as being a vasculitis. Vasculitis also occurs in the brains of Down syndrome and Parkinson's patients when they reach the stage of being demented.

Under specialized microscopic examination, the tissues of the blood vessels in this condition appear to be less dense and deformed. Researchers also find that amyloid protein accumulates along the vessels affected the most. The combination of the tissue being less dense, along with the accumulation of amyloid, leads to leakage or small hemorrhages of the vessels at normal or low blood pressures.

The three important points to remember about vasculitis are: the tissue being less dense, which means that it is weak and prone to leaks; that amyloid protein deposits occur along the affected blood vessels; and that it is associated with rheumatic conditions. My conclusion is that vasculitis is, in effect, the reaction of blood vessels to a long-term condition of a shortage of cholesterol molecules.

15-3   Low Cholesterol and the Lungs

Vance Wolff had several instances where fluid accumulated in and around his lungs. The doctor called it pleural effusion. It can progress to pulmonary edema, a dangerous state where a great amount of fluid accumulates in the lungs.

If vessels and tissues contain cells with defective membranes, it will lead to leakage of fluid across the membranes. Edema is the result of inappropriate fluid accumulation in tissues.

One of the signs of people suffering from starvation and protein-calorie malnutrition is an increase in edema in the body.

There is a condition called adult respiratory distress syndrome in which breathing becomes difficult. The changes that occur within the lungs in this syndrome include damage to the membranes of the capillaries, capillary leakage, small hemorrhages, and edema. In a 1990 paper, researchers noted that patients suffering from adult respiratory distress syndrome also showed significant decreases in blood cholesterol levels.

In a 1975 study of people with amyloid accumulation from various causes, edema was one of the most common findings.

In experiments to lower the blood cholesterol of rats, an unexpected effect was the development of edema in the lungs of the rats.

Chronic low cholesterol levels can lead to edema in various tissues in the body, as well as in the lungs. It is interesting to note that the treatment for fluid in and around the lungs involves the use of steroids. Steroids quickly raise the blood cholesterol levels.

15-4   Zinc and Cholesterol

At least thirty different enzymes are involved in the manufacture of cholesterol molecules. Scientists believe that some of these enzymes need zinc in order to function properly. Consequently, the belief is that the integrity of cell membranes depends, in part, on an adequate amount of zinc in tissues.

In both animals and human studies, increased consumption of zinc led to higher blood cholesterol levels.

In a 1987 experiment with laboratory animals, feeding a diet that lacked zinc caused cholesterol levels to decrease by 50 percent, compared to the animals whose food included sufficient zinc.

Up until about five years ago, there was some research interest in a possible connection between Alzheimer's disease and a deficiency of zinc in the body, including the brain. There were studies that showed that the amounts of brain tissue death, neurofibrillary tangles, etc., did indeed seem to correspond to shortages of zinc. One of the findings of the ongoing studies of elderly nuns ("The Nun Study") was that those ladies with the least amounts of amyloid plaque and neurofibrillary tangles in their brains also had normal blood levels of zinc before death, not deficiencies. The conclusion to be drawn is that an adequate amount of zinc in the body protects against Alzheimer's.

As stated earlier in this book, the production of amyloid segments occurs when there are shortages of cholesterol molecules.

The enzymes and proteins that generate amyloid segments need zinc to function properly, just as they do when they are processing cholesterol. This should not lead one to conclude that zinc, especially excess levels of it, cause Alzheimer's disease.

Researchers used zinc dietary supplements in a group of Down syndrome patients who were experiencing the early deaths of red blood cells in circulation. In this 1997 experiment, the zinc acted to prevent the early deaths of these cells. The cells avoided early death because the zinc acted to boost the cholesterol levels in these Down syndrome patients.

15-5   Apoptosis

Apoptosis is the explanation given whenever cells die with no obvious identifiable cause. Such causes are normally bacterial or viral infections, extreme heat or cold, harmful chemicals or metals, adjacent cancer tumors, and so forth.

The logic behind the use of the term apoptosis is that the cells in question died because they must have been genetically programmed to die when they did. This concept appears in a number of situations, from the death of neurons in the brain, to the death of red blood cells in Down syndrome patients.

Many cases presumed to be instances of apoptosis, or programmed cell death, may actually be cell deaths from shortages of cholesterol in the membranes of the cells.

As has been discussed previously, cells with membranes that are not intact are cells that eventually will die. I found four journal articles in which statin drugs caused apoptosis in living cells. Statin drugs block the manufacture of cholesterol molecules.

CHAPTER 16
Your Doctor

Prior to entering medical practice, your doctor spent four years in college, four years in medical school, then from two to five years or more in a residency program.

But after the practice is established, how does your doctor keep up with the developments in medicine?

There are typically four avenues for doctors in this regard: attending continuing education seminars, reading medical journals, communicating with other doctors person-to-person, and listening to drugmakers' sales representatives.

At first glance, it would appear that only one of the four avenues would involve a drugmaker's attempt to influence your doctor. But that would not be true, for the following reasons.

Formal continuing education seminars are almost always sponsored by a drugmaker, and the particular seminar's topic will usually involve a condition for which the drugmaker is marketing a medication.

Medical journals contain articles written by doctors and researchers. Much more often than not, these authors working in medical schools and university research labs will usually be receiving financial aid from one or more drugmakers.

Naturally, it is hoped that the readers of medical journals will believe that the opinions, conclusions, and recommendations put forth in the articles are free of drugmakers' bias.

You may ask, why don't doctors simply read the research themselves, and then make decisions accordingly? Aren't doctors smart enough to derive the critical key bits of information, and to filter out the things that really would not improve the medical conditions of patients?

Many doctors do just that, and the patients of those doctors are fortunate.

But there are only 24 hours in a day. Doctors have families and businesses that require their attention. It's easy to understand why many doctors' decision-making might be based solely on information provided by drugmakers, either directly or indirectly.

I will not say whether this is good or bad. Simply, it's just the way it is in today's medical environment in the U.S.

Today, the medical care available is better than ever. The medicines we have at our disposal are better than ever, and that is positive testimony for drugmakers.

But on the other hand, is it possible for drugmakers to occasionally be completely wrong about something? Could they be in error regarding what's in the patient's best interest on a particular subject, and for that to result in doctors making decidedly unhealthy decisions?

The answer is absolutely yes, and here is one example.

Research has shown that people in their seventies and beyond do not gain any health benefits from lowering their blood cholesterol levels. Despite this fact, many doctors continue keeping these older patients on medicines that lower blood cholesterol levels. There may be millions of elderly patients in the U.S. that are in this category.

Another issue that can be troubling is the manner in which drugmakers utilize and analyze numbers and statistics in attempts to show a particular new medication's effectiveness. There are several consumer "watchdog" groups that monitor this issue, so we won't debate it here. However, in Chapter 17, I look at the statistics used by some drugmakers regarding statin drugs and heart attacks.

Please realize that my comments in this chapter are not intended to get people to start ignoring their doctors' decisions.

What would be beneficial is for patients to simply be a little more inquisitive, simply by asking questions.

"Is this newer and much more expensive medication really an improvement over my current cheaper generic medicine?"

"Do I really need this medication?"

"Are the side effects of this medicine going to bother me more than the symptoms of the ailment we're trying to control?"

Here's the best question. "Doctor, if you had what I've got, and you weren't wealthy, or didn't have a good insurance plan, would you take this medicine that you're prescribing for me?"

CHAPTER 17
Cholesterol and Atherosclerosis

17-1   Cholesterol, Atherosclerosis and Heart Attacks

Atherosclerosis is a disease process in which plaques of fat, cholesterol, oxidized cholesterol, and cell debris accumulate in the walls of arteries. (This is yet another use of the word plaque). Atherosclerosis occurs in the large and medium size arteries, not smaller ones. The walls become thickened and hard as calcium accumulates in them. This is the origination of the term "hardening of the arteries".

As the wall becomes thicker, the space inside the artery becomes smaller. It is like the wall of a pipe getting thicker in places and bulging inwards.

The space inside of an artery through which blood flows is the lumen. As an atheroma, which is the name used for the lesion, gets larger, the lumen becomes smaller. This naturally results in less blood flow reaching the tissues served by the artery.

A heart attack occurs when an area of heart muscle dies after the blood flow serving it is severely restricted or blocked altogether. The medical term is myocardial infarction, or MI. Heart attacks result from blood clots, air bubbles, a severe constriction of a coronary artery, or atherosclerosis processes. They also result from various combinations of these factors and others.

The atheroma that forms in an artery in the atherosclerotic process does not develop overnight in humans. In most cases, it takes from 30 to 60 years or more for atherosclerosis to cause symptoms in a patient. Of course, there are some exceptions to this, such as in the cases of rare genetic diseases.

If it takes 30 to 60 years or more for coronary heart disease to cause symptoms, what does this tell us? This indicates that humans, in most instances, are very resistant to the development of atherosclerosis. However, think of all of the diseases, infections, and cancers that can kill a person in time periods of just a few weeks to one or two years.

In western countries, more deaths and disability are due to atherosclerosis than any other disease. There is no doubt that cholesterol plays a role in coronary artery disease. For proof of this, we only need to look at studies of people born with a condition called familial hypercholesterolemia. About one person in every thousand is born with one gene for this genetic disease in which the removal of cholesterol from the bloodstream does not occur very well. Even rarer are the people born with two genes for familial hypercholesterolemia, about one in a million.

Those with one gene develop atherosclerosis usually by the age of fifty. Their blood cholesterol levels may be up to 500 mg/dl.

Those very rare and unfortunate people born with two genes for this disease will have blood cholesterol levels of up to 1,000 mg/dl. They may develop a fatal case of coronary artery disease before the age of twenty.

The consensus is that blood cholesterol levels of 500 to 1,000 mg/dl, as are found in such rare conditions, are enough to cause atherosclerosis regardless of other influences. However, what about the person with average cholesterol levels? First, let us review some of the history of how the debate on cholesterol began.

In the 1950's, researchers in Europe noticed that there seemed to be fewer heart attacks from atherosclerosis during and immediately after the years of World War II. They thought that the food shortages of the war years might have been the reason.

Later, researchers linked the apparent increases in rates of heart attacks in the 1950's to cholesterol, which was in the meats, eggs, butter, and other dairy products that people were again able to eat. Researchers began to proclaim that "high" blood cholesterol levels were the primary cause of heart attacks.

We can trace the beginnings of the "war" on cholesterol to those early researchers in the 1950's. Apparently, they ignored the effects of smoking, obesity, genetics, lack of exercise, and other factors. Researchers believed that simply measuring total blood cholesterol levels would indicate who would and who would not develop atherosclerosis and suffer a heart attack. However, there were people with "high" cholesterol levels who were healthy with no signs of atherosclerosis. There were also people with "low" cholesterol levels who were having heart attacks.

Researchers realized that they must try to factor in other influences, such as things like heredity, being male or female, age, blood pressure, cigarette smoking, sedentary lifestyle, obesity, and mental stress.

Development occurred regarding the more detailed analyses of blood cholesterol into its components: HDL, LDL, and triglycerides. The experts then issued the next set of "simple rules to avoid a heart attack." A high LDL count meant that a person would have a heart attack eventually. Again, however, people with a high LDL, also referred to as bad cholesterol, were living healthy lives. There also were people with a low LDL suffering heart attacks.

Next came the focus on HDL, referred to as good cholesterol. The belief was that a high HDL would protect you, and a low HDL meant an increased risk for atherosclerosis.

This was another guideline that turned out to be not always accurate, so researchers then began to develop ratios of these numbers to develop risk patterns. Some of these ratios include HDL to LDL and HDL to total cholesterol. They simultaneously figured into the risk picture the influences of smoking, obesity, genes, blood pressure, etc.

One of the final factors was being male or female. Men have more heart attacks than women do, and at an earlier age. However, women then catch up after menopause.

There are now studies of such things as lipoprotein (a) and homocysteine.

Currently, researchers have identified over 200 risk factors for cardiovascular disease. The issue is so complex that physicians have begun making decisions based only on total blood cholesterol levels again, just as it was decades ago. Some doctors factor in HDL and LDL levels, too, but few go beyond that.

If 65-year old Mr. Smith, who happens to have a total cholesterol reading of 240 mg/dl, suffers a heart attack, his doctor will probably conclude that the cause is the "high" cholesterol count. However, what about Mr. Jones, Mr. Johnson, and Mr. Williams? They too are over 65 and have total blood cholesterol readings of 240 or higher, but have not had heart attacks. The chances are good that Mr. Smith's doctor will never even see them in his office, so he probably will not be wondering how they escaped heart disease.

A previous chapter mentioned The National Cholesterol Education Program, or NCEP, which has put forth guidelines for treatment considerations in coronary artery disease. Briefly, these guidelines use total cholesterol levels of 160, 200, and 240 mg/dl and LDL levels of 100, 130 and 160 mg/dl as benchmarks. The doctor then factors in other influences, such as smoking and previous heart attacks. The tailoring of treatment recommendations occur according to each person, based on these criteria.

The first recommendation is always supposed to be controlling cholesterol with diet and exercise. Several months later, the physician will make the decision regarding medications, such as taking at statin drug.

There are many references listed for this section. I encourage every treating physician and allied health professional to look them up. There are some studies where close examinations of the statistics and measurements can lead to conclusions other than the ones listed in the abstracts by the authors. Keep in mind that there is still a tremendous bias against cholesterol in the medical world, in spite of the actual statistics. Some scientists have been brave enough to speak out against the tide. You will find some of their studies in the list of references.

When the notion that "heart attacks were caused purely by high blood cholesterol levels" began developing in the 1950's, the first recommendation made was for people to limit their intake of foods containing cholesterol. If you eat foods containing cholesterol, we call it dietary cholesterol. The item that comes to mind is the egg, of course, but there are other things also high in cholesterol content.

Even today, the constant recommendation is to eat foods with little or no cholesterol in them. A trip to the average grocery store in the United States will indicate aisles well stocked with items that proudly state their lack of cholesterol.

Many different studies, going back several decades, provide the truth for the next statement. <u>For the typical healthy person, eating foods that contain cholesterol does not cause blood cholesterol levels to become high enough to cause heart disease.</u>

We are continuously bombarded every day with the message that eating foods containing cholesterol causes unnaturally high blood cholesterol levels, which in turn causes people to have heart attacks.

This is totally wrong, if you accept the published scientific documentation regarding this issue.

Those scientists familiar with this issue know that <u>in humans, eating cholesterol only raises the blood cholesterol levels in people that have levels that are already below normal at the beginning.</u> In healthy people with normal cholesterol levels, dietary cholesterol has no influence whatsoever in raising blood levels further.

Some people's blood cholesterol levels respond more than others to dietary cholesterol. These folks obviously had lower-than-normal levels at the beginning.

Let me state it again in simple terms. <u>In the average, healthy human, eating cholesterol does not cause one to have blood cholesterol levels high enough to cause heart disease.</u>

Nevertheless, what about the animal experiments, many used as references in this book, in which putting cholesterol in the feed caused atherosclerosis? Does this not supply conclusive evidence regarding humans and dietary cholesterol?

The answer is no, and the reason is based on the choice of animals used in the experiments. Rabbits are the preferred choice by experimenters wanting to show that consuming cholesterol causes heart disease. These experimenters neglect to state that rabbits are herbivores, or pure vegetarians. By nature, they never eat foods with cholesterol in them. "Sneaking" cholesterol into their rabbit chow causes them to develop very high blood cholesterol levels and heart disease because they are rabbits. These kinds of experiments do not apply to atherosclerosis in humans.

Does feeding cholesterol in such a manner cause laboratory dogs and cats to develop heart disease? No, because dogs and cats are carnivores.

In humans, dogs, cats, lions, tigers, and other carnivores and omnivores, there exists the liver/cholesterol feedback mechanism. This is a system whereby consuming cholesterol causes the liver to decrease the production of cholesterol. This acts to control the blood levels of cholesterol, as well as conserve energy and materials for use in other liver functions. We will review this mechanism in a later chapter.

What foods do cause blood cholesterol levels to be high? The answer is carbohydrates, also known as starches or sugars. All breads, cakes, cookies, potatoes, rice, vegetables high in starch content, candies and other sweets fall into this group, as well as all types of pasta. The word that ties all of these foods together is glucose. They all readily and easily are broken down into glucose, or blood sugar.

You must be physically active in order to burn up all glucose that results from eating carbohydrates. Any glucose not burned up by your body turns into fat and cholesterol by the liver. There is no feedback mechanism at work here. Unburned glucose from eating excess carbohydrates will raise blood cholesterol levels into the high ranges. It will do the same for triglycerides, or fats in the blood. Weight gain occurs in the form of body fat. Body mass index, or BMI, increases.

Eating carbohydrates also causes the pancreas to produce insulin, which is the hormone that allows cells of the body to take in glucose for energy or fat production.

What about eating fats and oils?

According to the experts, we should avoid fats and oils from animals, for they are saturated and supposedly unhealthy. However, how does one explain the fact that Eskimos who still eat their traditional diet have low rates of heart disease? After all, the traditional Eskimo diet consists purely of meats, cholesterol, and fats.

The experts counter this by saying that the consumption of fish oils helps to protect against heart disease. However, the evidence regarding fish oils is mixed.

What is the magic blood cholesterol number that will prevent the development of atherosclerosis and yet avoid diseases associated with low cholesterol levels? The answer is that there is no magic number.

Average blood cholesterol levels vary widely between people and between countries around the world. Similarly, blood cholesterol levels at which heart disease and heart attacks occur also vary between people and countries around the world.

In fact, many studies have proven that blood cholesterol levels by themselves are not reliable in pinpointing who will develop heart disease and suffer a heart attack.

The United States government recommends that people should strive to get their blood cholesterol levels under 200 mg/dl. If someone achieves this, is there assurance of avoiding a heart attack from atherosclerosis?

The answer is definitely no. In fact, more than 20 percent of heart attacks occur in people with total blood cholesterol levels of 200 mg/dl or lower. Statistics also show that most heart attacks occur in people with levels of 225 mg/dl or less.

The one hard, cold fact that the medical world seems to ignore is that many millions of people in the United States and elsewhere with blood cholesterol levels of 240 mg/dl or higher are healthy and growing older without being afflicted with atherosclerosis. Remember that the "healthy old" have high cholesterol levels.

We shall now discuss the four simplest ways to minimize your risks of developing atherosclerosis. They are simple, though they may not be easy to accomplish.

First, do whatever you can to avoid high blood pressure, or hypertension. Regardless of blood cholesterol levels, hypertension causes atheromas to form in coronary arteries and elsewhere. If your doctor says to take a medication to lower your blood pressure, do it, even if there are some annoying side effects. We will discuss hypertension in detail in a later section.

Second, you must participate in regular physical exercise that is strenuous enough to raise your heart rate. I like the term 'moderately vigorous exercise'.

Third, avoid excess body weight. High blood cholesterol levels almost always lead to atherosclerosis in people who are medically obese.

Fourth, do not smoke cigarettes. Smoking cigarettes causes atherosclerosis and heart attacks. It also causes cancers of the mouth, throat, and lung. Smoking leads to emphysema, as well.

Smoking may slightly lower blood cholesterol levels, in spite of the fact that it causes atherosclerosis.

How then does it increase the formations of atheromas in coronary arteries?

The answer is because nicotine from smoking causes small blood vessels throughout the body to constrict. Small blood vessels everywhere that are constricted causes blood pressure to be slightly higher than it normally would be on a constant basis. Higher blood pressures increase the risks of heart disease and heart attacks, regardless of the blood cholesterol levels.

Heart attacks can occur in people whether they have low, medium, or high blood cholesterol levels. We have just discussed some of the factors that are more important for the development of atherosclerosis than are cholesterol levels. The conclusion drawn from this is simply that screening and testing people for high cholesterol levels is not of any real medical benefit in the vast majority of people.

There are researchers who have been brave enough to state that cholesterol screening is not worthwhile, so I am by no means a pioneer on this issue. The exception is in the cases of people who have had a heart attack in the past. Screening of these patients should occur routinely. I would guess that in these heart attack survivors, however, another factor played a role, such as smoking, obesity, or hypertension.

Another concept that is a proven fact is that cholesterol levels considered normal in one society, country or ethnic group may not be normal in another. With the mixing of cultures and shrinking of the planet because of modern methods of transportation, trying to establish normal cholesterol levels is probably a wasted effort.

There is one category of people who should actually be trying to maintain what are considered high blood cholesterol levels. These are the elderly. Numerous studies have shown that people aged 70 and beyond remain healthier if they continue to possess higher levels. If a doctor places a healthy 75 year-old patient on medication to lower cholesterol, he is acting opposite to what the research recommends.

Lastly, let's review the main points of this section.

Eating cholesterol does not give you blood cholesterol levels high enough to cause heart disease.

Eating carbohydrates (starches) can lead to blood cholesterol levels that are very high. Body fat may increase. Diabetes may develop.

Average, healthy cholesterol levels vary widely from person to person and between countries.

Atherosclerosis and heart attacks occur at all ranges of blood cholesterol levels.

There is evidence that shows that blood cholesterol levels must remain well over 350 mg/dl before a consistent relationship to atherosclerosis formation develops. At 500 mg/dl and above, as in the cases of a rare genetic disease called familial hypercholesterolemia, heart disease will almost always occur. Below the 350 level, however, there is no definite relationship between blood cholesterol levels and atherosclerosis, except where other factors are involved.

Since you cannot change your genetics, here are things you can do to help prevent atherosclerosis.

First, control high blood pressure, even if the medication has side effects.

Second, engage in moderately vigorous physical activity every day.

Third, avoid becoming obese. Medically obese people usually have cholesterol levels high enough to contribute to heart disease.

Fourth, do not smoke. Cigarettes cause heart disease even if your blood cholesterol levels are well into the low ranges.

Many authorities consider family history and mental stress as heart disease risk factors. However, you cannot change your genes. Secondly, regular vigorous exercise tempers the effects of stress.

Remember that humans are actually resistant to the development of atherosclerosis, unless one or more of these four factors are also involved.

So, who is at the highest risk of developing atherosclerosis and suffering a heart attack? This is easy to answer: an overweight smoker with high blood pressure who never gets any exercise. His cholesterol levels no doubt will be high, but it would be a mistake to just focus on cholesterol during his rehabilitation after the heart attack.

Finally, it is a mistake to be measuring cholesterol levels in young adults and children. Growing up is hard enough without another point of stress being developed.

17-2   Statin Drugs and Heart Attacks

The key enzyme in the production of cholesterol molecules in cells is HMG-CoA reductase. Drugs that lower cholesterol levels by blocking the action of this enzyme are called statins.

Doctors place patients on statin drug therapy in the hope that heart attacks will be prevented. We are going to analyze this concept in this section.

At the time this was written, not all statins were shown in medical studies to have an effect on the numbers of patients suffering heart attacks. The other statins are marketed to doctors based on their being less expensive to the patient, or the ability to decrease cholesterol levels to a great extent.

We shall focus on two statins that have been the subjects of large medical studies involving several thousand patients. These large studies are listed in the references for this section. I will use the actual statistics found in these studies for my analysis. My interpretation, however, may be different from that given by the drug companies' sales representatives.

First, we need to discuss a concept that seems to be used frequently with these drugs. It goes by three slightly different terms that still mean the same thing. The three are "risk reduction," "reduction in risk," or the one that is the most precise, "relative reduction in risk."

They are used in contrast to the simple term "reduction." I shall create an example to show the differences between these terms.

Let us say that a drug company has produced a new medicine for the treatment of toenail fungus. In a research trial of the medicine are utilized 200 patients with active cases of toenail fungus. They are divided into two groups, with 100 patients receiving the real medicine and 100 receiving a placebo, which means something that appears to be genuine to the patient but actually has no medical properties.

After two weeks of treatments, the entire group receiving the placebo still has active cases of toenail fungus. Of the one hundred people receiving the real medicine, however, fifty have seen their toenail fungus totally healed. By calculation in our example, the medicine has produced a 50 percent "reduction" in cases of toenail fungus.

Let us now imagine that a drug company has produced a new medicine that is supposed to prevent cases of toenail fungus from developing. In this medical study, 200 people are chosen who do not have any signs of toenail fungus present. They are divided into two groups, with 100 receiving a placebo and 100 receiving the real medicine that is supposed to prevent the development of toenail fungus.

Instead of two weeks, however, this study lasts five years. At the conclusion of the five years it was determined that six cases of toenail fungus developed in the 100 people receiving the placebo, while three cases developed in the 100 receiving the real medicine that is supposed to prevent toenail fungus.

In other words, six percent of the people receiving the placebo developed cases of toenail fungus during the five years, and three percent developed toenail fungus in the group receiving the real medicine. Subtracting three percent from six percent results in a difference of three percent as the benefit. Remember, though, that to obtain that three percent benefit, over 100 people had to take the medicine for five years.

The drug company that produced this medicine for the prevention of toenail fungus has decided to make public the results of the five-year study. However, the company has chosen to use the term "risk reduction" in their advertising to doctors and the public. How does this work? The ads will state that in the "landmark trial lasting five years, their new medicine for the prevention of toenail fungus <u>produced a risk reduction of 50 percent in new cases</u>." Somewhere in the ad it may have printed "placebo-6, their medicine-3." Going down from six to three is mathematically 50 percent! You now know the difference between the simple term "reduction" and a precise, statistical definition of something called "risk reduction."

There is nothing wrong with this use of statistics in advertising placed in medical and scientific journals that are meant to be read by doctors as long as the terms "reduction in risk," "relative reduction in risk," or even just "risk reduction" appear with the numbers. I hope that the doctors reading the ads or listening to sales representatives understand fully what the terms mean.

If an ad is placed on television or in a magazine that is read by the general public, however, the situation is different. One ad placed in a popular weekly magazine states a particular statin drug demonstrated "42 percent fewer deaths from heart disease." The term "risk reduction" or either of the other terms did not appear in the ad. This seems to be a good place to begin our analysis of statin drug advertising.

We all should be mindful of two important facts regarding statin drugs. First, statins block the production of cholesterol molecules in every cell of the body that the drugs enter. In other words, all the cells in every tissue can be affected, including the brain. There may be a statin that supposedly does not readily cross the blood-brain barrier, but that is not relevant. This is because in adult humans the cholesterol levels in the brain are related to the levels in the rest of the body.

The other fact to keep in mind is that the studies show it takes three to five years of continuous statin therapy before any benefit appears regarding heart disease.

The first statin study we shall look at is the Scandinavian Simvastatin Survival Study. It is abbreviated as 4-S. A study of 4,444 patients, who already were shown to have coronary heart disease, took place. In 4-S, there were 2,223 patients in the placebo group and 2,221 in the group receiving the real statin drug. The study lasted five years.

Those receiving the real statin saw their blood cholesterol levels fall in varying but still significant amounts.

In 4-S, there were 189 coronary deaths after five years in the placebo group. Of those receiving the real statin, 111 people died. In summary, the "relative reduction in risk" after five years is 42 percent. We obtain this figure by subtracting 111 from 189, which equals 78. Dividing 78 by 189 gives us 0.413. Remember that in an advertisement placed in a popular magazine, this particular statin drug demonstrated over five years "42 percent fewer deaths from heart disease."

Let us look at these same numbers from the 4-S research in a slightly different way. After five years, there were 189 coronary deaths among the 2,223 patients in the placebo group. That computes to about 8.5 percent. After five years, there were 111 coronary deaths among the 2,221 patients receiving the real statin drug. That computes to about 5.0 percent. Is that a real difference after five years? The answer is yes, according to statistical analysis. However, let us divide that 3.5 percent difference by five years, which is the length of time of the study. We now have a difference in the number of coronary deaths per year of 0.7 percent, which is less than one percent. If you are a doctor who is thinking of writing prescriptions for statin drugs for your patients, this should help you put things in perspective. In other words, for every 100 patients (with existing heart disease) placed on statin drugs for at least five years, your best hope is that you will reduce the number of coronary deaths by less than one percent per year. That is the real bottom line. In addition, remember also, doctor, compare this to 100 other patients in your practice with coronary heart disease that you did not place on statin drug therapy.

Produced by a different drug company, pravastatin is the other statin that has been the subject of extensive medical studies. We shall look at some of the claims in ads for this statin and the data used by the company.

One ad states that pravastatin is proven to "reduce the risk" of a first MI, or heart attack, by 31 percent. The basis of this is the results of a study of 6,595 men who had never had a heart attack but who were labeled as having high blood cholesterol levels. Their average reading was 272 mg/dl, which they classify as being high. The men also had at least one or more additional cardiovascular risk factors, such as smoking or high blood pressure.

The study lasted five years. There were 31 percent fewer heart attacks in the statin group compared to the placebo group. The 31 percent included both those that died from coronary heart disease and those that survived their heart attacks. Remember that this is technically a 31 percent "reduction in risk," though the ads do not emphasize that very important point.

Let us analyze the study regarding their statistics of those that had a heart attack and survived or died from coronary heart disease. There were 3,293 patients in the placebo group. After five years, 248 either had a nonfatal heart attack or died from coronary disease. There were 3,302 patients in the group receiving the real statin drug. After five years, 174 either had a nonfatal heart attack or died from coronary heart disease. A reduction from 248 to 174 after five years is a "reduction in risk" of 31 percent. By my calculations, the difference between 248 and 174 is 74, which computes to be 30 percent, but there is no need to be splitting hairs here.

Let us analyze these figures from a different perspective. The study involves 6,595 men with cholesterol levels averaging 272 mg/dl, which they classify as being high. They have never had a heart attack, but they each have risk factors such as smoking or high blood pressure.

There were 248 nonfatal heart attacks or deaths out of 3,293 patients in the placebo group after five years. This calculates to about 7.5 percent.

There were 174 similar "coronary events" in the group of 3,302 patients receiving the real statin drug for five years. This calculates to be about 5.3 percent.

In summary, this study shows that; in a group of men with average cholesterol levels of 272 mg/dl and cardiovascular risk factors such as smoking or high blood pressure, placing them on statin drugs for five years can reduce their risk of a coronary event by 2.2 percent! We obtain this by subtracting 5.3 from 7.5.

In other words, the statin drug reduces the number of nonfatal heart attacks or coronary heart disease deaths by 2.2 percent over five years. That computes to be less than one half of 1 percent per year as the best benefit a doctor can hope for in placing patients like these on this particular statin drug.

In the references for this section are studies involving stroke, transient ischemic attacks, and other medical problems that statin drugs are supposed to be able to help. Interested readers may wish to analyze these studies in the same ways that I have.

There are also references regarding the debate over the true effectiveness of statin drugs in the larger picture of things. Included are studies that show that statins do not reduce the overall death rate in patient populations. I am not the first to raise questions on this issue. However, the debate seems to be over.

Millions of people are now taking statin drugs, and the health officials of the United States government seem to think that it is entirely justified from both the economics of the issue and the supposed health benefits.

Let me remind the reader that my investigation began with a simple question. My father-in-law developed Alzheimer's disease after years of reducing his weight and eliminating fat and cholesterol from his diet. He also was taking a statin drug. The question I asked was, "Is cholesterol related to the brain in any way?" After years of studying the medical research, the published literature revealed that cholesterol relates to not only the brain, but to every system and tissue in the human body.

One researcher that is very well known in the study of heart disease and is an enthusiastic proponent of statin drug therapy wrote that, "statins proved to be safe over the five years of each trial. Furthermore, clinical experience with these drugs over a decade has failed to uncover common, major side effects."

My response is simply to read the side effects listed in the advertisements for statin drugs. You will read not only of headaches, but also things like rash, myopathy, arthralgia, diarrhea, dyspepsia, and so on. You may remember that statin drugs are associated with cataracts in animal experiments.

As for the side effects listed for statins, the reader may wish to review the earlier sections of this book that dealt with muscle problems, rheumatoid arthritis, psoriasis, etc.

Let me point out one final aspect of the side effects of statin drugs to which the manufacturers readily admit. In the very fine print that is part of the magazine ads for statin drugs you will see a list of "adverse reactions" that were seen in patients using the particular statin. Next to side effects such as rash, gastrointestinal, diarrhea, muscle and joint pain, headache, etc., will be the percentages of patients affected. The percentages always seem to range between 2 and 10 percent of all that are on the statin drug. The company considers various adverse side affects that occur in from 2 to 10 percent of all who are taking the statin to be insignificant.

However, we have just found out through an analysis of two of the major medical trials of statins, that after five years there were reductions in heart disease "events" of only 3.5 percent with one statin and only 2.2 percent with another. These reductions average out to be less than one percent per year for each statin.

It seems to me that statins may be more successful at causing harmful side effects than in reducing coronary heart disease problems.

Those in favor of statin drugs claim that there is no downside risk whatsoever in lowering blood cholesterol levels. However, this book documents that there most definitely are risks, with some being very serious.

17-3   Blood Pressure and Atherosclerosis

People who have inherited a disease called familial hypercholesterolemia are genetically programmed to have high blood cholesterol levels. It is the result of biochemical alterations, and the cholesterol they eat in food plays no role in their condition. These patients readily develop atherosclerosis, thereby providing proof that cholesterol levels, if very high, play a part in coronary heart disease.

As we recently learned, however, people can have heart attacks at all ranges of blood cholesterol levels. We found out that other factors besides cholesterol levels have a great influence in the disease process. These factors include high blood pressure, smoking, obesity, lack of physical activity, and so on.

One should also be conscious of the fact that in most cases, it takes from 30 to 60 years or more before someone has a heart attack from atherosclerosis. Though coronary artery disease is common, it is still hard to die from it when thought of in these terms.

The purpose of this book is to make people aware of the fact that low blood cholesterol levels are definitely linked to diseases such as Alzheimer's, rheumatoid arthritis, and all of the others mentioned earlier.

I personally want to maintain an adequate blood cholesterol level but I also want to avoid heart disease. I decided to take a different approach regarding this tissue. Instead of investigating groups of people that may (or may not) be more successful in avoiding heart disease, I looked for those who always develop atherosclerosis and have heart attacks. We have mentioned the genetic disease familial hypercholesterolemia, but these rare people have cholesterol levels far higher than those found in normal populations.

There is a category of people who satisfied my desire for a group who will definitely develop heart disease. The people in this group will not only develop the disease, but they will predictably do it within five to ten years.

Who makes up this unfortunate group that will predictably develop heart disease in only five or ten years? It is those people who have previously undergone coronary bypass surgery for heart disease.

In other words, someone who has just had heart bypass surgery is almost guaranteed within five to ten years to develop atherosclerosis in the blood vessels that were newly grafted around the heart. This person will then need another bypass, or will die from this second episode of heart disease.

Each year in the United States, over 100,000 bypass operations are performed, so there is ample evidence to show that what I just said is indeed true. People who have had one bypass operation will usually need another even if they keep their blood cholesterol levels in the low ranges with diet and medications. Therefore, why do they still get atherosclerosis in the new blood vessels placed around the heart? In addition, why does the disease process happen so fast? The answers to these questions led me to conclude that one factor is more important than all others in the development of heart disease. That factor is blood pressure.

All of the larger arteries in the body are subject to the development of atherosclerosis, including the neck, arms, brain, and leg arteries. In a heart bypass operation, the surgeon takes veins from the leg of the patient and grafts them to blood vessels of the heart.

The question I asked myself related to the large veins in the body. Only arteries develop atherosclerosis. Why is it that a heart surgeon can depend on being able to utilize leg veins to replace the blocked heart arteries? Why is it that the large veins serving the heart never develop blockages from atherosclerosis? In other words, why is it that we never hear of someone undergoing a coronary vein bypass operation?

Let us briefly discuss the differences between arteries and veins. Arteries carry blood away from the heart to the tissues of the body. Coronary arteries are those that feed the muscle tissue of the heart. The blood in them has just left the pumping chamber of the heart and makes a sharp turn in these arteries towards the surface of the heart. The blood pressures in these arteries are, therefore, very high.

Veins carry blood back to the heart from tissues throughout the body. Arteries have oxygenated blood while veins carry blood with carbon dioxide. The only exceptions to this are the arteries and veins to the lungs, in which the reverse is true.

The walls of arteries have layers of muscle, the purpose of which is to provide the ability to contract or relax their size depending on the activity level of the person. Veins do not have layers of muscle tissue.

Most components of blood are the same in both arteries and veins, except for the oxygen status. The amounts of glucose, wastes, electrolytes, etc., are equal. This includes cholesterol and the various cholesterol fractions, such as HDL and LDL. If the cholesterol levels are the same, why does atherosclerosis block arteries, but not veins?

The difference is due to the blood pressures of the pumping heart!

As the larger arteries, which are closer to the heart, branch into smaller arteries and eventually into capillaries, pressure from the pumping heart decreases and dissipates. There is literally no pressure to speak of on the return trip to the heart through the venules, small veins, and then the large veins. If there is no pressure in the veins, how does blood flow through them? The answer is that there are one-way valves in veins. As muscles of your body contract during physical activity, veins are squeezed. The valves permit blood to flow in only one direction, which is back to the heart.

Veins are not subjected to blood pressure, as are arteries. I do not pretend to know why the pressure from the pumping of the heart leads to atherosclerosis in the larger arteries. It seems the basis of this are the observations by researchers of microscopic injuries to the walls of arteries. As these tiny injuries repair, there can occur the development of the beginnings of small atheromas. Higher blood pressures seem to cause greater injuries in the wall of arteries, which can probably lead to more atheromas as the years go by. This seems to be a logical explanation as to why arteries develop atherosclerosis while veins do not.

The references listed for this section discuss this concept in greater detail. The bottom line is that hypertension causes heart disease, regardless of cholesterol levels.

You now know the one exception to the rule about veins never developing atherosclerosis. Those leg veins used in bypass surgery develop the disease within only five to ten years. They place these veins next to the heart and ask them to withstand pressures that they never had to previously. These veins used in bypasses do not have muscle layers as arteries do, so there is less protection from the microscopic injuries caused by the pressures of the pumping heart.

In conclusion, you must avoid high blood pressure in order to prevent heart disease, regardless of your blood cholesterol levels.

17-4   Can Atherosclerosis Be Reversed?

If you or a loved one develops narrow or blocked coronary arteries, can we reverse the situation? In other words, can changes in diet or lifestyle and the possible use of medication result in the unclogging of those arteries?

The short answer is no. Arteries with atheromas cannot be brought back to a clear condition. If someone survives a heart attack from atherosclerosis at the age of fifty and does not have bypass surgery, how would their arteries appear when they eventually did die, say, at the age of eighty? The answer is that the arteries would still be diseased with atheromas. This would be the case even if the person had become a strict vegetarian, eating no cholesterol or other animal products.

This has been a factor in the confusion over the causes of Alzheimer's disease. At autopsies of Alzheimer's patients, the arteries may show signs of obvious coronary artery disease. The investigators quickly conclude that atherosclerosis must have played a role in the development of Alzheimer's. They follow this with another conclusion, which is that high blood cholesterol levels must also be involved with Alzheimer's, because cholesterol causes atherosclerosis, right?

There are two errors here. First, Alzheimer's patients almost never die from a classic heart attack, which is the end result of atherosclerosis.

The second error is based on the failure to know that arteries with atheromas never return to a clear, healthy condition in humans. The atherosclerotic clogging of arteries may have occurred two years or thirty years before the death of the patient.

Can the progression of atherosclerosis be stopped, even if it cannot be reversed? The short answer is yes. To some degree, it is possible to halt the progression of coronary heart disease.

Although the atheromas can only be removed with surgery, the function and flexibility of the arteries can be improved in areas free of major deposits.

Can the opening, or lumen, in a diseased artery be made to open up without using a balloon or similar procedure? The answer is yes, but the actual amounts of arterial opening are very small. The research I have seen lists increases of 0.1 to 0.3 mm of opening, which is very small.

Why do some researchers proclaim that they have proof of the reversing of clogged arteries? I do not know. Improvements seen are due mainly to the improved function in areas of arteries not heavily clogged. There is also evidence that even a very small widening of the opening of an artery is beneficial to the tissue served by that artery.

17-5   Eggs and Heart Disease: The True Facts

If asked, the typical American would say that heart attacks result from eating foods containing cholesterol. This same individual would then say that eating eggs is bad for you, because they are high in cholesterol.

These two notions are part of the accepted medical knowledge taught to the public by professionals in the medical community. As an example of how successful this campaign has been, most grocery stores now carry an egg substitute in the dairy section. I believe this substitute consists of the whites of eggs, to which they add yellow food coloring. By not eating yolks, one avoids eating the cholesterol of eggs.

Incidentally, each egg typically has about 250 to 300 mg of cholesterol, and all of it is in the yolk.

Is blood cholesterol level a factor in heart disease? Yes, but it is not a major factor, unless it is very high. The major factors are smoking, hypertension (high blood pressure), obesity, and lack of physical activity. Remember also that heart attacks can occur at all levels of blood cholesterol and not just at the high ranges.

If you have very high blood cholesterol levels, is it the result of eating foods containing cholesterol, such as eggs? The answer is no! It is very important to understand that eating cholesterol does not cause one to have blood cholesterol levels high enough to cause heart disease.

Of course, it does sound logical for such a connection to be true, but it is not. Furthermore, and you may find this hard to believe, <u>there has never been an accepted medical study which shows that eating cholesterol raises blood cholesterol levels high enough to cause heart disease.</u>

The Framingham Study is the most famous ongoing research project concerned with heart disease. Framingham studies documented the connections between high blood cholesterol levels and increases in the risk for heart disease. However, Framingham research never concluded in any study that dietary cholesterol caused blood cholesterol levels to become high enough to cause heart disease.

Somehow, over the years, it just became accepted that eating foods with cholesterol causes heart disease. As stated earlier, it sounds logical, but it is just not true.

The reason for this is that humans possess something called the liver/cholesterol feedback mechanism. A later chapter will discuss this. Briefly, it means that your digestive system will retain cholesterol found in food only if your body is lacking it. If the liver senses that your body has a sufficient amount of cholesterol, it will not allow you to absorb any more from the food you eat.

There have been studies that conclude that people can be grouped into categories regarding the effects of dietary cholesterol upon blood cholesterol levels. These various research projects found that a similar amount of cholesterol in food would raise the blood cholesterol levels of some patients but not others. Researchers then classified these people as hyper-responders to dietary cholesterol or hypo-responders.

What is actually occurring here? If dietary cholesterol caused a significant increase in blood cholesterol levels, than those folks in whom this occurred had levels lower than what their bodies actually needed. In the people whose blood cholesterol levels failed to increase a significant amount, then they must already have been at a satisfactory level.

In summary, eating foods containing cholesterol will raise blood cholesterol levels only if those levels are lower than what the body needs. If the liver senses that the body is not in need of cholesterol, eating more of it will not raise blood levels because it will not be absorbed.

Incidentally, eggs happen to be low in fat content, even though they are high in cholesterol. In fact, one would be consuming a low-fat, high-cholesterol diet if one ate only eggs every day. Would a diet consisting only of eggs lead to blood cholesterol levels high enough to cause heart disease? The answer is no.

Have eggs been unjustly and unfairly accused of causing heart disease and heart attacks? The answer is yes.

In other words, is it correct to say that eating eggs has no connection whatsoever to heart disease and heart attacks? The answer is yes.

Let me state it as bluntly as possible, so that there is no way to misunderstand. Eating eggs does not cause heart disease. Eating eggs does not cause heart attacks.

The references listed for this section provide the basis for my conclusions.

In a 1979 paper, 116 men consumed two eggs each day in addition to their regular diet. There was found to be no significant association of dietary cholesterol with their blood cholesterol levels.

There are a number of papers listed that point out the connection between a high-fat diet and heart disease risk. Basically, they conclude that as far as diet alone is concerned, recommendations for lowering the risk of heart disease should concentrate on a reduction in fat and not cholesterol intake.

In a 1975 paper regarding the treatment of people who had suffered severe burns over large parts of their bodies, researchers fed the patients thirty-five (35) eggs each day! The patients consumed the eggs in a variety of forms, both cooked and raw. In almost no instances could diarrhea, vomiting, or allergic reactions, if they appeared, be attributed to the high intake of eggs in these burn patients. Additionally, none of the patients developed a dislike for the taste of eggs. This diet proved to be beneficial for the healing of the patients' burns. Significant to our current discussion, high blood cholesterol levels of the kind associated with heart disease did not occur in these patients who were eating 35 eggs each day.

In a 1982 paper, researchers presented the results of an investigation regarding egg consumption and heart disease. In an analysis of 912 people in the Framingham Study, they found no relationship between egg intake and the incidence of coronary heart disease. <u>Furthermore, they discovered that egg consumption was unrelated to blood cholesterol levels</u>.

Let me conclude by stating that if you like eating eggs but are afraid to tell people that you do, relax. The real medical research shows that eating eggs does not cause coronary artery disease and does not cause heart attacks. It is safe for closet egg-eaters to come out and sit at the table in public view. Do not be ashamed to eat eggs. Those people who state that it is unhealthy to eat eggs are ignorant of the true facts on this issue.

It is time to stop beating up the egg.

17-6   Corticosteroids and Atherosclerosis

In previous sections, we discussed cortisol, a steroid hormone that originates from molecules of cholesterol. Cortisol raises blood levels of cholesterol, proteins, fats, and other substances by forcing cells throughout the body to "donate" them. Other cells can then utilize these various components for rebuilding and repairing their own membranes.

The actions of cortisol do not last very long, as it quickly neutralizes. If, for whatever reason, your body keeps producing cortisol, there can be some serious damage done to tissues. The most obvious example of this is starvation. The weight loss of starvation is actually the result of body tissues being consumed in order to maintain the actions of organs and systems.

A corticosteroid is a synthetic version of cortisol. We will also use the term steroids, which shall mean the same thing as corticosteroids. If you hear or read of people receiving steroid anti-inflammatory therapy for some type of medical condition, what they are receiving is a synthetic version of cortisol.

Note: The term steroid as used in this book does not refer to the types of steroids used by some athletes and bodybuilders.

Two important differences exist between the cortisol your body makes from cholesterol molecules and the synthetic steroids produced by the drug industry. First, cortisol does not last as long in your body as will steroids. Second, steroids may have actions that are ten to one hundred times stronger than the cortisol produced by your body. Because of these reasons, the effects of steroids can be fast and dramatic.

In this section, we will briefly discuss one aspect of steroid therapy, that of the raising of blood cholesterol levels. Again, steroids raise blood cholesterol levels the same way that cortisol does, by forcing cells in tissues throughout the body to donate cholesterol molecules. Steroids, as we just discussed, are stronger and last longer than cortisol. A number of chronic illnesses include long-term steroid therapy as one of the treatment options. Patients treated with steroid therapy exhibit high blood cholesterol levels. Doctors usually state that this is an undesirable side effect of steroid therapy. I hold the opinion that the higher blood cholesterol levels are, in fact, the primary source of the benefits of steroid anti-inflammatory therapy.

If steroid therapy produces continuous high blood cholesterol levels, and if high blood cholesterol is one of the factors of atherosclerosis, do people receiving this therapy have higher rates of heart disease? The answer is yes.

The diseases in which premature atherosclerosis from steroid therapy occurs include rheumatoid arthritis and psoriasis. It is my opinion that any condition treated with steroid therapy over a long period will be, therefore, associated with premature atherosclerosis. This includes organ transplantation. People with transplants may be receiving steroid therapy to control rejection of their new organ.

It is, therefore, unfortunate that organ transplant recipients, who have been granted more years of life, must by virtue of steroid therapy, be subjected to premature heart disease. The same situation holds for the people on steroid therapy for lupus, rheumatoid arthritis, and various other conditions. It is a cruel fate for someone to be able to control the symptoms of a disease like lupus, only to die young of a heart attack.

17-7   Statins Will Not Prevent Alzheimer's
(Written in the spring of 2005)

I finished the text of *Alzheimer's Solved* in 2000, and copyrighted it in October, 2000. Beginning in January, 2001, I self-published some copies and distributed them to several select Alzheimer's researchers.

Alzheimer's disease is caused, in most instances, by shortages of cholesterol in the brain. And back in 2000 and 2001, I assumed it would only be a short time before mainstream Alzheimer's researchers would be reaching the same conclusion.

However, in the October, 2000 issue of the journal *Archives of Neurology*, an Illinois scientist, Dr. Benjamin Wolozin, published a paper in which he concluded that cholesterol-lowering statin drugs seemed to lower the incidence of Alzheimer's disease. Dr. Wolozin had looked at the computer databases of patients in three hospitals for the period October 1, 1996, through August 31, 1998, a time of twenty-three months. His conclusion was based on some statistical analyses in this purely observational study.

Dr. Wolozin's objective from the very beginning of the study, as stated in the published paper, was to determine if statins would cause patients to have a statistically lower incidence of Alzheimer's disease.

Incidentally, on November 13, 1998, forty-five days past the August 31, 1998 date in which his study period ended, Dr. Wolozin filed for a patent on the use of statins in treating Alzheimer's disease. (His research paper wasn't accepted for publication by *Archives of Neurology* until later, on June 28, 2000.) Dr. Wolozin, in association with a company called Nymox Corporation, eventually received a patent in October, 2002 for "Methods for treating, preventing, and reducing the risk of the onset of Alzheimer's disease using an HMG CoA reductase inhibitor" (statin).

After *Archives of Neurology* published his paper in that October, 2000 issue, a number of scientists pointed out the shortcomings and possible statistical flaws of Wolozin's purely observational study.

However, the major effect of his paper was to cause a big increase in the amount of additional research that supposedly showed that excess cholesterol causes Alzheimer's, and that using statins to lower blood cholesterol levels would be a method for preventing or treating the disease.

Obviously, if statins could be used to prevent or treat Alzheimer's, then millions of people could be saved from the disease, and many billions of dollars would flow to the drug companies that produce statins.

However, when the Wolozin paper came out, my years of studying the research caused me to conclude the exact opposite to his position. Here are some of the reasons.

First, which patients do doctors place on statin therapy in the first place? It is those patients with consistently high blood cholesterol levels. Brain cholesterol metabolism is slow and is measured in many months or years, so over the short term, these are the folks who are not going to develop Alzheimer's disease, anyway.

Secondly, people with lower blood cholesterol levels over a long period of time are not going to be placed on statins. Elderly folks with low blood cholesterol levels are going to be, on average, the first ones to start showing signs of Alzheimer's. Hence, you have here a group of folks not taking statins who are then developing symptoms of the disease, and this can be used as some sort of proof that taking statins protects against Alzheimer's.

Thirdly, if statins can supposedly prevent Alzheimer's by lowering blood cholesterol levels, then the disease must therefore be caused by high cholesterol levels, or hypercholesterolemia.

For decades we have been told that high blood cholesterol levels cause heart disease and heart attacks. In following this line of thinking, we should, therefore, be seeing Alzheimer's patients having heart attacks on a large scale. There should be an epidemic of heart attacks among Alzheimer's patients, right? Is this the case? Are Alzheimer's patients dying from classic heart attacks?

The answer is no. In fact, Alzheimer's patients almost never die from a classic heart attack. These patients seem to survive for many years. They may suffer a stroke, but it is the kind of stroke the occurs at low blood pressure, not high blood pressure, or hypertension. This evidence also argues against Alzheimer's as being caused by high blood cholesterol levels.

When Alzheimer's patients do finally die, the usual cause of death is pneumonia. Now they may have had active atherosclerosis and suffered a heart attack years earlier in life, and before developing Alzheimer's, and this fact causes confusion among some Alzheimer's researchers.

Fourth, and along this same line of thinking, let us consider Down syndrome patients. These folks always eventually develop Alzheimer's disease. However, Down syndrome patients never develop classic atherosclerosis, and never have heart attacks. (They may be born with a heart defect, but it has no connection to heart disease.) The hypothesis that high blood cholesterol levels causes Alzheimer's disease simply falls apart completely when one looks at Down syndrome patients.

Lastly, Vance Wolff was taking a statin to lower his cholesterol, and he still went on to develop Alzheimer's disease. Obviously, the statin did not protect Vance.

There has been another bit of research that supposedly shows that statins might prevent Alzheimer's. Some researchers in Europe placed neurons in a laboratory culture, to which was added a statin drug. The neurons produced amyloid for a while, then stopped. Since beta amyloid is thought by some to be the primary cause of the disease, then this experiment also supposedly shows that statins might prevent Alzheimer's.

However, the scientists in this experiment admitted that they had to remove so much cholesterol from the neurons' cell membranes in order to achieve the desire effect, that the neurons began to die.

Additionally, it should be noted that not all scientists believe Alzheimer's is caused simply by a build-up in the brain of beta amyloid. Remember that in Alzheimer's, there are neurons dying even in places in the brain without nearby amyloid plaques.

As stated earlier, Vance Wolff was taking a statin to lower his cholesterol levels, and he still went on to develop Alzheimer's. Does this mean that all people taking a statin will develop Alzheimer's disease? No, and this is because of at least three reasons.

First, normal blood cholesterol levels are different among individuals. Someone may take a statin and achieve lower blood cholesterol levels, but the new levels may not be low enough to cause neuron damage in the brain.

Secondly, brain cholesterol metabolism is slower than the rest of the body's cholesterol metabolism. Someone taking a statin may end up dying of some other cause before any Alzheimer's symptoms are recognized. Remember also that true Alzheimer's symptoms may be present for four or five years before a family member or physician suspects that the patient has the disease.

Thirdly, and this is important, many people taking a statin will, for lack of a better word, cheat on their diet. They will continue to eat the things that maintain cholesterol levels high enough to prevent Alzheimer's disease. People are human.

In conclusion, statin drugs will not prevent Alzheimer's disease. In fact, with so many millions of people now taking statins, it may end up causing an increase in the numbers developing Alzheimer's. Now that's a scary thought.

CHAPTER 18
The Cholesterol U

Throughout this book, I have explained the links between cholesterol levels and human health. Shortages of cholesterol molecules are the direct cause of many diseases, depending upon which particular body tissues are most affected. Defective uses of an adequate supply of cholesterol molecules can also cause disease, most notably in the cases of genetic conditions. There are diseases that take cholesterol away from normal tissues, and this in turn causes additional symptoms.

Finally, there are diseases that are the result of an excess amount of cholesterol.

Measuring blood cholesterol levels is one of the most commonly performed medical tests today. It is unfortunate, however, that concern is expressed only when someone is judged by an arbitrary standard to have "high" blood cholesterol. The medical community focuses only on heart disease, and ignores any other conditions regarding blood cholesterol levels. The constant message is that the lowest possible blood cholesterol levels will automatically result in the highest degrees of health. There are some cardiologists, in fact, who religiously believe that your blood cholesterol level cannot be too low. This book disproves that notion.

There is no ideal measure of blood cholesterol level that is right for everyone. There is no perfect number. The optimal blood cholesterol for someone is that level which seems to satisfy most of the tissues, most of the time.

The conclusions regarding blood cholesterol levels and disease organize into a relationship shaped like a U. Think of a simple horizontal line graph with low cholesterol levels on the left side and higher levels to the right. To the left of this U are diseases and conditions that are associated with low blood cholesterol levels. To the right, those linked to high levels. In the middle of the U is the safe area. The highest degrees of health occur when someone can maintain blood cholesterol levels in this safe zone over long periods.

Therefore, the bottom middle point of the U is the ideal blood cholesterol level point on a graph that has low levels to the left and high levels to the right.

Furthermore, in each person there is a cholesterol U for each tissue of the body. The hope is that someone's average level will satisfy the cholesterol U of each tissue.

We can now list some of the diseases and conditions that fall outside of the safe inner zone of the cholesterol U.

To the right of the U are the familiar diseases that are associated with high blood cholesterol levels. These include atherosclerosis and classic heart attacks, hypertension (high blood pressure), and strokes that occur in association with high blood pressure. (It is very important to remember that higher blood cholesterol levels are only a true risk factor for heart disease when high blood pressure is present.) I would add vascular (or multi-infarct) dementia to the list of diseases occurring at higher blood cholesterol levels. The symptoms of vascular dementia are different from those of Alzheimer's, though many doctors are not aware of this.

We would also place NIDDM on the right side of the cholesterol U, because it is associated with high blood cholesterol levels in the vast majority of cases. NIDDM stands for non-insulin dependent diabetes mellitus.

In the low blood cholesterol area to the left of the U are conditions that are the result of the low cholesterol levels. There also are those illnesses not caused by low levels, but over time result in low cholesterol. This, in turn, leads to more symptoms.

What follows is the list of diseases and conditions on the left side of the U that are associated with low cholesterol levels (either directly or indirectly). It includes Alzheimer's and Parkinson's diseases (except cases due to brain injury/surgery), hypotension (low blood pressure), stroke at low blood pressure, cerebral amyloid angiopathy, various amyloidoses, some cataracts, some types of epilepsy, some types of heart arrhythmias, vasculitis, and some cases of rheumatoid arthritis and psoriasis.

Some types of true medical depression are placed on the left side of the cholesterol U. We will discuss the reasons for this in a later chapter.

Also to the left of the U are diseases and conditions that eventually cause the patient to have low cholesterol levels in tissues. These low levels then can lead to the development of Alzheimer's disease. This list consists of Down syndrome, long-term kidney dialysis, long-term alcoholism, HIV/AIDS, anorexia nervosa, hereditary cerebral hemorrhage with amyloidosis-Dutch type (HCHWA-D), some types of cancer, and of course, long-term semi-starvation.

In Chapter 12, we discussed genetic defects of cholesterol metabolism. These are placed to the left of the U in the low cholesterol area. The conditions we covered were cerebrotendinous xanthomatosis, Smith-Lemli-Opitz syndrome, mevalonic aciduria, and Niemann-Pick Type C disease. Fetal alcohol syndrome is also placed on the left side.

By thinking in terms of the cholesterol U, it is easier to grasp the relationships between cholesterol, tissues, disease and health. It shows us that we must think in terms of cholesterol shortages as well as excesses.

We have one final aspect to consider. In the (year 2000) original version of *Alzheimer's Solved*, I wrote about the thymus gland's effect on cholesterol metabolism (though the thymus is normally thought to be involved only with our immune system). Thymus gland extract blocks the production of cholesterol in the liver, and this is one way that nature controls cholesterol production in our bodies. In fact, in the 1970's, some researchers considered using thymus gland extract (from animals or synthetic origin) to lower patients' cholesterol levels in the effort to possibly prevent heart disease. In other words, the extract could be considered to be our bodies' natural "statin".

As we age, the thymus gland shrinks and withers away. Consequently, a point is reached when no more thymus gland extract is produced in our bodies. This results in the liver producing more cholesterol (in someone who is adequately nourished), which gradually raises blood cholesterol levels. We now have the natural, physiological reason as to why the "healthy old" have "high" cholesterol levels, as was discussed in an earlier chapter. This is actually what nature intended. Consequently, this has an effect on the position of the cholesterol U, in that as we get older into the senior years, the U moves to the right of the graph, towards the high cholesterol area.

What exactly does this mean? It means that elderly folks need to maintain a higher blood cholesterol level compared to younger people of similar genetic backgrounds. Again, this is the natural way of things. For example, a 45 year old woman may do fine with a total blood cholesterol level of, say, 210 mg/dl, but if her 78 year old mother has that same 210 mg/dl level, it might open the door to health problems at some point. It might even lead to Alzheimer's disease.

CHAPTER 19
Alzheimer's and Cardiovascular Disease

19-1   Alzheimer's and Atherosclerosis

Researchers who have looked at the relationships between Alzheimer's disease and atherosclerosis believe that if there is a connection, it must be that atherosclerosis causes one to develop Alzheimer's. The reasons:

First, autopsies of Alzheimer's patients frequently reveal the signs of classic heart disease in their major arteries. We refer to these as atherosclerotic plaques or atheromas.

Second, there was research done by one particular team of scientists that utilized rabbits in a manner that supposedly proved that atherosclerosis caused amyloid deposits to form in arteries. This particular team pumped cholesterol into rabbits by mixing it in with their food pellets. Remember that rabbits are pure vegetarians and do not normally consume cholesterol. These laboratory rabbits quickly developed atheromas in their aortas and brain blood vessels. Traces of amyloid were found at the points where the brain vessels showed damage. These researchers then concluded that the processes of both atherosclerosis and Alzheimer's disease were the same. This particular research team's results and conclusions have continuously been cited as proof that atherosclerosis leads directly to the development of Alzheimer's disease in patients.

There is a third reason behind the belief that atherosclerosis can cause Alzheimer's. It is that in both heart disease patients and Alzheimer's victims, the apo E 4 gene is thought to exert an influence. We shall briefly analyze all three reasons.

Regarding the autopsy evidence of atheromas in blood vessels, I remind the reader that once an atheroma develops in a blood vessel, it is there forever. The damaged areas remain, even if the patient undergoes lifestyle, diet and medication therapies in an effort to avoid heart attacks.

Regarding the evidence gathered from feeding cholesterol to laboratory rabbits, I once again remind the reader that amyloid is part of the body's normal repair process. Therefore, it is not surprising to find traces of amyloid at points of damage cause by atherosclerosis processes. However, in true Alzheimer's disease, they find amyloid plaques in continuous association with the small blood vessels in the brain, and not just at isolated points of damage. In fact, other researchers using careful microscopic analysis have found that classic Alzheimer's amyloid plaques do not occur in the areas of classic atherosclerotic deposits.

The processes leading to atherosclerosis and Alzheimer's are different. My conclusion is easily understood if you think in terms of the cholesterol U explained in the previous chapter. The evidence found in the references, combined with my concept of the cholesterol U, provide the basis for the opinion that follows.

The disease processes of both Alzheimer's and atherosclerosis can occur in the same person, but not at the same time. The only exceptions are in those people with a history of head injury or brain surgery, people on long-term steroid therapy, Cushing's disease patients, and in some rare genetic conditions.

During the development of atherosclerosis, the patient is on the right side of the U in the high cholesterol range. For the moment, we are ignoring the important factors of high blood pressure, smoking, obesity and lack of exercise. After making changes in lifestyle, diet, and medications, the patient moves to the left and into the safe zone of the cholesterol U. The atherosclerotic disease processes stop.

If the patient stays in the safe zone of blood cholesterol levels, then a healthier future lies ahead. However, at some point the patient may go further to the left and cross into the low cholesterol area of diseases and conditions we discussed in the previous chapter. If the patient is in their senior years, Alzheimer's may be one of the results.

My late father-in-law, Vance Wolff, is an example of a former heart disease patient who successfully halted the process of atherosclerosis, but later went on to develop Alzheimer's.

Regarding the third reason that involved apo E 4, we will discuss this factor in more detail in Chapter 20.

The references listed for this section highlight the fact that very rarely will you find a true Alzheimer's patient dying of a classic heart attack. One would think that if atherosclerosis and Alzheimer's disease link directly, then Alzheimer's patients would be dying almost exclusively as the result of classic heart attacks. Epidemiology researchers, in fact, discovered that the exact opposite situation exists. Alzheimer's patients seem to be healthy (physically) and never have heart attacks or high blood pressure. They are healthy in terms of heart disease only, of course.

It is true that clogged brain arteries from previous atherosclerotic processes can contribute to the later Alzheimer's processes of under-nutrition and cholesterol shortages to brain cells. Narrowed arteries allow fewer things to pass through, and only surgery can "unclog" the major brain arteries.

In addition, some researchers believe strongly that other characteristics of atherosclerosis, namely high blood cholesterol and hypertension, are direct risk factors for developing Alzheimer's disease. However, the typical patient developing Alzheimer's exhibits lower blood cholesterol levels and low blood pressure. As a result, these researchers have "developed" data which supposedly proves that high cholesterol and high blood pressure in the midlife years causes one to develop Alzheimer's decades later.

The reader should be skeptical of research studies that put forth conclusions like this. Instead, one should focus on the more definitive evidence, which shows that the typical patients who develop Alzheimer's have the following characteristics:

1) Lower blood cholesterol levels.
2) Low blood pressure.
3) Do not suffer heart attacks from classic atherosclerosis/heart disease after full Alzheimer's symptoms appear.

The most important fact to remember is that people do not develop Alzheimer's disease until *after* their cholesterol levels decrease. Their blood pressure decreases along with the decreases in blood cholesterol.

You will remember a discussion earlier in this book about the genetic condition familial hypercholesterolemia, abbreviated as FH. Patients with FH have extremely high blood cholesterol levels and go on to develop classic heart disease. There have been a large number of studies performed regarding patients with FH. There have also been thousands of studies of Alzheimer's disease. In my years of searching the medical literature, I have not been able to find a study showing that patients with FH go on to develop Alzheimer's disease. One would think that Alzheimer's would be common in FH patients, if atherosclerosis and Alzheimer's disease were directly connected.

Autopsies of patients dying with Alzheimer's will sometimes show evidence in their brains of vascular dementia, as well. Researchers frequently label patients with signs of both Alzheimer's and vascular dementia as having "mixed dementia." This has been another mystery in the world of Alzheimer's research, but it also is resolved if we think again in terms of the cholesterol U.

Vascular dementia brain damage occurs as part of atherosclerosis, which we consider to be on the right side of the U in the high cholesterol area. This damage remains forever in the brain. At some point, the patient moves to the left side of the U into the low cholesterol area, and Alzheimer's damage develops.

We should note that the opposite situation is also possible. By that, I mean a situation where an Alzheimer's patient begins a phase of overeating to the point of becoming obese and prone to the development of atherosclerosis. However, this is not commonly the case. These cases may be patients who developed Alzheimer's as a result of a previous brain injury or brain surgical procedure.

19-2   Stroke

Neurons need a continuous supply of various nutrients in order to continue functioning. Interruptions of these nutrients will eventually lead to poor neuron health or the possible death of cells as time goes on.

If oxygen deprivation occurs in neurons as a result of a loss of blood flow, they will die within a few minutes. This is a simple explanation of what occurs in a stroke, or cerebrovascular accident.

Major strokes are frequently fatal. If the patient has managed to survive the episode, there may be paralysis of those functions controlled by the part of the brain that dies. Strokes affect skeletal muscle movements, speech, and other processes of the body. Therapy after the stroke involves a long period of training to compensate for the defects.

There are two primary causes of stroke. The blood supply stops by either a blockage in a brain artery or by the artery opening up some type of hole, causing bleeding (hemorrhage).

When an object becomes stuck in a brain artery, strokes from the blockage occur. The object is usually either a blood clot that formed in another part of the body or a piece of atherosclerotic plaque that broke off of an atheroma in another artery.

In a bleeding, or hemorrhagic stroke, an aneurysm may have first developed in the affected artery. Aneurysms are weak areas in the walls of arteries that balloon outward and eventually burst. They are common in people who have had hypertension (high blood pressure) for a long period.

There are also many cases of stroke occurring in people with normal or even low blood pressure. The brain artery just opens up and starts to hemorrhage.

Why are we discussing strokes at this point? Because in medicine today, the terms stroke and cerebrovascular accident are clustered together with heart disease, atherosclerosis, and hypertension in an indiscriminate manner. There should be much more emphasis placed on the distinctions between the types of strokes and their causes.

My suggested terms would be simple and descriptive.

Blood clot stroke: Caused by a blood clot that usually originates in a vein and becomes lodged in a brain artery.

Atheroma stroke: Caused by a piece of atherosclerotic plaque breaking off from a larger atheroma in another artery and becoming lodged in a brain artery.

Hemorrhagic stroke associated with hypertension (high blood pressure): This is self-explanatory. Brain aneurysms usually fall into this category.

Hemorrhagic stroke at normotension or hypotension: The patient suffering the stroke had normal or even low pressure.

Investigations reveal that Alzheimer's patients who suffer strokes fall into this last category. They incur hemorrhagic strokes at normal or low blood pressures. The discussion regarding the association between Alzheimer's disease and low blood pressure is in an earlier chapter.

Insufficient blood cholesterol levels over a long period will result in a weakening of artery walls. Eventually a break in the artery occurs and bleeding begins. A stroke occurs when the neurons in the part of the brain served by the broken artery die.

It is apparent that unless medical investigators are more precise in these situations it becomes easy for doctors to group Alzheimer's patients who suffer strokes into the same category as those who have active atherosclerosis and high blood pressure. It is a mistake for this to continue to happen.

Confusion occurs to researchers performing autopsies on Alzheimer's patients, because they sometimes find atherosclerotic plaques in the larger arteries in spite of the fact that the patient had low blood pressure when the hemorrhagic stroke occurred. Some will mistakenly conclude that this is proof that atherosclerosis causes Alzheimer's.

We must keep in mind that once an atherosclerotic plaque has formed in an artery, it remains there forever, even if the person begins a long period of a low-cholesterol lifestyle in an effort to stop heart disease.

19-3   Usual Causes of Death in Alzheimer's

It is correct to say that a patient dies <u>with</u> Alzheimer's disease, and not from it. A precise way of looking at it would be to say that the death was attributed to Alzheimer's.

In a recent study, an analysis of 1995 death statistics revealed that they could attribute about 170,000 deaths to Alzheimer's disease. This estimate suggests that 7.1 percent of all deaths that year were linked to the disease, which places it as the third leading cause of death in the United States.

Regarding the actual specific events in their demise, pneumonia is the most common immediate cause of death in Alzheimer's patients. Sometimes the cause listed is simply respiratory failure. Why is pneumonia the most common cause of death in these patients? I address the answer to this question back in Chapter 15, in the section on low cholesterol and fluid accumulation in the lungs. Briefly, the reason behind the fluid buildup is the lack of strength in the walls of lung vessels. They are weak and literally falling apart because of a long-term shortage of cholesterol molecules.

Several researchers have noticed that Alzheimer's patients never die as the result of a classic heart attack. If atherosclerosis causes Alzheimer's, as some believe, it seems that the opposite would be true.

Patients with vascular dementia, on the other hand, frequently have active heart disease. This fits well into out cholesterol model.

Alzheimer's patients rarely die from growing cancer tumors. My explanation for this is that growing tumors need an ample supply of cholesterol molecules, which is something that Alzheimer's patients do not have.

Some Alzheimer's patients choke to death on food that they forgot to swallow. Caregivers must always be sure that the patient does not have food remaining in the mouth when mealtime is over.

Regarding my father-in-law, Vance Wolff, pneumonia was the final cause of death, just as it is in the majority of Alzheimer's cases.

19-4   How Could Someone So Healthy Develop Alzheimer's?

One of the things commonly observed by health professionals experienced in the field of Alzheimer's is that most of these patients seem to be so fit and healthy (except for their minds, of course).

The reason for this is that we currently only measure health status in terms of risk factors for heart disease. If someone is obese and has high blood pressure and high blood cholesterol, we automatically classify them as having significant health risks.

On the other hand, if someone is thin, energetic, has low blood pressure and low blood cholesterol, we automatically judge him or her to be in excellent physical health.

If two patients just described were each 70 years old, which one would be at a greater risk of developing Alzheimer's disease? People who have read this book would immediately say the second person.

Alzheimer's patients seem to be healthier than others at the same age because we base opinions on whether someone has the signs and symptoms of atherosclerosis.

How would I describe the person at age 70 who is at low risk for heart disease and simultaneously at low risk for developing Alzheimer's? It is simple: normal or slightly above normal weight for their height; normal blood pressure; and physically active. Most important of all, blood cholesterol levels in the ranges that many would consider as being too high.

Back in Chapter 6, we discussed the fact that people who are old and still healthy seem to have high blood cholesterol levels. If one desires to age with both mind and body intact, he or she must have a balance. Any error should be on the side of high cholesterol. The reason for this is the fact that we have good treatments for heart disease, such as angioplasties and bypass surgery.

However, there is no treatment for Alzheimer's. Neurons in the brain do not reproduce. If they die, it is permanent.

CHAPTER 20
Apo E 4

(Average readers may wish to skip this somewhat technical chapter.)

20-1   The Genes for Amyloid, Presenilin and Apo E

Researchers have identified several genes that have an influence on the development of Alzheimer's disease. The amyloid gene is on chromosome 21, the presenilin-1 gene on chromosome 14, and the presenilin-2 gene on chromosome 1. If any of these three genes mutate in an undesirable way, it can lead to increased amounts of amyloid circulating in the bloodstream.

Only a very small percentage of people with Alzheimer's developed the disease as a result of having one of these three mutated genes. However, most folks with these gene mutations do not develop the disease, which tells researchers that something else must be exerting an influence.

That something else, of course, is the cholesterol level of the person with the mutated gene. If the mutation has resulted in higher levels of amyloid circulating in the bloodstream as well as what is being produced by individual cells, then shortages of cholesterol molecules result in faster accumulations of amyloid plaques in the brain.

A gene on chromosome 19 controls Apolipoprotein E or simply apo E. This gene has three alleles. They are apo E 2, apo E 3, and apo E 4. You inherit one from each parent, so there are six possible combinations that can result. The six are apo E 2,2, apo E 2,3, apo E4,2, apo E 3,3, apo E 3,4, and apo E 4,4.

Around 1993, some researchers discovered that people with the apo E 4 allele seemed to develop Alzheimer's at a slightly higher rate than those with apo E 2 or 3.

Most people (up to 80 percent) have the apo E 3 allele. From 10 to 15 percent carry one or two apo E 4 gene alleles. The apo E 2 is the most rare.

Earlier in this section, we learned that mutations in the amyloid and presenilin genes could increase the risk for Alzheimer's by slightly raising the amounts of amyloid in cells and the circulating blood. However, in the case of apo E 4, the mechanism that seems to increase the incidence of Alzheimer's disease is still unknown. In other words, the only thing researchers can say at this point is that the apo E 4 allele is more associated with Alzheimer's than is the apo E 3 allele.

The one thing that most researchers seem to agree on is that the apo E 4 allele causes someone <u>that is going to develop Alzheimer's,</u> to do so about five years earlier than a person with the apo E 3 allele.

Can someone with the apo E 4,4 combination live to the age of 100 without developing Alzheimer's disease? The answer is yes.

Can someone with the apo E 3,3 combination develop Alzheimer's at the age of 70? The answer is yes.

The only thing that is certain is that when considering large groups of people, those who happen to develop Alzheimer's disease and have the apo E 4,4 combination will do it about five years earlier than someone with the apo E 3,3 combination.

Since millions of people develop Alzheimer's disease without having an apo E 4 allele, researchers universally conclude that something else is a factor in the disease.

Let me emphasize again the fact that Alzheimer's researchers do not know why having an apo E 4 slightly increases the chances of developing Alzheimer's at an earlier age. In the last section of this chapter, I will explain how it does, and of course, it involves cholesterol.

Returning to the discussion about the presenilin genes, scientists recently identified an enzyme called gamma-secretase. This enzyme cuts the long precursor amyloid protein into smaller amyloid fibrils, which in turn can condense in large numbers into amyloid plaques. Gamma-secretase associates with presenilin protein in producing amyloid fibrils. Some researchers believe they may be one and the same.

Scientists in Germany discovered that the activity level of gamma-secretase increases as cholesterol content in a cell membrane decreases. In other words, cholesterol shortages cause the gamma-secretase enzyme to work harder, which results in increased production of amyloid fibrils. As has been stated numerous times, amyloid is used as a temporary substitute for cholesterol.

20-2   Apo E 4 in Down Syndrome and Twins

Some researchers believe that all people possessing the apo E 4,4 combination will eventually develop Alzheimer's disease.

We learned in an earlier chapter that all people with Down syndrome will develop Alzheimer's if they survive to at least the age of forty and beyond.

Based on these two bits of information, it seems logical to conclude that most, if not all, Down syndrome patients probably possess the apo E 4,4 allele combination. Is this the case?

The answer is definitely no. In fact, studies of Down syndrome patients who have already developed Alzheimer's disease reveal that there is no connection between the apo E 4 gene and the disease. There is a study of forty Down patients with Alzheimer's in which there were no subjects having the apo E 4,4, combination.

Regarding identical twins, a study revealed that there was a concordance rate of fifty percent for identical twins with the apo E 4,4 allele combinations. In other words, if one identical twin had Alzheimer's disease, they found the partner had the disease only half of the time. This again proves that other factors are involved (cholesterol levels).

20-3   Apo E 4 and the Very Old

The purpose of this section is primarily for those researchers who still believe that possessing the apo E 4 allele almost guarantees that one will develop Alzheimer's.

The references for this section clearly show that people can live to be very old having the apo

E 4,4 combination and not develop Alzheimer's. By very old, I mean the ages of 90-100 years and beyond.

20-4   Additional Information Regarding Apo E 4

This section is also primarily for the benefit of medical professionals. Here is a brief summary of the information found in the references listed for this section.

The progression of the disease does not differ between those patients with the apo E 4 allele and those that lack it. In other words, having an apo E 4 does not mean that one will have a faster and more aggressive form of Alzheimer's. After a diagnosis has occurred, one's apo E status does not affect the rate of decline.

Research shows that the metabolism of glucose in the brain is the same regardless of whether or not the patient with Alzheimer's has the apo E 4 allele.

There is little or no difference between apo E 3 and apo E 4 regarding the ability to transport amyloid.

Once a patient receives a diagnosis of Alzheimer's, there is no difference in the numbers of neurons that die between those with apo E 3 and those apo E 4.

As was stated in an earlier section, possessing an apo E 4 allele, especially two of them as in the apo E 4,4 combination, only means that if one is going to develop Alzheimer's because of other factors, it will occur a few years earlier. The reader already knows that the primary "other factor" is low cholesterol levels.

20-5   Apo E 4, Alzheimer's and Cholesterol

As was stated in previous sections, the apo E 4 allele can cause a person to develop Alzheimer's disease several years earlier than in a person with the apo E 3 allele.

Ignoring the low cholesterol factor for a moment, since only readers of this book are aware of it, there has never been a clear reason put forth by Alzheimer's researchers as to why this relationship between apo E 4 and the disease exists. I will now proceed to give an explanation, after covering some necessary background information.

There exists a blood-brain barrier as part of the arteries bringing blood to the brain. There are fewer substances able to pass across this barrier than in the rest of the body. For oxygen, glucose, and cholesterol molecules to reach neurons, passage across the barrier must occur.

Cholesterol molecules travel in the bloodstream as part of lipoproteins. The cholesterol going from the liver to tissues in the body is carried on LDL particles. Cholesterol moving from tissues throughout the body back to the liver for either reuse or disposal is carried on HDL particles.

The large protein that makes up the core of an LDL particle is called apolipoprotein B, or apo B. For a cell to receive cholesterol molecules from the bloodstream, the LDL particle must first bind to the surface of the cell at an LDL-receptor protein. The LDL particle is then pulled into the cell and the needed cholesterol molecules are removed and then placed wherever the cell desires.

Cells in our bodies do not normally just absorb cholesterol molecules. They must be brought into the cells as part of lipoprotein molecules. This is in contrast to some viruses, bacteria, and organisms which do seem to be able to just absorb cholesterol molecules in a simple manner.

Apolipoprotein E lipoproteins also transport cholesterol molecules, but an apo E is smaller than an LDL. Both the liver and the brain make apo E particles. In the brain, this occurs on the brain tissue side of the blood brain barrier. Throughout the body, apo E carries cholesterol in lesser amounts compared to the major carrier, LDL particles.

In brain tissue, however, apo E particles act as the primary mover of cholesterol molecules. There are no LDL particles in the brain tissue side of the blood-brain barrier. There are LDL-receptors in brain tissue, just no LDL particles. The apo E particles bind with these LDL-receptors in order to deliver cholesterol molecules to brain cells.

As we learned in earlier chapters, in old age our brains depend on the blood in general circulation for bringing fresh cholesterol molecules to the neurons and other brain cells that are in need. However, this fact is not widely known.

LDL particles bring cholesterol to brain arteries. The cholesterol molecules are shuttled across the tissue wall of the artery and collected by apo E particles. The apo E particles bind to the surfaces of neurons (or other brain cells) and are pulled inside. The cells can now utilize the cholesterol molecules.

In earlier sections, we learned that there are three forms, or alleles, of apo E. They are apo E 2, apo E 3 and apo E 4. About 80 percent of the population carries the apo E 3 allele, 15 percent have apo E 4, and only 1 to 5 percent have the apo E 2 allele.

Over the past twenty years, various researchers have discovered characteristics about apo E that are important in our current discussion.

First, apo E 3 particles tend to associate with HDL particles in the blood in general circulation. Apo E 4 particles, on the other hand, tend to associate with LDL particles. Apo E 3 is in 80 percent of the population and apo E 4 is in 15 percent. It is for this reason, that we consider apo E to be an HDL in most people and an LDL in that smaller percentage of the population. In the brain and spinal cord, all apo E particles (E 2, E 3, and E 4) act as both an HDL and an LDL.

The first studies of apo E alleles were in association with blood cholesterol levels and atherosclerosis. People carrying the apo E 4 allele had slightly higher LDL cholesterol levels and slightly higher rates of heart disease, compared to people carrying the apo E 3 allele. You now know the reasons behind these findings.

The second characteristic we are concerned with is the finding that the actual amounts of apo E produced in the brain vary according to the allele. Those with the rare apo E 2 allele have the highest concentrations of particles in brain tissue, and those with the apo E 4 allele have the fewest. The apo E 3 group falls in the middle.

The third and last characteristic deals with the actual ability of apo E particles to bind to the surfaces of neurons in the brain. Remember that this is the only way that neurons can receive fresh cholesterol molecules. Research shows that apo E 3 particles bind much more readily to the neuron cell surface than do apo E 4 particles.

Let us summarize these three characteristics. First, apo E 3 associates with HDL particles and apo E 4 associates with LDL particles. Second, a person carrying the apo E 3 allele will have more particles available for transporting cholesterol to neurons in the brain than will a person with the apo E 4 allele. Lastly, apo E 3 particles are far better than apo E 4 particles at attaching themselves to the cell surfaces of neurons in order to deliver the needed cholesterol molecules.

We can now answer the two major questions regarding the associations between apo E 4 and heart disease, and apo E 4 and Alzheimer's disease.

Why does research link apo E 4 to slight increases in blood LDL cholesterol levels and he associated slight increases in heart disease rates that follow? Because in time of adequate nourishment, the apo E 4 will add to the capacity of LDL to carry cholesterol molecules. The ate of heart disease may increase slightly, but this helps to protect against the development of Alzheimer's.

Why has apo E 4 been linked more closely to Alzheimer's disease than has apo E 3? Because n times of long term semi-starvation, in which there are shortages of cholesterol molecules, he lower numbers of available apo E 4 particles and their decreased ability to attach to the cell surfaces of neurons in the brain act to magnify the cholesterol shortage.

Let us answer the same two questions, but this time in regards to apo E 3.

Why is apo E 3 considered a factor that protects against higher LDL cholesterol levels and, therefore, helps to insure slightly lower incidences of heart disease? Because apo E 3 particles in the general circulating blood associate with HDL particles, and we know that a higher HDL cholesterol level is protective against heart disease.

Why is apo E 3 considered a factor that protects against or at least delays the development of Alzheimer's disease? Because even if there are shortages of cholesterol as a result of long periods of semi-starvation, the greater numbers of apo E 3 particles in the brain, and their better ability at binding to the cell surfaces of neurons, combine to offer some protection. Though less cholesterol may be available, these two factors regarding apo E 3 create a more efficient use of the dwindling supply.

Regardless of whether someone carries the apo E 3 allele or the apo E 4 allele, shortages of cholesterol molecules from long periods of semi-starvation will still result in the death of neurons. The only difference is that the onset of Alzheimer's will be delayed somewhat in those with the apo E 3 allele.

For those who believe that amyloid plaque accumulations are the most important factor in Alzheimer's disease, two things are critical to consider. First, amyloid protein can be transported almost equally as well between any of the three apo E alleles. Second, remember that neurons are dying in the brains of Alzheimer's patients even in places where there are no accumulations of amyloid.

CHAPTER 21
Estrogen

21-1   Estrogen

Studies have shown that women develop Alzheimer's disease at a higher rate than men. There are also studies that show a slight decrease in this higher rate in those women given estrogen over long periods as part of therapies to lessen the impact of menopause.

In addition to providing a degree of protection against Alzheimer's, women receiving estrogen also displayed lower rates of osteoporosis.

On the negative side, estrogen therapy can increase the risks for various cancers.

There are actually three estrogens present in the blood of the human female. They are estradiol, estrone, and estriol. Estradiol is the primary form. When we use the term estrogen, it usually refers to estradiol.

In a female that is not pregnant, most of the estrogen comes from the ovaries. The adrenal glands produce smaller amounts. In a pregnant woman, the placenta becomes a source of large quantities of estrogen.

Males produce small amounts of estrogen. This occurs in the testes.

There is a third reason for discussing estrogen in this book, and it relates to the actual chemical production of estrogen. The body produces estrogen molecules from molecules of cholesterol.

21-2   Estrogen and Cell Growth

Estrogen promotes the development of female secondary sex characteristics as one grows from childhood into sexual maturity. The uterus, vagina, and all of the other components increase several times in size. Estrogen also causes the growth and development of the breasts to occur.

During the menstrual cycle, estrogen causes the endometrium, which is the tissue lining the uterus, to thicken and become filled with blood vessels. The high estrogen levels are preparing the uterus for implanting a fertilized egg.

If fertilization does not occur, then the estrogen levels decrease. The result is the drying up of the tiny blood vessels in the endometrium, which then shrivels and sloughs off (menstrual bleeding).

If fertilization does take place and the implanting of the fertilized egg occurs, estrogen levels increase further as the pregnancy progresses. The placenta that surrounds the developing baby grows and produces large quantities of estrogen during the months of gestation. (Progestins and other hormones are important in these processes, too.)

Therefore, the principal function of estrogen is to cause cells to grow in size and reproduce. We normally relate this property to just the tissues of the female sex organs and other reproductive tissues, but estrogen influences other parts of the body as well.

Estrogen acts to make cells grow and reproduce by plugging into the DNA of the nucleus in each cell via specific estrogen receptors. The details of how this happens are not important in our discussion. What you need to remember is that estrogen promotes cell growth and, therefore, the growth of tissues. Increased amounts of protein form and cell membranes grow larger. Of course, if cell membranes are growing, then the cells must make cholesterol molecules, or obtain them from the bloodstream.

In summary, estrogen makes cells grow, which requires cholesterol molecules. Cells can make some of the cholesterol molecules needed, but they also obtain them from the bloodstream. As a general rule, estrogen tells cells to take in cholesterol. This benefits cells that are growing in size, cells growing in number, and cells in stressful environments that are just trying to maintain a condition of optimum health.

The last situation refers to neurons in the brain, of course. Estrogen can act in the brain to tell neurons, which do not reproduce or grow in number, to take in cholesterol molecules for optimum maintenance in a stressful environment.

21-3   Estrogen and Blood Cholesterol Levels

Growing and/or multiplying cells can produce cholesterol molecules, but they also pull them from the circulating blood.

Numerous studies have shown that women receiving estrogen replacement therapy are characterized by decreasing blood cholesterol levels.

Women of menopausal age and beyond experience decreases in the amount of estrogen produced in their body. These women simultaneously will have gradual increases in their average blood cholesterol levels if they maintain adequate nutrition.

Researchers normally conclude that the decreasing blood cholesterol levels in women receiving estrogen replacement therapy are due to the uptake of cholesterol from the blood by the liver. I believe that researchers are forgetting the fact that various tissues throughout the body are triggered by estrogen to take in cholesterol from the blood. The focus should not be totally on the liver on this aspect of estrogen metabolism.

There is one situation where estrogen increases will not result in blood cholesterol decreases, and that is in the case of pregnancy. Blood cholesterol levels increase throughout the nine months as the uterus and placenta increase in size in support of the growing baby. Incidentally, you will remember that the growing baby uses cholesterol molecules from the mother for body tissues other than in the developing brain. Glucose is used to manufacture the cholesterol for the brain, which is why it is important for the mother to maintain adequate blood glucose levels.

In conclusion, estrogen lowers blood cholesterol levels by causing cells to take in cholesterol from the bloodstream.

21-4   Estrogen as an Antioxidant

Antioxidant molecules protect the normal molecules of a cell by being oxidized themselves as a type of sacrifice.

Estrogen molecules have an antioxidant effect. There are several sites on the ringed structure where oxygen atoms can attach, thus protecting molecules such as cholesterol and phospholipids. In fact, estrogen is even more effective than vitamin E when it comes to protecting cholesterol from oxidation. Remember that vitamin E is the primary antioxidant found in the brain.

21-5   Estrogen and Alzheimer's

Women develop Alzheimer's at a higher rate than do men. After menopause, circulating estrogen levels drop sharply in women. Though estrogen levels are lower in women after menopause, some will have slightly more estrogen in circulation than others. Studies show that these women with slightly higher levels (though still lower than before menopause) have a decreased rate of Alzheimer's disease.

Women who have been taking estrogen for long periods for help with the symptoms of menopause also show a slightly decreased rate of Alzheimer's.

Many Alzheimer's researchers conclude that estrogen provides a degree of protection against the disease, based on the facts and observations just listed.

Part of the protection, according to researchers, is due to the antioxidant properties of estrogen. Nevertheless, the primary mechanism by which estrogen acts against the development of Alzheimer's is still unknown in the medical research world.

In my opinion, estrogen protects against Alzheimer's by signaling cells in the brain to take in more cholesterol molecules. Neurons possessing the optimum amount of cholesterol in their cell membranes are better able to resist the damage caused by oxidation, waste accumulation, and temporary fuel (glucose) shortages.

Over a long period of semi-starvation, even estrogen will not prevent the deaths of neurons in the brain of an elderly woman. Similarly, one who is maintaining adequate nutrition, that includes eating foods containing cholesterol, will be resistant to developing Alzheimer's even if there is very little estrogen in the bloodstream.

Astrocytes and other cells perform supporting functions for neurons. Researchers have found that estrogen in the brain area causes the astrocytes and other supporting cells to produce more apo E proteins. The primary purpose of apo E protein is to deliver cholesterol to neurons.

Does administering estrogen to someone who has already fully developed Alzheimer's disease act as a cure? No, it does not, because the symptoms of the disease are due to the deaths of neurons. Neurons do not reproduce, unfortunately, so estrogen does not reverse the disease.

21-6   Estrogen and Heart Disease

Before menopause, women have lower rates of heart disease compared to men. During the years after menopause, a time of sharply lower estrogen levels, the rates of heart disease in women begin to catch up to the rates seen in men.

Many studies have found that women after menopause seemed to maintain slightly lower rates of heart disease if they were taking estrogen on a regular basis.

Unfortunately, taking estrogen will not protect against heart attacks in women who already have heart disease.

Estrogen will lower blood cholesterol levels by telling cells in the body to take in cholesterol molecules. This helps cells in tissues, in addition to reducing the amounts of oxidized cholesterol floating around in the blood.

Estrogen itself is an antioxidant, which helps prevent the oxidation of cholesterol in the bloodstream.

By taking in more cholesterol through the influence of estrogen, fibroblasts and other cells associated with protection of heart and blood vessels can function better.

A factor that causes some confusion in this topic has to do with the typical women who receive estrogen for the symptoms of menopause, for they tend to be individuals who practice healthier habits of lifestyle. Perhaps the healthier lifestyles are the primary reason for the protection against heart disease, and not the estrogen therapy. Then again, perhaps it is a combination of both.

21-7   Estrogen and Cancer

Estrogen therapy might provide some protection against Alzheimer's and heart disease in women after menopause. In light of these possibilities, should we place all women on estrogen replacement therapies after reaching menopause?

The answer is no, because research shows an association between estrogen and cancer. I am speaking primarily about cancer tumors, not things like leukemia.

A cancer tumor consists of normal cells that have somehow changed into cells that multiply and grow uncontrollably.

The basic role of estrogen is to tell cells to grow and/or multiply. In so doing, the cells take in cholesterol and other substances.

Will estrogen tell cells that have somehow changed into cancer cells to grow and/or multiply? The answer is yes.

You may be thinking that estrogen promotes only those cancers particular to females, such as cancers of the breast, ovaries, or endometrium. However, estrogen also stimulates cancers of the colon, prostate, liver and brain.

Estrogen's relation to the different kinds of breast cancers can be confusing. Estrogen stimulates some breast cancers to grow. Some will stop growing if exposure to estrogen is blocked. Still other breast cancers will stop growing if estrogen is present.

Other research shows that the risks of cancer may decrease if the estrogen is combined with progestin.

One study demonstrated that estrogen replacement therapy was associated most strongly with an increased risk of invasive breast cancer with a favorable prognosis. In other words, estrogen increases your risk of breast cancer that spreads, but if caught in time, you can be cured. I do not find that to be very reassuring.

Estrogen tells cells to grow and/or multiply. This applies to both normal, healthy cells, and those that somehow have become cancerous.

21-8   Estrogen and Rheumatoid Arthritis

Cholesterol shortages and/or inefficient use of cholesterol are present in some cases of rheumatoid arthritis. And we know that estrogen tells cells to take in cholesterol.

There are times in the female menstrual cycle when high levels of estrogen are present in the circulating blood. Therefore, do women with rheumatoid arthritis have an easing of their symptoms whenever the estrogen levels are at a high point in their monthly cycle? Are there scientific studies that demonstrate such a connection?

The answer to both questions is yes. We can also add psoriasis in cases of psoriatic arthritis. Of course, the studies linking estrogen to the easing of symptoms in rheumatoid arthritis do not mention cholesterol, but we know that it is the critical factor.

21-9   Estrogen and Your Skin and Bones

Cells function at their optimum level when their membranes have sufficient amounts of cholesterol molecules. Estrogen tells cells to take in cholesterol molecules. Therefore, estrogen acts to help cells perform their functions at optimum levels.

It is in this way that estrogen can help to prevent osteoporosis in women. The cells that maintain bone tissue perform at their best through the actions of estrogen.

Estrogen does not make bone any harder than what it is normally. Estrogen helps primarily to prevent loss of bone tissue. Of course, adequate nutrition is absolutely necessary in order to maintain strong bone tissue. There must be adequate amounts of calcium, vitamin D, cholesterol, and various proteins present in order for estrogen to exert an influence in the maintenance of bone tissue. Is it necessary for a woman after menopause to take estrogen supplements in order to maintain strong bones?

The answer is no. Women throughout history have lived into their nineties without suffering osteoporosis, and they have done this without estrogen supplements. If women maintain complete nutrition through old age, then adequate amounts of calcium, vitamin D, cholesterol, and various proteins will be available for maintaining bone strength. Regular physical exercise is also important.

Regarding skin, estrogen again helps by telling skin cells to take in cholesterol molecules. The key to maintaining more elasticity and fewer wrinkles is by insuring a high water content in and around skin cells. What is the best way to prevent loss of water from skin? Insuring that the membranes of skin cells have the optimum amounts of cholesterol molecules.

21-10 Estrogen, Cortisol and Vitamin D

One of the things that vitamin D does is to tell cells that are multiplying to slow down or stop. A consequence of this is that the cells influenced by vitamin D would slow down or stop any processes involved with the taking in of cholesterol molecules.

In another of the earlier chapters, we learned that cortisol forced cells to donate cholesterol molecules for the benefit of other cells in the body that are in need of cholesterol. Cortisol also tells these cells to stop making new cholesterol molecules. Cortisol does this by blocking the action of HMG-CoA reductase.

In the references for this section are research papers on some interesting experiments relative to our current discussion. In working with cultures of breast cancer cells, adding estrogen caused the cells to multiply. Adding vitamin D then caused the cells to stop multiplying.

Keratinocytes and fibroblasts are cells that form skin. Exposing them to estrogen promoted growth activity, while vitamin D caused them to stop, just as in the experiments with breast cancer cells.

Estrogen causes cells to grow and take in cholesterol molecules. Vitamin D causes cells to slow down or stop growing, which means that they stop taking in cholesterol molecules. Cortisol causes cells to donate cholesterol molecules, and to temporarily stop making any new ones. It is interesting that all three, estrogen, vitamin D, and cortisol, are made from cholesterol molecules.

CHAPTER 22
The Amyloid Crossover Effect

The pancreas is an organ that produces various digestive enzymes and bicarbonates. It also produces the hormones called insulin and glucagon. They regulate the blood glucose (sugar) levels.

Insulin and glucagon work together but in opposite ways. If blood glucose levels are low, glucagon stimulates the liver to convert glycogen to glucose, which raises the levels. Insulin facilitates the diffusion of glucose across cell membranes and into the cells for the production of either energy or conversion into fat for storage. Therefore, insulin acts to lower blood glucose levels.

In an earlier chapter of this book, we learned that people with non-insulin dependent diabetes mellitus (NIDDM) generally do not develop Alzheimer's disease. Most people with NIDDM are or were obese. In addition to hypertension and heart disease, they usually maintain high blood cholesterol levels. It is the high cholesterol levels that prevent Alzheimer's in these people.

An endocrinologist might point out that amyloid protein is found in the pancreatic tissues of people who die with NIDDM. What is the explanation for this if cholesterol shortages over a long period cause amyloid deposition? Is the pancreatic amyloid of NIDDM patients the same amyloid found in the brains of Alzheimer's patients?

The answer is no. The amyloid material that accumulates in the pancreas of a patient with NIDDM comes from amylin, which is a third pancreatic hormone. The technical term for amylin is islet amyloid polypeptide. Amylin will coalesce into a type of amyloid plaque deposit if continuously produced in large amounts. This is what occurs in the pancreas organs of patients with NIDDM.

To try to minimize confusion, I will refer to the deposits in the pancreas of NIDDM patients as amylin-amyloid, and will refer to the deposits in the brains of Alzheimer's patients as beta amyloid. Though closely related chemically and structurally, they are of different lengths and fulfill different roles in the body.

As stated in earlier chapters, beta amyloid is integral to repair processes, acting as a temporary cell membrane bandage until adequate amounts of cholesterol molecules become available.

There are studies that show that amylin acts as an appetite suppressant. Amylin administered to laboratory animals caused them to stop eating, resulting in weight loss. Perhaps the pancreas produces amylin as part of an effort to naturally prevent obesity.

However, if produced continuously in large amounts, amylin coalesces and condenses into what we have termed amylin-amyloid around cells in the pancreas. This material, when condensed, becomes toxic and kills cells in the pancreas. At autopsy, the pancreas of a patient who has died with NIDDM exhibits these accumulations of amylin-amyloid and pockets of dead cells.

Amylin acts in the brain to curb appetite. There may be amylin receptors in the hypothalamus, because eating patterns are thought to originate there.

Amylin is very similar to the glycoprotein that condenses and accumulates in the brain as beta amyloid, which makes up the plaques of Alzheimer's.

It is my conclusion that the amyloid material deposited in the brains of Alzheimer's patients may be triggering the receptors for curbing appetite that amylin affects.

Alzheimer's disease is the result of cholesterol shortages from long periods of semi-starvation (in most cases). As beta amyloid is deposited in the brain, it is possible that it acts similar to amylin to cause further loss of interest in eating.

This is what I call the "amyloid crossover effect." The beta amyloid of Alzheimer's can act in the brain like pancreatic amylin as an appetite suppressant.

Another bit of evidence in support of my theory is that both the beta amyloid of Alzheimer's and amylin from the pancreas are transported by apo E!

Many diseases and conditions besides Alzheimer's cause patients to gradually lose weight and appear to waste away, despite efforts to maintain nutrition. Some of these include various cancers, advanced tuberculosis, AIDS, liver disease, massive chronic infections, anorexia nervosa, and so on.

Why would someone whose body is wasting away seem to lose the desire to eat, which happens so frequently? I believe that the "amyloid crossover effect" plays a part. In conditions where there is weight loss, the blood cholesterol levels decrease. Low cholesterol levels cause beta amyloid to deposit wherever cell membranes need instant repairing, and this includes the brain. I believe that the beta amyloid protein can trigger receptors for curbing appetite in the way that amylin from the pancreas is supposed to do.

The result? The patient has less interest in eating, even though they are losing weight. I believe that in such situations one factor may be the "amyloid crossover effect."

CHAPTER 23
Humans are Omnivores

23-1   Introduction

Heart disease is a major killer in industrialized societies. Over the past forty years, it seems that cholesterol has been targeted as the major villain responsible.

In any book or magazine article that discusses heart disease and diet, you will probably find one or more of the following sentences:

"Your body makes all of the cholesterol it needs."

"Humans are naturally meant to be vegetarians."

"Human teeth are designed for eating plants, not animals."

"The human digestive system is designed for digesting plants, not animals."

"Never eat anything that had a face or had a mother."

The theme presented is that the vegetarian lifestyle must obviously be the healthiest lifestyle for people.

Is there any scientific evidence behind the notion that humans are naturally meant to be vegetarians?

The answer is no, even though some doctors, scientists, and celebrities may sincerely believe that people should only eat foods from plants and not from animals.

I shall now define my use of the terms carnivore, herbivore, and omnivore. We will only be considering larger mammals, and not mice, squirrels, etc.

A carnivore eats meat and other parts of animals. Tigers and lions are carnivores.

A herbivore is a strict vegetarian, eating only plant materials. Cows and deer are herbivores.

An omnivore is an animal that eats both plants and other animals. Raccoons and bears are omnivores.

Humans are omnivores, and we will discuss the evidence behind this fact.

We begin our review of the evidence by mentioning the fact that human breast milk contains significant quantities of cholesterol. And baby formula will have glucose, but not cholesterol.

Remember that the brain in an infant makes its cholesterol from glucose molecules, sparing the cholesterol in breast milk for use in skin and other tissues during the critical first months and years.

Are there studies that show any differences between breast-fed and formula-fed babies? The answer is yes. Breast-fed babies seem to attain larger sizes in body measurements on average.

A question on this topic would be about early prehistoric man. What foods did our human ancestors eat while the evolutionary processes leading to modern man were occurring?

The study of coprolites, which are fossils of ancient human feces, answers that question.

Analyses of coprolites reveal that man evolved while consuming an omnivorous diet, based more, in fact, on foods from animals than plants.

There also is fossil evidence demonstrating that the transition from human ancestors with small brain size to later ancestors with a much bigger brain occurred at the same time as when animals became a larger part of the diet.

What about the human of today? A pure vegetarian is likely to have lower blood cholesterol levels than is an omnivorous person. (The exception is in the cases of those who consume large amounts of carbohydrates to the point of being obese.) Are there any studies that directly show some kind of danger from consuming a pure vegetarian diet?

The answer is yes, but they usually relate to some type of vitamin or mineral deficiency that can be overcome with nutritional supplements. This is not new information, so there are no references about it listed for this section.

Indirectly, of course, this entire book is a study of the potential health risks of a diet that lacks things found only in animals, especially cholesterol.

These health risks may not be identified as being dietary in origin. There was a study, however, which demonstrated directly that if a woman follows a pure vegetarian diet, it might cause her to stop ovulating. If you happen to be a woman who refuses to eat meat or eggs, and you are failing in efforts to become pregnant, you may want to ask your doctor about the references listed for this section. And perhaps you should start your days with some bacon and eggs for breakfast.

23-2   Human Teeth and Jaws

The discussion in this section pertains to the teeth and jaws of humans and animals. There are no drawings for this section, so those readers who wish to see some will need to consult an encyclopedia or computer.

The teeth of a pure carnivore are pointed and sharp. Their design is for grasping and tearing the flesh of another animal. A cat's teeth do not look like the teeth of a cow.

If a paleontologist discovered the fossilized skull of a previously unknown animal and saw that its jaw contained only sharp, pointed teeth, he would conclude that this fossilized specimen was a carnivore.

The teeth of a pure herbivore, on the other hand, are broad and flat. They act like millstones, grinding plant matter as the first step in deriving the nutrients.

Herbivores usually have just a few front incisor teeth used only for grabbing vegetation. Some herbivores have front teeth on only one jaw. In addition, some just use the tongue to grab plants, thereby rendering front teeth as nonessential entirely.

Again using our example of a paleontologist, a fossilized skull bearing only rows of broad, flat teeth would fall into the classification of a plant-eating herbivore.

If the paleontologist found a fossilized skull with both types of teeth, the animal's classification would be as an omnivore.

Humans have both types of teeth. I am a dentist, and know this to be a fact. Therefore, humans evolved as omnivores, at least as far as their teeth are concerned.

The typical adult human has 32 teeth, with 16 on each jaw. There are 20 of these 32 teeth that are carnivore-type teeth in that they are pointed or have sharp edges. The design of these 20 teeth, called the incisors, canines, and bicuspids, are for biting off pieces of animal flesh and crushing small, hollow bones and cartilage.

Only 12 of our 32 teeth are broad and flat for grinding plant matter. They are the molars. It is interesting that in many cases, four of these 12 molars will not be able to fit in the spaces of our jaws designated for posterior teeth. These are the wisdom teeth or third molars, and surgical removal of these may be necessary for many people, due to lack of room. Human evolutionary patterns may be showing us that only eight molars are sufficient for grinding the plant portions of the natural human diet.

Full size mammals that are herbivores usually have upper and lower jaws that are very long in relation to the rest of the skull. Picture in your mind the head of a cow, horse, or deer. The long jaws provide room for the large, flat molar teeth necessary for grinding tremendous quantities of plant matter. Long jaws also allow for the attachment of broad muscles that must work for many hours each day.

Though the jaws of a typical herbivore are long, they do not open very wide in relation to the size of the skull. Herbivore jaws open only wide enough to get the plant matter into the mouth.

In contrast, full-size mammals that are carnivores usually have shorter jaws in relation to skull size. These jaws open very wide in relation to skull size. The reason for the wide opening ability is that it is necessary in order for the carnivore to adequately bite the leg, neck, or trunk of whatever unfortunate animal was caught. Imagine a lion or tiger opening its mouth.

We shall also discuss the jaw joint, which is the hinge area where the upper and lower jaws connect.

In full-size mammals that are herbivores, the lower jaw makes circular motions during the many hours spent each day grinding plant matter. Think of a cow "chewing its cud." These circular motions result from the sliding movements of the connecting points in the hinge. These connecting points of the lower jaw are sliding forwards and backwards in alternate movements. As the left connecting point slides forwards, the right point slides backwards. Then the opposite occurs. This alternately sliding forwards and backwards creates the circular motion that we see.

In a typical full-size carnivore, however, a different movement occurs. A carnivore's jaws open straight up and down like a pure hinge. There is no circular, side-to-side movement as in "chewing cud." Think of a lion opening and closing its mouth.

The drawback to this type of pure hinge movement is that very little actual chewing can occur. The carnivore instead swallows its prey in chunks.

Let us review. In relation to its skull, the typical herbivore has long jaws that do not open very wide. In chewing, the creation of the circular motion occurs when the connecting points of the lower jaw alternately slide back and forth.

In contrast, the typical carnivore has shorter jaws that *do* open wide in relation to skull size. The jaw opens straight up and down like a pure hinge. The typical carnivore does not have a circular chewing motion because its jaw connecting points do not slide.

The herbivore's jaw joints slide, and the carnivore's jaw joints work like a hinge.

How do we classify the human jaw joint? Remarkably, the human jaw joint does *both* the sliding movement *and* the pure hinge motion. In fact, the human jaw joint, referred to as the TMJ, actually has the medical label as a sliding/hinge joint.

Remember that humans evolved before the invention of knives and forks, so a wide jaw opening was necessary in order to take a bite of meat from the limb or trunk of the animal serving as dinner. Then for chewing bites of either animal or plant foods the jaw joints create the circular motion by alternately sliding forwards and backwards.

Regarding jaw length in relation to skull size, a human more closely relates to the typical carnivore.

From the evidence of jaw length, jaw opening, and jaw movement, one can easily conclude that this is further proof that humans evolved as omnivores. Also, this evidence tips the scales for the consideration of humans as more carnivorous than herbivorous.

Now that we have learned that the teeth, jaws, and jaw joints place humans in the category of being omnivores, let us look at our digestive system.

23-3   The Human Digestive System

Full-size mammals like cows and deer are herbivores that we also happen to call ruminants. A ruminant receives all of its nutrition from plants, which are in reality very difficult to digest (except for plants with a high carbohydrate content, such as potatoes).

Ruminants have complex stomachs made up of three or four chambers. There are specialized enzymes and bacteria in these chambers for digesting plant matter. In addition, ruminants must periodically regurgitate plant matter back up into the mouth for additional chewing ("chewing its cud").

Humans, as you can see, differ greatly from ruminants in that we do not have stomachs with three or four chambers, do not have the special enzymes and bacteria for digesting plant matter, and we do not regurgitate food for additional chewing.

Another important factor is that a pure herbivore must consume very large amounts (in relation to body size) of plant matter every day. Carnivores, on the other hand, eat a much smaller amount (in relation to body size) of food from animals. In addition, full-size carnivores do not necessarily need to eat every day.

We shall now review some of the enzymes and secretions found in the human digestive tract.

Ptyalin (in saliva) and pancreatic amylase are the enzymes that digest starches. (Amylase is not the same thing as amyloid or amylin). The plant starches turn into glucose and glycogen, which in turn immediately become an energy source or convert into fat.

In the stomach, hydrochloric acid and various pepsinogens are produced by cells in the lining and act together to form pepsin. The purpose of pepsin is to digest collagen, which is the substance that makes up the connective tissue of meats. Also produced in the stomach are tributyrase, which digests butterfat, and gelatinase, which liquefies the proteoglycans of meats.

Collagen, butterfat, and meat proteoglycans are not in plants, yet humans have special enzymes for digesting them. Let us continue.

Pepsin in the stomach only begins the meat digesting process. In the small intestine are secretions from the pancreas that continue the work. These secretions are trypsin, chymotrypsin, and carboxypolypeptidase. They take the complex meat proteins and break them down into smaller protein pieces.

Elastase, another enzyme, is specialized for the digestion of elastin fibers that help hold meat cells together.

Various other peptidases secreted from cells lining the small intestine perform the final work in breaking down the smaller meat proteins into amino acids, which are then passed into the blood.

Various enzymes digest triglycerides, which are primarily fats from animals. The process involves the emulsification of fats by bile acids and lecithin. The resulting free fatty acids and monoglycerides transport in the blood as micelles.

Finally, humans have an enzyme called cholesterol ester hydrolase for the sole purpose of digesting cholesterol. The cholesterol molecules then transport via bile salt micelles. Remember again that cholesterol is not found in plants.

If the design of humans were to just use plants as a food source, why are there so many enzymes for digesting the parts of animals in the normal human digestive system?

Because humans are omnivores with more emphasis towards the carnivore side.

Plant cell walls are rigid. They consist of cellulose, which we know of as fiber. This fiber is useful in some people for helping to keep the contents inside intestines moving along.

This is actually the only benefit that humans derive from fiber. Because we do not have an enzyme for digesting the cellulose of plant cell walls, we must thoroughly chew or previously cook all plants eaten in order to obtain their nutrients.

If humans were designed to primarily eat plants, why doesn't our digestive system have an enzyme for digesting cellulose, the primary building block of vegetation?

Some readers at this point may be thinking about gorillas, which are very closely related to humans and are pure herbivores. It is true that they do not eat animal-based foods. However, the typical adult male gorilla weighs 400 pounds and must eat 60 pounds of plant matter each day to maintain an adequate level of nutrition. This corresponds to an adult man weighing 200 pounds eating almost 30 pounds of lettuce, vegetables, and fruit each day. I do not know of any man or woman willing to eat 30 pounds of plants every day.

The gorilla is a close relative of modern man, but the chimpanzee is even closer. In the areas of animal intelligence, humans are first, chimpanzees are second, and gorillas are in third place. Chimpanzees are pure vegetarians, just like gorillas, *or are they?*

We now know that chimpanzees are omnivores, though they are leaning towards the herbivore side. They kill and eat a variety of small mammals, but not on a daily basis. They may also consume carrion at times.

Chimpanzees will even kill and eat other chimpanzees.

In third place on the earth's ladder of animal intelligence is the gorilla, a pure herbivore. In second place is the chimpanzee, which is an omnivore that leans toward the herbivore side. At the top on the ladder of animal intelligence is man, who is an omnivore with leanings towards the carnivore side. *Do you see a pattern?*

Many people believe that dolphins are somewhere in this top three list. Dolphins are pure carnivores.

Think of the tastes and aromas associated with grilled steaks, hamburgers, roast turkey, baked ham, sizzling bacon, sausage, pepperoni pizza, barbecued pork and beef, hot dogs, fried chicken, spare ribs, bratwurst, chili and anything else you think should be on this list. Why are these tastes and aromas so appealing to the vast majority of humans? I think you know the answer.

23-4   Liver/Cholesterol Feedback Inhibition

Cells throughout the human body are able to manufacture some but not all of the cholesterol molecules they need. Proof of their need for additional molecules lies in the simple fact that there exists an elaborate system for transporting cholesterol in the bloodstream using LDL, apo E, etc.

The major site for manufacturing cholesterol molecules for shipment to other body tissues is the liver. The intestines also make cholesterol in addition to what is absorbed from food, but the liver has ultimate control over shipping it in the blood.

If blood cholesterol levels fall below a genetically determined level, then the liver will release enough cholesterol into the bloodstream to make up the shortage.

The amounts of cholesterol stored in liver cells are also genetically determined. This is where the liver/cholesterol feedback inhibition mechanism is at work.

The liver performs many different tasks. Included is the manufacturing of cholesterol molecules, which requires raw materials, enzymes, and energy. Humans and other animals with carnivorous diets have livers that can sense the amount of cholesterol absorbed from food and use it to supply the needs of other body tissues. This is a tightly regulated mechanism. It allows the liver to save on energy, enzymes, and materials.

Pure carnivores, such as lions and tigers, must have very strong liver/cholesterol feedback inhibition mechanisms. If they did not, then they would quickly develop very high blood cholesterol levels and die of heart attacks. Remember that a pure carnivore eats only meat, animal fat, and cholesterol.

A pure herbivore, on the other hand, eats no meat, cholesterol, or animal fat when in its natural environment. Pure herbivores, therefore, genetically lack a liver/cholesterol feedback inhibition mechanism, because cholesterol is not found in any plant.

What happens when cholesterol is mixed into the plant material consumed by an animal that is a pure herbivore? The animal's blood cholesterol levels increase tremendously, for its liver is not capable of regulating the amount of cholesterol absorbed by the intestines and added to the bloodstream. Atherosclerotic lesions form quickly in the herbivore's major arteries.

Heart disease researchers actually make use of this technique. By mixing cholesterol into chow pellets, they can cause atherosclerotic plaques to form in the aortas of laboratory rabbits in just two to ten weeks. The rabbits are pure herbivores and therefore lack the mechanism that controls cholesterol absorbed from food.

Some breeds of rats and hamsters do not readily develop atherosclerosis after the mixing of cholesterol into plant chow pellets. Also, at least one breed of rabbit is resistant in this manner. The explanation, of course, is that some types of rats and hamsters and one type of rabbit have genetically developed a liver/cholesterol feedback inhibition mechanism. This now places them in the category of being slightly omnivorous.

Therefore, there is a direct relation between the degrees of resistance to the development of atherosclerosis from eating cholesterol, and the degrees of "carnivorousness" of an animal. Though heart disease is the major killer in western societies, it is still a fact that it takes from 30 to 60 years for it to cause illness in most people. Therefore, we must consider humans as being resistant to atherosclerosis.

As learned in an earlier chapter, no scientific studies prove that simply eating foods containing cholesterol will raise blood cholesterol levels high enough to promote heart disease. This is because most healthy people have functional liver/cholesterol feedback inhibition mechanisms at work in their digestive systems.

On the other hand, a diet lacking foods with cholesterol can dramatically lower blood cholesterol levels, especially if the diet is also very low in fats and carbohydrates. It is my opinion that this means humans are naturally meant to eat at least some foods containing cholesterol.

What foods, when eaten, will raise blood cholesterol to very high levels? The answer is those foods that are primarily carbohydrates from plants and some kinds of saturated fats. Humans did not evolve in an environment with limitless amounts of foods containing flour and other carbohydrates. The "caveman grocery store" did not stock great quantities of breads, cakes, cookies, potatoes, rice, pasta and other starchy foods and sugars.

CHAPTER 24
Risks and Recommendations

24-1   Risks

We know that lifelong cigarette smokers are at much higher risk for developing heart disease, stroke, lung cancer, and emphysema. Is it possible to list in a similar manner those who are at risk for developing Alzheimer's disease? The answer is yes.

All people born with Down syndrome will eventually develop Alzheimer's disease if they live past the ages of 35 or 40.

Those people who have experienced a serious head injury or undergone brain surgery at some point in their life are at slightly higher than average risk for developing Alzheimer's. This may be true even if they maintain adequate or even high blood cholesterol levels.

Unfortunately, there are a small number of people genetically programmed to develop Alzheimer's at some point in their lives. Less than 5 percent of all cases of the disease fall into this category.

People who have a disease or medical condition which happens to steal cholesterol molecules from normal tissues are at increased risk for developing dementias that I maintain are identical to Alzheimer's. In this category are cases of AIDS/HIV, long-term kidney dialysis, and cancer tumor patients who experience extensive weight loss over a long period.

Untreated Cushing's disease patients will develop Alzheimer's symptoms.

Young people who have anorexia nervosa will develop brain shrinkage and some memory problems. Fortunately, the brains in younger bodies are better able to cope with and bounce back from periods of semi-starvation, providing they regain proper nutrition.

Older people who are chronic alcoholics are at increased risk for developing the disease. This is primarily due to the malnutrition that goes along with being an alcoholic.

The majority of people who go on to develop Alzheimer's disease have the following characteristics. They are in their sixties or older; they are not obese; they seem to be active and full of energy; they have blood pressures that fall into the lower ranges; and most important of all, their blood cholesterol levels are in the lower ranges.

The picture of the person most at risk for developing Alzheimer's is, unfortunately, the current profile of the ideal healthy older person.

Remember that in the semi-starvation mode, the blood cholesterol levels may temporarily elevate due to the actions of cortisol. Also increased in the semi-starvation mode are the levels of epinephrine, and this may make the person seem to have boundless amounts of energy.

How can an older person prevent the development of Alzheimer's disease and at the same time, decrease the risks for heart disease and atherosclerosis? The answer is simple. If you are not obese, prevent any weight loss by eating adequately. Eat animal-based foods regularly, which will provide dietary cholesterol (remember that plants do not contain cholesterol). Control high blood pressure. If you are obese, lose some weight, but not so much as to become underweight. Exercise regularly. Don't smoke cigarettes.

As I have stated previously, eating foods that actually contain cholesterol will not raise blood cholesterol levels high enough to the point where the risks for developing heart disease are increased.

One final point about blood cholesterol levels needs to be emphasized. Current thinking in the medical profession is now at the stage where "lower is always better," without any lower limits. Many doctors want their patients, including the elderly, to have total blood cholesterol levels significantly below 200 mg/dl, even if the patient has no signs or symptoms of heart disease. This is not the best approach if one wants to avoid developing Alzheimer's disease in the senior years.

24-2   Recommendations for Those on Cholesterol-Lowering Therapies

Patients should have several medical tests performed when beginning therapies to lower blood cholesterol levels, especially if statin drugs will be involved. An MRI or some other scanning image of your brain is necessary, so that a baseline standard picture will be in your records. This will make it easier to detect any signs of brain atrophy (shrinkage) at a later date.

Testing for amyloid is confusing because doctors presently are unaware of its natural purpose in the body and its relationship to cholesterol levels. Blood levels of amyloid generally increase over time in Alzheimer's patients, though overlapping with healthy people occurs. The true reason behind this is the relationship between blood platelets, which store amyloid, and blood cholesterol levels. As the levels decrease, the fluidity of platelet membranes increases, which causes the release of amyloid.

If a patient manages to eat more nutritiously for several days or weeks, their blood cholesterol will rise. Platelet membrane fluidity will decrease as a result, causing a drop in amounts of amyloid released. Remember that blood platelets are on a ten-day turnover cycle. We can now see why levels of amyloid in blood increase at times and then seem to decrease at other times.

In testing for amyloid, cerebrospinal fluid (CSF) might be utilized. As opposed to blood, however, CSF amyloid levels decrease in Alzheimer's patients over time. Why? As brain tissue cholesterol decreases, amyloid from CSF is used up as a substitute.

Perhaps the best test is one for measuring tau protein levels in CSF. If decreasing cholesterol levels in the blood results in the deaths of neurons in the brain, the levels of tau protein in CSF will increase.

Blood pressure readings are a way of keeping track of the effects of lowering cholesterol levels. Eventually, blood pressures drop so low that it can be seen as a sign that arteries are literally falling apart. A stroke at low blood pressure may then occur.

These tests are necessary for any patient beginning therapy to reduce blood cholesterol levels, especially if it involves the use of a statin drug.

Periodic eye exams should take place, to check for development of cataracts.

There are other medical tests that involve the measuring of levels of cortisol, nitric oxide, prolactin, growth hormone, tumor necrosis factor, and interleukins.

The references listed for this section include studies that provide some very interesting information about statin drugs. It would be helpful for prescribing doctors to know the information listed in these references.

CHAPTER 25
Depression and Cholesterol

(Average readers may wish to skip this somewhat technical chapter.)

25-1   Depression in Alzheimer's

Depression is a condition where the patient has feelings of sadness, melancholy, dejection, emptiness, worthlessness, and hopelessness that are exaggerated and out of proportion to reality. We are not talking about the depression one might briefly feel over the cancellation of a favorite television show.

Many published studies confirm that depression is common in Alzheimer's patients. There is not uniform agreement as to whether depression first appears before, after, or at the same time as when full Alzheimer's symptoms are recognized. The important thing to remember is that depression is associated with Alzheimer's disease.

Physical aggression that includes true assaults against others is common in Alzheimer's patients.

Some of the more commonly prescribed antidepressant medications provide a measure of relief for some of the depression symptoms in Alzheimer's patients. We will discuss antidepressants later in this chapter.

Low cholesterol levels over a long time in an elderly brain causes Alzheimer's. Is low blood cholesterol a common finding in people diagnosed with depression?

The answer is in the next section. First, let me mention two papers providing us with clues.

Amyloid protein, which I maintain is a temporary substitute for cholesterol, deposits in the brains of Alzheimer's patients. The laboratory sign that this is happening is a decrease in the cerebrospinal fluid levels of amyloid. Researchers in Switzerland discovered that amyloid levels in patients with depression decreased similarly to that seen in Alzheimer's patients.

As you are aware, brain atrophy (shrinkage) occurs in Alzheimer's patients. Researchers in New York found that older patients with depression also displayed atrophy on brain scans. These researchers theorized that this might be a sign that Alzheimer's disease may develop later in these patients.

25-2   Depression and Blood Cholesterol Levels

Is low blood cholesterol a common finding in people diagnosed with depression?

The answer is yes. There are many studies which conclude that depression is associated with low blood cholesterol levels. I have listed only a representative sample for this section, but there are many more.

The studies also show that the association between depression and low blood cholesterol levels persists across all variables; male or female, young or old, slender or obese, smoker or non-smoker, physically active or not, and so on.

Depression can even reach a point severe enough as to cause the patient to contemplate or attempt suicide. Several studies exist which show that patients with depression who are suicidal have low blood cholesterol levels.

There are various explanations as to the reasons behind the association of depression with low blood cholesterol levels. I base my opinion for the association on the myelin insulation layers surrounding nerve fibers in the brain and the cholesterol content in the membranes of neurons.

Shortages of cholesterol molecules result in myelin that does not insulate as well. In turn, this slows the nerve impulses throughout the brain. Cholesterol shortages in the cell membranes of neurons, especially in the synapses, also effect the transmission of nerve signals. These two effects are the primary reasons for the symptoms of depression in these patients.

As an aside, the evidence showing an association between low blood cholesterol levels and depression is further proof that brain cholesterol levels link to cholesterol levels in the blood.

Older people have a lesser ability to recover from depression, because it is more difficult for the older brain to recover from periods of low cholesterol content.

In the *Merck Manual* is a table listing various illnesses and conditions known to be associated with depression. This list includes Parkinson's disease, rheumatoid arthritis, seizure disorders, head trauma, Cushing's disease, and AIDS. Of course, this table does not list the connection of low cholesterol to these illnesses and conditions, but we know of its existence.

Medical professionals reading this can learn of the debate regarding depression, suicide, or other mental disorders, and the use of statin drugs for lowering blood cholesterol levels. You will find it to be very interesting.

Will they find low blood cholesterol levels in every patient diagnosed with true medical depression? No, but a blood cholesterol test may be a good (and inexpensive) screening step to take when a patient first develops symptoms of depression.

25-3   Depression and Semi-Starvation

Long periods of semi-starvation will naturally lead to lower blood cholesterol levels. Remember, however, that the body increases cortisol production when it is in the starvation mode, and the cortisol may temporarily support blood cholesterol levels near the normal ranges.

Is depression a common finding in patients who are losing weight because of a condition marked by long periods of semi-starvation?

The answer is yes. There are many studies on the subject of weight loss and depression. I have listed just a few of them for this section, but there are many more.

There is some minor debate as to which comes first, the depression or the weight loss. This is usually in connection with anorexia nervosa in young people. Overall, however, researchers in this field agree that depression is associated with the weight loss resulting from long periods of semi-starvation. This association also holds true across all of the variables, such as young or old, male or female, etc.

Weight loss from advanced cancer tumors is also associated with depression.

And there are studies showing that brain atrophy (shrinkage) occurs in people experiencing severe weight loss from long periods of semi-starvation.

25-4   Antidepressants, Serotonin and Cholesterol

Millions of prescriptions are written every year for depression. The most popular of these antidepressant medications are serotonin reuptake inhibitors. These drugs block the uptake of serotonin in the brain. Serotonin molecules signal feelings of calm and relaxation. These drugs supposedly work by making serotonin last longer in the brain.

However, we have just learned that many cases of depression are associated with low blood cholesterol levels. We know that low blood levels lead to lower levels of cholesterol in brain tissues, which in turn results in the appearance of the symptoms associated with depression.

Is it possible, therefore, for these antidepressant drugs to also influence the amounts of cholesterol in brain tissues?

The answer is yes.

Making molecules of cholesterol requires materials, energy, and at least thirty enzymes. The key enzyme in the process is HMG-CoA reductase. Statin drugs lower cholesterol levels by artificially "turning off" this enzyme.

There are several enzymes in cells that naturally act to "turn off" HMG-CoA reductase, thereby halting the production of cholesterol molecules. One of these is called protein kinase C.

In a living cell, HMG-CoA reductase must be actively controlled in either the "on" mode or the "off" mode. Protein kinase C is a natural enzyme that actively controls HMG-CoA reductase in the "off" mode.

Researchers have found that one of the effects of these antidepressant drugs is the ability to "turn off" protein kinase C. In fact, the most widely prescribed of these drugs (Prozac) is also the most effective at "turning off" protein kinase C.

What is the ultimate result of this action? If you "turn off" the enzyme that "turns off" HMG-CoA reductase, you are, in effect, artificially "turning on" the process that causes cholesterol molecules to be manufactured in living cells.

The unrecognized effect of these types of antidepressant drugs (such as Prozac) is to artificially increase the production of cholesterol molecules in living cells.

This effect occurs not only in the brain, but also in skin, muscle, and other tissues.

If the cholesterol levels rise in brain tissues, then the easing of the symptoms of depression are to be expected. These antidepressant drugs are effective in decreasing the symptoms of depression primarily because they artificially cause increases in the production of cholesterol molecules in the brain and elsewhere. The influence of these drugs over serotonin actions plays a part, but it is not the major reason behind the improvements seen in people with depression.

CHAPTER 26
In Closing

26-1   Preventive Dietary Suggestions

Simple dietary changes can prevent or at least manage most of the diseases and conditions discussed in this book. However, do not make changes in your diet without first consulting your personal physician.

The goal is to somehow maintain blood cholesterol levels that will be high enough to keep you in the safe middle area of the cholesterol U.

The easiest and most natural way to do this is by eating foods that contain cholesterol, while minimizing the consumption of foods that are primarily carbohydrates (starches).

Eating foods containing cholesterol will not cause you to have blood cholesterol levels high enough to increase the risks for heart disease. The liver/cholesterol feedback inhibition mechanism will protect against it.

For those readers who believe that some type of plant-derived carbohydrate is absolutely necessary, my response is that the design of humans is such that they can actually do quite well with minimal amounts of starch in the diet. Obtaining glucose (blood sugar) from animal proteins and animal fats through the process of gluconeogenesis is part of the human design.

Some health and medical professionals believe that a diet high in animal protein places extreme stress on the kidneys. However, no real medical research provides a basis for this notion. As long as you drink plenty of water every day, your kidneys will be able to handle all of the animal protein you eat.

What follows is a brief outline of what I believe is a natural dietary plan for humans. It is important to eat sensible portions and perform regular exercise every day.

Any kind of meat is acceptable.

Also acceptable are eggs, cheeses, milk, yogurt, butter, and ice cream.

Soups made with animal bones are acceptable.

All vegetables are acceptable. However, try and limit consumption of starches, such as potatoes, rice, breads, cakes, donuts, cookies, bagels, nachos, pizza, etc.

Eat fruits with a high sugar content sparingly.

Now comes some good news. If you are not obese, engage in moderately vigorous exercise every day, do not smoke, and do not have high blood pressure, you can eat anything you want. It is still important, however, to regularly eat foods containing cholesterol. This is especially important as you enter the senior years.

As far as nutritional supplements are concerned, I recommend taking the following every day: a multivitamin that has all of the trace items, vitamins C and E, calcium (for those who do not like milk), and vitamin D for calcium absorption and help in minimizing cancer risk. There are some brands of orange juice with calcium added, which helps those who cannot swallow large pills.

Remember to eat sensible portions.

A pure vegetarian diet, with absolutely no foods derived from animals, is not a natural diet for humans, especially as you get older. Can you find a society of people someplace on Earth who all reach the age of 100 or beyond, and yet eat no foods whatsoever that are derived from animals? The answer is no.

If you believe that you may be at risk for one or more of the diseases and conditions in this book, it becomes imperative that you consume foods with cholesterol. The easiest method is by eating eggs every day or almost every day. (Remember to consult your physician before making dietary changes).

I do not know if the amounts of cholesterol obtained from eating eggs change according to the way they are prepared. If there are differences, then it is probably a scale with raw eggs providing the most and hard fried or hard-boiled providing the least amounts of cholesterol. Those eggs softly scrambled, once over lightly, and sunny-side-up are probably somewhere in the middle of the scale.

A quick and easy way to obtain a maximum amount of cholesterol is by drinking eggnog. What follows is my recipe. I prepare this eggnog in the same glass I drink it from, using an electric mixer with a beater blade that reaches down into the glass. I mix it in a very tall glass.

The ingredients are: four ounces of milk that has vitamins A and D added, three eggs, one teaspoon of vanilla extract, one packet of artificial sweetener, and a few sprinkles of nutmeg. Mix thoroughly, then drink it. It will usually total up to be about nine ounces in all. (Underweight folks should use whole milk.)

It is a mistake to think that the consumption of eggs is only for their cholesterol contribution. The egg possesses all components necessary for the construction of a warm-blooded vertebrate. The materials in an egg can create skin, muscle, bone, cartilage, brain, nerves, blood vessels, and eyes. These materials are almost exactly the same chemically as those that are found in the human body.

Finally, there are some individuals who believe that the only way to deal with Alzheimer's is through a strategy labeled "prevention through delay." It seems to be based on the premise that some people are destined to develop the disease sooner or later. In this strategy, one follows specified lifestyle, dietary, medication and medical testing recommendations, which supposedly will delay the development of full Alzheimer's disease. This delay then provides time for the patient to die of some other cause before full Alzheimer's symptoms appear.

I do not think this is a good strategy. First, some of this plan's dietary and medication recommendations might actually cause one to develop Alzheimer's sooner, instead of delaying the disease.

More importantly, because you have read this book, you now know the true cause of the disease. You are now prepared to prevent Alzheimer's by actually preventing Alzheimer's.

26-2   Treatment and Research Proposals

The following are suggestions for products based on cholesterol Those health and medical companies that have the necessary capabilities should develop them.

I recommend the development of intravenous fluids containing cholesterol formulated as LDL, HDL, and apo E, just as is found normally circulating in blood. It would not be safe to inject pure cholesterol into the vein of a patient. The goal is to be able to provide an immediate boost in the cholesterol amount available to tissues and yet do it in a safe, natural way.

We shall refer to these formulations of LDL, HDL, and apo E collectively as "I.V. cholesterol."

There is no need to worry about atherosclerosis in this proposal. Several days or weeks on I.V. cholesterol will not cause a heart attack to occur.

The following are proposals for treating and preventing the diseases and medical conditions discussed in this book.

The arrangement of my list of proposed treatments is in groups that are somewhat similar to or have at least one thing in common with each other.

Group A: This is for those in whom Alzheimer's disease or Parkinson's disease is already fully developed. The symptoms result from neurons having died in the areas of the brain dealing with memory (Alzheimer's) or motor control (Parkinson's). Neurons do not reproduce, so the symptoms already displayed are permanent.

The only hope available is to arrest the process as soon as possible. A diet high in food containing cholesterol is mandatory. Consuming the eggnog drink once or twice each day is necessary. The prescribing of anticonvulsant drugs should occur, even if the patient has not had any seizures. However, if a considerable amount of beta amyloid material has already accumulated in the brain, a problem will still exist. This is because beta amyloid has an adhesive property towards cholesterol molecules in membranes.

Medical research needs to develop a drug or chemical that will remove beta amyloid. Your body has cells that can remove it, but only when it is in very small amounts. Natural metabolic processes do not remove large accumulations of beta amyloid in plaques.

There are substances that remove beta amyloid. They are in the references for this section. There is hope for those in whom only the first symptoms of Alzheimer's or Parkinson's are appearing. The diseases that are noted by accumulations of amyloid, yet are not Alzheimer's or Parkinson's, will also benefit when a drug is perfected that can dissolve and remove amyloid that is in plaques.

The best way to prevent Alzheimer's and Parkinson's is to eat foods containing cholesterol every day, especially as you enter your fifties.

There are drugs approved for treating the symptoms of Alzheimer's disease. One of them has advertisements in many magazines and journals on a regular basis. However, these drugs don't stop the disease. Any benefits are temporary, if they occur at all. Side effects can include nausea and vomiting, which may possibly speed up the progression of Alzheimer's because of the effect on the nutritional status of the patient. The drugs are very expensive, and again, they do not halt the disease.

Group B: There are a large number of medical conditions and diseases in this group. Patients diagnosed with one of these should eat foods containing cholesterol every day. The eggnog drink, or eggs prepared another way, is best for satisfying this requirement. Anticonvulsant drugs may help in some cases. <u>Please remember that it may take from three to six months or longer before seeing improvements in health.</u> For acute attacks of symptoms of one of these diseases, the ideal treatment would be I.V. cholesterol. I hope that someone will develop this soon. The medical conditions and diseases that fall into my Group B are rheumatoid arthritis, psoriasis, some cases of depression, and some cases of atrial fibrillation. Cataracts are also in group B, though they are not subject to acute episodes as are the others in this group. Gold therapy would provide additional (and safe) benefits for rheumatoid arthritis patients.

Group C: This is about cancer tumors in general. Let me first remind you that vitamin D is your body's natural cancer fighter, though everyone normally only considers it in connection with calcium and bone metabolism.

There are many types of cancer tumors because there are many different types of tissues in our bodies. All tumor cells need cholesterol for maintenance and growth, just as normal cells do. Consider attacking all tumors from the aspect of cholesterol as an additional weapon in the war against cancer. Here are some of the strategies to utilize. Let me stress that their use is in addition to currently employed strategies, such as surgery, chemotherapy, and radiation. <u>My proposals are not meant to be substitutes.</u>

All cancer tumors patients should receive large doses of oral vitamin D. If a patient is receiving I.V. chemotherapy, the doctor can add vitamin D to the I.V. solution, as long as it does not affect the cancer drugs.

Something that has already begun is the preparation of anticancer drugs in association with a cholesterol "vehicle." As the tumor cells absorb the cholesterol, they bring in the anticancer drug as well. In the list of references for this section are some reports on this developing science.

It would be a good idea for the drug companies to prepare a statin in gel form for injection purposes. Surgeons would use it with removal of tumors. The areas around the sites would receive an injection with the statin gel so that it would kill any hidden tumor growths. There may be a slight delay in healing, but that is a small price to pay.

The injection of statin gel into cancer tumors not surgically removable because of their size, location, or large numbers, would also occur. This may not be a cure for patients in these situations, but their comfort and time remaining may be increased.

A statin gel may help a patient with an inoperable brain tumor. The doctor could use three-dimensional computer imaging in real time to direct a long needle to the site of the brain tumor. The needle could even remain in place for a period as they continuously administer the statin gel.

I keep saying statin gel, because a gel would remain in the area where it's placed.

Group D: This group consists of folks with Down syndrome, who have a metabolism that produces excesses of hydrogen peroxide on a continuous basis. A larger-than-average supply of beta amyloid is in circulation in these patients as well. The hydrogen peroxide violently oxidizes and, therefore, removes cholesterol molecules from the brain and all body tissues, and it does this at all times.

Our strategy, therefore, is to feed cholesterol and carbohydrate (glucose) to Down syndrome patients continuously from the time they are born and for the rest of their lives. In addition, they should take large doses of antioxidants, such as vitamin E, every day. After the age of twenty, they can scale back the amounts of carbohydrates they consume each day. However, they must not decrease their cholesterol intake. In other words, people with Down syndrome must eat eggs in some form every day.

Group E: This covers the treatments that are involved with estrogen. My recommendation for those taking estrogen for any reason is that they should also take large doses of vitamin D every day. This is to minimize the risks of various cancers. Remember that estrogen causes tissues to grow, and that holds true for cancer tissue, as well as healthy tissue.

Group F: These are the people undergoing surgery, or who have suffered a head injury that affects the brain. Placing these patients on I.V. cholesterol should occur. This is especially important for cases involving the brain. The amounts of amyloid deposited at surgical sites in the brain can be minimized if the tissue can be made to heal quickly. Smaller amounts of amyloid in the brain now may keep the patient from developing Alzheimer's disease decades from now.

In surgical removal of cancer tumors, statin gel should be injected or painted in the immediate area. There may be a delay in healing, but that is not of prime importance in these cancer cases.

Group G: These are people with burns or minor sunburn. In my opinion, I.V. cholesterol is the perfect treatment for people hospitalized for burns over their bodies. This is the fastest way to reestablish the barrier function that prevents loss of body fluid. Until I.V. cholesterol is developed, however, burn patients should consume a large number of eggs every day. The eggnog is also beneficial for people with sunburned skin.

Group H: These are heart bypass surgery patients and balloon angioplasty patients. These are people with established atherosclerosis, of course.

The patients should have I.V. cholesterol administered for several days after surgery to promote quick healing.

After discharge, the patients must change their lifestyle, of course. Stopping smoking, losing weight, regularly exercising, and controlling high blood pressure are the most important things for these patients.

To avoid developing Alzheimer's disease, even bypass patients and angioplasty patients need to eat foods that contain cholesterol if they are in their sixties or older. I shall remind all readers once again that eating foods containing cholesterol will not raise blood cholesterol levels high enough to promote heart disease. Even the mountain of Framingham research does not refute this principle.

Group I: These are people on kidney dialysis. Three or four times each week, these patients undergo dialysis, receiving a large dose of heparin each time. Heparin removes cholesterol from all tissues, including the brain. A dementia identical to Alzheimer's may eventually develop in these patients. It is for this reason that I recommend all kidney dialysis patients eat two or three eggs every day if they are experiencing weight loss as the months pass. Many of these patients have lost the use of their kidneys in association with obesity, hypertension, diabetes, atherosclerosis, or a combination of these. It is for this reason that egg consumption should only be increased in the dialysis patients who are experiencing weight loss and obvious malnutrition.

Dialysis patients would benefit from receiving I.V. cholesterol for several minutes at the end of dialysis. This would help to counteract the effects of the heparin.

Group J: These are people infected with HIV, the virus that causes AIDS. This virus must have cholesterol molecules in order to survive. It takes them from the tissues and fluids of the infected person. As the disease progresses, the cholesterol levels of the patient decrease, though the gradual wasting away of the body contributes to the decrease. In the late stages of AIDS, a dementia develops that is identical to Alzheimer's. The brain shrinkage in AIDS dementia results from the decreasing cholesterol levels that accompany the disease. The proof of this is the finding that some AIDS dementia patients have almost no viral particles in their brains.

I recommend the utilization of two strategies with this disease. The first is for those newly infected with HIV, but have no symptoms of AIDS. The virus requires cholesterol, so the strategy should be to limit the availability of cholesterol. The physician should place them on an I.V. statin medication for several weeks while administering anti-AIDS drugs.

Incidentally, some researchers are combining these drugs with cholesterol so that the virus will pull the anti-AIDS medications close into direct contact.

Although the patient may never fully eliminate all signs of the virus, perhaps it can be controlled and prevented from progressing into full AIDS. A strategy involving a week or two of I.V. statins, along with anti-AIDS drugs every three months may be one solution.

The second situation involves the patient with full AIDS and little time left. Keeping such a patient as comfortable and free of pain as is possible is the prime concern. Eating may be difficult, so the use of I.V. nutrition is necessary with these patients at times. Simultaneous administering of I.V. cholesterol would benefit these terminal patients, even though the virus would also gain.

One benefit of boosting the cholesterol levels of a terminal full-AIDS patient would be a decrease in the growth of Kaposi sarcoma tumors. These blood vessel tumors grow only when cholesterol becomes scarce in tissues.

Group K: These are epilepsy and atrial fibrillation patients. I believe that some cases of each of these conditions have a connection to low cholesterol levels. These patients need to consume more cholesterol (eggnog, etc.). The I.V. cholesterol product would be of benefit to epileptics. Hospital emergency rooms and emergency ambulances could keep a supply of I.V. cholesterol on hand for these types of patients. Incidentally, I.V. cholesterol would also be of benefit for people with physical injuries that produce a great amount of bleeding.

Group L: These are pregnant women abusing alcohol. Alcoholic mothers-to-be run the risk of delivering babies afflicted with Fetal Alcohol Syndrome. My advice for women who continue to drink while pregnant is to eat a lot of potatoes, bread, and starchy snacks. The developing baby's brain needs glucose, and this strategy will help.

Group T: These people are those who have had organs transplanted into their bodies. The anti-rejection drugs these patients must continuously take can dramatically raise blood cholesterol levels in many instances. I believe the success of these drugs is due to the increased cholesterol. However, there is another aspect to this, and it involves cancer. I believe the increased cholesterol levels from anti-rejection drugs may increase the risks for the development of various cancer tumors (though I have no studies to back me up on this). In my opinion, these patients should be receiving large doses of vitamin D in order to minimize this cancer risk.

Though I have stressed in this section the benefits of raising blood and tissue cholesterol levels through the consumption of foods with cholesterol, we should not forget the need for various vitamins and minerals as well. Total nutrition should also include zinc supplements, because some of the enzymes in cells involved in making cholesterol molecules need zinc.

This section consists of a list of various diseases and conditions. My preliminary investigations indicate that cholesterol is a possible factor in some way in each of them. I leave it to others to fully investigate these possibilities.

In this list are chronic fatigue syndrome, corticobasal degeneration, cystic fibrosis, dermatomyositis, fibromyalgia, Huntington's disease, inclusion body myositis, polychondritis, polymyalgia rheumatica, polymyositis, sarcoidosis, scleroderma, eczema, connective tissue disorder, Sjogren's syndrome, progressive supranuclear palsy, frontotemporal dementia, and ALS (Lou Gehrig's disease).

People with Down syndrome have shortages of cholesterol molecules. Cancer tumors need cholesterol to grow. It would be interesting to learn if these patients exhibit lower-than-expected rates of the more common cancers, such as lung, breast, colon, and ovarian cancers.

26-3   Closing Comments

I have researched a number of population groups, both past and present, in terms of diet, culture, and longevity. I placed emphasis on periods before the 1970's, because major advances against illnesses and disease seemed to accelerate in that decade.

In other words, I studied people who lived before the age of modern medicine and analyzed what they ate, what they did, and how long they lived.

One of the groups of people I examined was the Eskimo, who happen to live in a cold, unforgiving climate. The present day Eskimo diet is similar to what the rest of North America consumes, in that it is high in carbohydrates. The rates of obesity and heart disease are increasing as a result, though nutritionists would lay the blame on the animal-based foods they eat.

In contrast, the basis of the traditional Eskimo diet of the past was on foods derived from animals. Vegetables do not grow very well in places that are dark and frozen for most of the year.

Today, experts in nutrition tell us that the healthiest way to eat is by following a low-fat, low-cholesterol, high-fiber diet. In direct contrast to this is the old, traditional Eskimo diet, accurately labeled as a high-fat, high-cholesterol, "no-fiber" diet. In view of this obviously harmful diet, just how long could the typical Eskimo hope to live in the times before the age of modern medicine?

By looking at official census statistics, I learned that there were Eskimos born before 1880 living to the age of 100 and beyond. One can assume that living to an advanced age in a climate like that which exists in the frozen North requires a brain that is still sharp and functioning well. The traditional Eskimo diet that was high in cholesterol but lacked glucose from plants was obviously an important element.

Previously, I mentioned that the one most-perfect food for babies in their first years, breast milk, contained significant quantities of cholesterol. However, we learned that babies still survive on manufactured baby formula that contains no cholesterol, but does have significant quantities of glucose from plants. As you will recall, the cholesterol in a growing baby's brain is made from glucose. The use of the cholesterol in breast milk is for the tissues in the rest of the body of the baby, not the brain.

I mention these two different subjects because they connect in an ironical way. To have a healthy brain in the first years of life requires glucose, but little or no cholesterol in the diet. In contrast, having a healthy brain in the last years of life requires cholesterol, but little or no glucose in the diet.

Finally, I would like to point out a few things for the benefit of those readers who remain skeptical about the connections between cholesterol and the medical conditions detailed in this book.

There are many different types of cells in the human body: brain, muscle, skin, intestine, liver, fat, blood vessel, and so on. Each cell type has a cell membrane with different types of molecules in it, because there are different roles to fulfill. The molecules in cell membranes are mixtures of fatty acids, phospholipids, sphingolipids, ceramides, and specialized proteins.

However, regardless of cell type, each cell must maintain a barrier against water and still remain flexible (except for bone tissue). What molecule do we find in the membranes of all cells that must maintain a flexible barrier to the passage of water molecules? The cholesterol molecule. Cholesterol is nature's universal waterproofing agent for flexible cell membranes.

Currently, the medical establishment is totally concerned with real or imagined excesses of cholesterol in the body. The medical establishment does not consider the possibility of cholesterol shortages. However, if one did accept the concept of tissue shortages of cholesterol, what signs and symptoms would appear in an affected patient? Would a person simply melt down overnight into a pool of "tissue pudding"?

I do not think so. Cholesterol shortages would instead manifest themselves gradually over time, affecting different organs and tissues in ways highlighted throughout this book. The genetic make-up, age, and lifestyle of a person will determine the tissue or organ affected first.

In conclusion, I believe that deficiencies of cholesterol play a significant role in many illnesses and conditions, beginning with Alzheimer's disease.

END OF TEXT

Chapter 2, Section 2, Diagram A
CROSS-SECTION OF HUMAN BRAIN

TOP OF
BRAIN

WHITE   CEREBRAL CORTEX   FISSURE   SULCUS
MATTER   GRAY MATTER

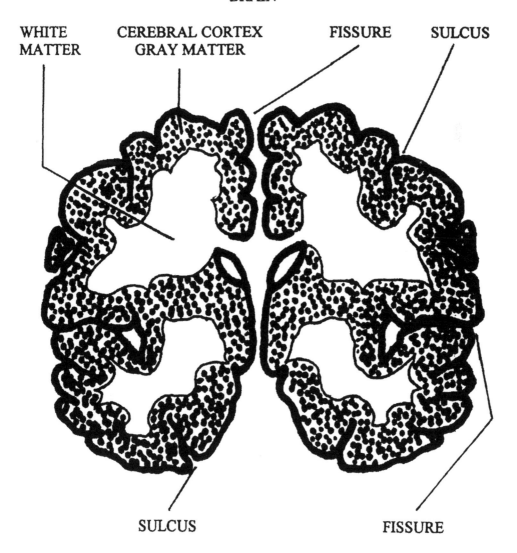

SULCUS   FISSURE

BASE OF
BRAIN

Chapter 2, Section 2, Diagram B
LIMBIC SYSTEM STRUCTURES OF THE HUMAN BRAIN

HUMAN BRAIN (LEFT SIDE)

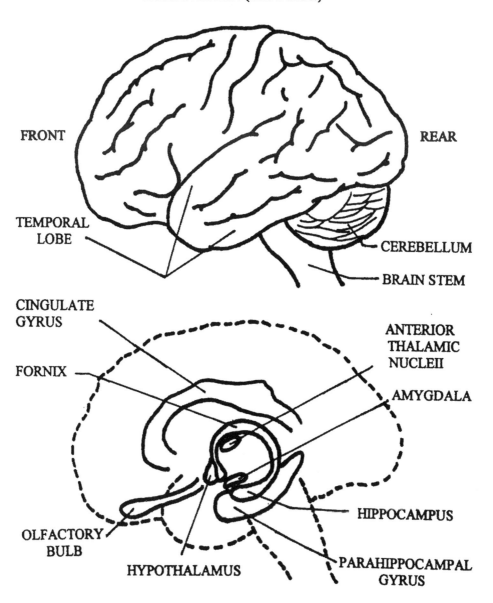

Chapter 3, Section 2, Diagram
THE CHOLESTEROL MOLECULE
(TWO TYPES OF DIAGRAMS)

(THE HYDROGEN ATOMS
ATTACHED TO EACH
CARBON ATOM ARE
NOT SHOWN)

**4 – RINGED STEROL
STRUCTURE**

**HYDROPHOBIC
(LIPOPHILIC)
AREA**

**HYDROPHILIC
(LIPOPHOBIC)
AREA**

Chapter 3, Section 3, Diagram A
TYPICAL PARTS OF A CELL

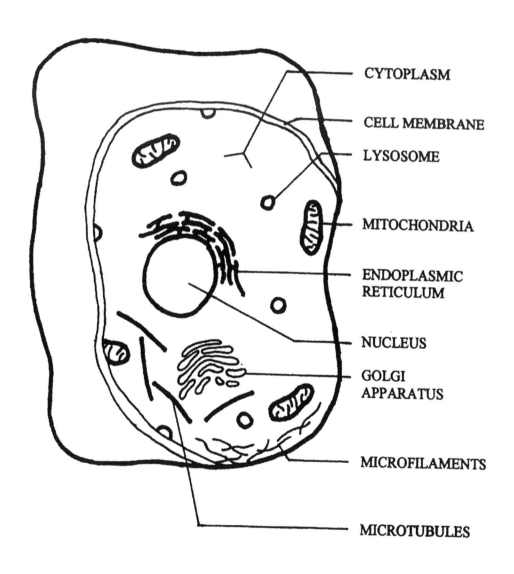

CYTOPLASM

CELL MEMBRANE

LYSOSOME

MITOCHONDRIA

ENDOPLASMIC
RETICULUM

NUCLEUS

GOLGI
APPARATUS

MICROFILAMENTS

MICROTUBULES

Chapter 3, Section 3, Diagram B
CHOLESTEROL AND PHOSPHOLIPID MOLECULES

CHOLESTEROL

HYDROPHILIC END   HYDROPHOBIC END

TYPICAL MEMBRANE PHOSPHOLIPID

OTHER TERMS FOR HYDROPHOBIC ARE LIPOPHILIC AND
NONPOLAR

OTHER TERMS FOR HYDROPHILIC ARE LIPOPHOBIC AND POLAR

Chapter 3, Section 3, Diagram C
TYPICAL CELL MEMBRANE BILAYER

CHOLESTEROL

PHOSPHOLIPID

HYDROPHILIC END   HYDROPHOBIC END

MEMBRANE BILAYER

CELL
EXTERIOR

CELL
INTERIOR
(CYTOPLASM)

PROTEIN

Chapter 4, Section 1, Diagram
NEURON AND SYNAPSE

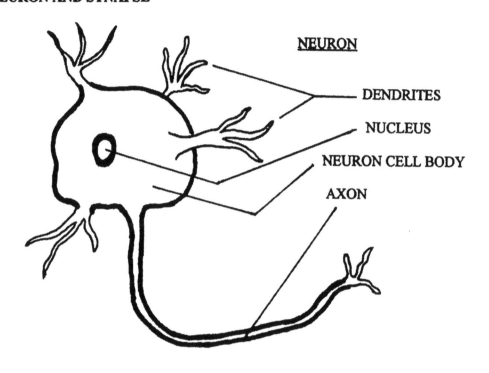

NEURON

DENDRITES

NUCLEUS

NEURON CELL BODY

AXON

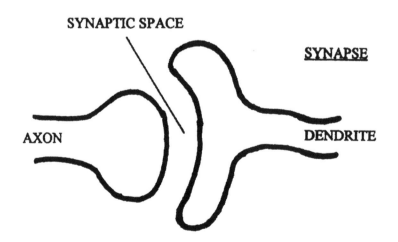

SYNAPTIC SPACE

SYNAPSE

AXON

DENDRITE

Chapter 4, Section 2, Diagram A
MYELINATED NERVES

MYELINATED CENTRAL NERVOUS SYSTEM NERVE
(BRAIN AND SPINAL CORD)

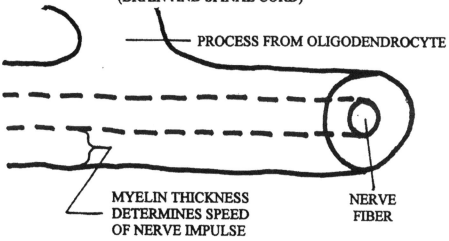

PROCESS FROM OLIGODENDROCYTE

MYELIN THICKNESS
DETERMINES SPEED
OF NERVE IMPULSE

NERVE
FIBER

MYELINATED PERIPHERAL NERVOUS SYSTEM NERVE
(OUTSIDE OF BRAIN AND SPINAL CORD)

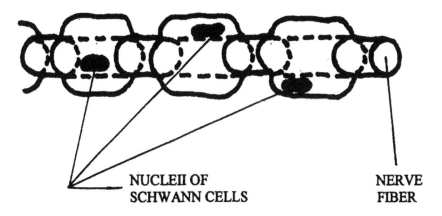

NUCLEII OF
SCHWANN CELLS

NERVE
FIBER

Chapter 4, Section 2, Diagram B
CROSS-SECTIONS OF MYELINATED NERVES

MYELINATED CENTRAL
NERVE (BRAIN AND
SPINAL CORD)

MYELINATED PERIPHERAL
NERVE (OUTSIDE OF BRAIN
AND SPINAL CORD)

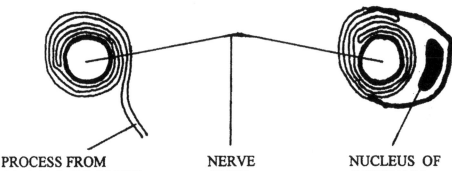

PROCESS FROM
OLIGODENDROCYTE

NERVE
FIBER

NUCLEUS OF
SCHWANN
CELL

PROCESS FROM
OLIGODENDROCYTE
TO SUPPLY MYELIN

OLIGODENDROCYTE

NERVE BUNDLE
SHEATH

MYELINATED
NERVE FIBERS

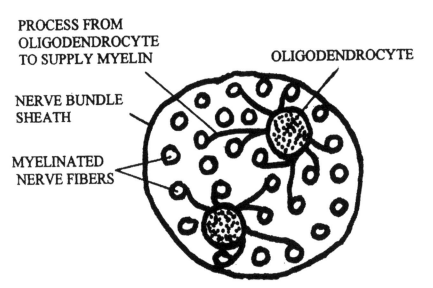

NERVE BUNDLE IN CENTRAL NERVOUS SYSTEM
(BRAIN AND SPINAL CORD)

Chapter 4, Section 4, Diagram
MICROTUBULE AND TAU PROTEIN

MICROTUBULE

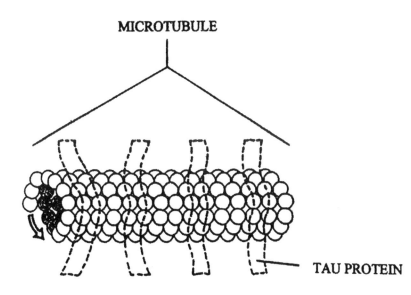

TAU PROTEIN

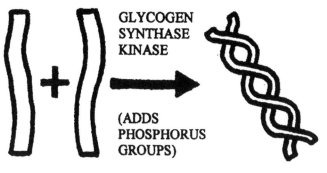

GLYCOGEN
SYNTHASE
KINASE

(ADDS
PHOSPHORUS
GROUPS)

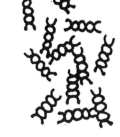

TAU
PROTEINS

PAIRED
HELICAL
FILAMENT
(PHF-TAU)

NEUROFIBRILLARY
TANGLES
(DRAWN TO
SMALLER SCALE)

Chapter 7, Section 2, Diagram
GLUCOSE AND GLYCOGEN

GLUCOSE
MOLECULE

(HYDROGEN
ATOMS ARE
NOT DRAWN)

GLYCOGEN
(BRANCHED CHAINS OF GLUCOSE MOLECULES)

Chapter 10, Section 10, Diagram
CHOLESTEROL AND VITAMIN D (CALCITRIOL)

CHOLESTEROL

HO

SUNLIGHT/
ULTRAVIOLET
RAYS, ENZYMES

VITAMIN D/
CALCITRIOL

OH

HO   OH

Chapter 10, Section 11, Diagram
VITAMIN D (CALCITRIOL) AND METHOTREXATE

**VITAMIN D/
CALCITRIOL**

METHOTREXATE

(LOWER PART POSSIBLY LOST DURING DRUG'S METABOLISM)

APPENDIX 2
References

Alzheimer's Solved

(Condensed Edition)

By Henry O. Lorin

Copyright 2005 Henry O. Lorin

<u>List of References</u>

Reference articles are listed according to author, source, and year of publication. Articles having several authors are listed by the name of the initial author only.

<u>Chapter 1</u>   —None

<u>Chapter 2</u>

<u>2-1</u>

1. Aevarsson, O. J. American Geriatrics Society 44:1455-1460. 1996
2. Braak, H. Neurobiology of Aging 18(4):351-357. 1997
3. Gilley, D. J. American Geriatrics Society 45:1074-1079. 1997
4. Howieson, D. J. American Geriatrics Society 45:584-589. 1997
5. Jost, B. J. American Geriatrics Society 43:1248-1255. 1995
6. Khachaturian, Z. American J. Medicine 104(4a):26s-31s. 1998
7. Larner, A. Dementia and Geriatric Cognitive Disorders 8(4):203-209. 1997
8. Lee, H. International Psychogeriatrics 8(3):469-476. 1996
9. Linn, R. Archives of Neurology 52(5):485-490. 1995
10. Meek, P. Pharmacotherapy 18(2 Pt 2):68-73. 1998
11. Payami, H. Neurology 46:126-129. 1996
12. Small, G. JAMA 278(16):1363-1371. 1997
13. Solomon,P. Archives of Neurology 55:349-355. 1998
14. Wahlund, L. Acta Neurologica Scandinavica, Suppl. 165:85-91. 1996

<u>2-2</u>

1. Armstrong, R. Acta Neuropathologica 88(1):60-66. 1994
2. Ball, M. Lancet 1(8419):14-16. 1985
3. Bobinski,M. Neurobiology of Aging 17(6):909-919. 1996
4. Braak, H. J. Neural Transmission 103:455-490. 1996

5. Brion, J. Biochimica et Biophysica Acta 1160(1):134-142. 1992

6. Brion, J. Acta Clinica Belgica 51(2):80-90. 1996

7. Carr, D. American J. Medicine 103(3a):3s-10s. 1997

8. Convit, A. Neurobiology of Aging 18(2):131-138. 1997

9. Cullen, K. Neuroscience 78(3):641-652. 1997

10. DeCarli, C. American J. Neuroradiology 15(4):689-696. 1994

11. De la Monte, S. Annals of Neurology 25(5):450-459. 1989

12. De Leon, M. Neurobiology of Aging 18(1):1-11. 1997

13. Detoledo-Morrell, L. Neurobiology of Aging 18(5):463-468. 1997

14. Dickson, D. Neurobiology of Aging 18(4 suppl):s21-26. 1997

15. Double, K. Neurobiology of Aging 17(4):513-521. 1996

16. Foundas, A. Neuropsychiatry, Neuropsychology, & Behavioral Neurology 10(2):81-89. 1997

17. Fox, N. Lancet 348(9020):94-97. 1996

18. Frisoni, G. American J. Neuroradiology 17(5):913-923. 1996

19. Heun, R. Dementia and Geriatric Cognitive Disorders 8(6):329-336. 1997

20. Kaye, J. Neurology 48(5):1297-1304. 1997

21. Lassman,H. Annals of the New York Academy of Sciences 695:59-64. 1993

22. Lippa, C. Archives of Neurology 50(10):1088-1092. 1993

23. Mouton, P. Neurobiology of Aging 19(5):371-377. 1998

24. Murphy, D. Biological Psychiatry 34(9):612-621. 1993

25. Nagy, Z. Dementia 6(1):21-31. 1995

26. Najlerahim, A. Acta Neuropathologica 75(5):509-512. 1988

27. Perlmutter, L. Molecular Neurobiology 9(1-3):33-40. 1994

28. Rusinek, H. Radiology 178(1):109-114. 1991

29. Skullerud, K. Acta Neurologica Scandinavica . Supplementum 102:1-94. 1985

30. Smith, A. British Medical Bulletin 52(3):575-586. 1996

31. Smith, C. Neuropathology & Applied Neurobiology 20(4):322-338. 1994

32. Tanabe, J. American J. of Neuroradiology 18(1):115-123. 1997

33. Terry, R. Annals of Neurology 10(2):184-192. 1981

34. Xanthakos, S. Progress in Neuro-Psychopharmacology & Biological Psychiatry 20(4):597-626. 1996

2-3

1. Benkovic, S. J. Comparative Neurology 339(1):97-113. 1993

2. Bjertness, E. Alzheimer Disease & Associated Disorders 10(3):171-174. 1996

3. Bjorkman, L. Community Dentistry & Oral Epidemiology 24(4):260-267. 1996

4. Breteler, M. International J. Epidemiology 20 Suppl 2:s36-42. 1991

5. Connor, J. J. Compartive Neurology 355(1):111-123. 1995

6. Connor, J. Glia 17(2):83-93. 1996

7. Deatly, A. Neuropathology & Applied Neurobiology 16(3):213-223. 1990

8. Dysken, M. International Psychogeriatrics 3(1):53-58. 1991

9. Fung, Y. J. Toxicology—Clinical Toxicology 33(3):243-247. 1995

10. Fung, Y. General Dentistry 44(1):74-78. 1996

11. Fung, Y. J. Toxicology—Clinical Toxicology   35(1):49-54. 1997

12. Gun, R. Alzheimer Disease & Associated Disorders 11(1):21-27. 1997

13. Hachinski, V. Archives of Neurology 55(5):742. 1998

14. Hock, C. J. Neural Transmission 105(1):59-68. 1998

15. Hyman, B. Annals of the New York Academy of Sciences 640:14-19. 1991

16. Kala, S. International J. Neuroscience 86(3-4):263-269. 1996

17. Kasa, P. Acta Neuropathologica 90(5):526-531. 1995

18. LeVine, S. Brain Research 760(1-2):298-303. 1997

19. Makjanic, J. Neuroscience Letters 240(3):123-126. 1998

20. Martyn, C. Epidemiology 8(3):281-286. 1997

21. Metcalfe, T. Neurochemical Research 14(12):1209-1212. 1989

22. Munoz, D. Archives of Neurology 55(5):737-739. 1998

23. Neill, D. J. Neuroscience Research 46:395-403. 1996

24. Pailler, F. Presse Medicale 24(10):489-490. 1995

25. Pendergrass, J. Neurotoxicology 18(2):315-324. 1997

26. Renvoize, E. Age & Ageing 16(5):311-314. 1987

27. Salib, E. British J> Psychiatry 168:244-249. 1996

28. Saxe, S. J. American Dental Association 130(2):191-199. 1999

29. Schlatter, C. Medicina del Lavoro 83(5):470-474. 1992

30. Scileppi, K. J. American Geriatrics Society 32(10):709-711. 1984

31. Smith, M. Proceedings/America 94(18):9866-9868. 1997

32. Storey, E. Medical J. Australia 163(5):256-259. 1995

33. Thomas, D. Acta Psychiatrica Scandinavica 76(2):158-163. 1987

34. Thompson, C. Neurotoxicology 9(1):1-7. 1988

35. Wisniewski, H. Ciba Foundation Symposium 169:142-154; discussion 154-164. 1992

2-4

1. Bergem, A. Archives of Gneral Psychiatry 54(3):264-270. 1997

2. Breitner, J. Archives Neurology 52(8):763-771. 1995

3. Creasey, H. Neurology 39(11):1474-1476. 1989

4. Gatz, M. J. Gerontology. Series A, Biological Sciences & Medical Sciences 52(2):M117-125. 1997

5. Geroldi, C. J. Neuroimaging 6(2):76-80. 1996

6. Heston, L. Progress in Clinical & Biological Research 317:195-200. 1989

7. Kumar, A. Archives of Neurology 48(2):160-168. 1991

8. Lautenschlager, N. Neurology 46(3):641-650. 1996

9. Luxenberg, J. J. Neurology, Neurosurgery & Psychiatry 50(3):333-340. 1987

10. Nee, L. Neurology 37(3):359-363. 1987

11. Raiha, I. Lancet 347(9001):573-578. 1996

12. Raiha, I. Biomedicine & Pharmacotherapy 51(3):101-104. 1997

13. Rao, V. American J. Human Genetics 55(5):991-1000. 1994

14. Renvoize, E. British J. Psychiatry 149:509-512. 1986

15. Small, G. Archives of Neurology 50(2):209-219. 1993

2-5

1. Bowler, J. Archives of Neurology 54:697-703. 1997
2. Cullum, C. JAMA 279(21):1689-1690. 1998
3. Hebert, R. Neuroepidemiology 14(5):240-257. 1995
4. Kase, C. Alzheimer Disease & Associated Disorders 5(2):71-76. 1991
5. Klatka, L. Archives of Neurology 53(1):35-42. 1997
6. Knuffman, J. J. American Medical Directors Association 2(4):146-148. 2001
7. Meyer, J. Stroke 26(5):735-742. 1995
8. Skoog, I. Dementia 5(3-4):137-144. 1994

Chapter 3

3-1

1. Bucht, G. Acta Medica Scandinavica 213(5):387-392. 1983
2. Concise Encyclopedia Biochemistry, Second Edition Published by de Gruyter 1988
3. Denke, M. Archives of Internal Medicine 153:1093-1103. 1993
4. Encyclopedia of Neuroscience edited by George Adelman published by Birkhauser 1987
5. Halter, J. J. American Geriatrics Society 44(8):992-993. 1996
6. Hendrie, H. International Psychogeriatrics 5(1):5-14. 1993
7. Landin, K. J. Internal Medicine 233(4):357-363. 1993
8. Nielson, K. J. American Geriatrics Society 44(8):897-904. 1996
9. Thouez, J. Arctic Medical Research 49(4):180-188. 1990
10. Uusitupa, M. Annals of Medicine 28(5):445-449. 1996

3-2

1. Arebalo, R. J. Biological Chemistry 256(2):571-574. 1981
2. Goad, L. in Biochemistry of Steroid Hormones (ed Makin, H.), 17-44 (Blackwell Scientific Publications, 1975)
3. Carr, B. J. Clinical Endocrinology & Metabolism 55(3):447-452. 1982
4. Kempen, H. Biochimica et Biophysica Acta 876(3):494-499. 1986
5. Orci, L. Cell 36(4):835-845. 1984
6. Soma, M. Toxicology Letters 64-65 Spec No:1-15. 1992
7. Triscari, J. Metabolism: Clinical & Experimental 29(4):377-385. 1980

3-3

1. Bloch, K. Current Topics in Cellular Regulation 18:289-299. 1981
2. Bloch, K. Steroids 53(3-5):261-270. 1989
3. Chong, P. Proceedings/America 91(21):10069-10073. 1994
4. Cooper, R. New England J. Medicine 302(1):49-51. 1980
5. Corvera, E. Biochimica et Biophysica Acta 1107(2):261-270. 1992
6. Cruzeiro-Hansson, L. Biochimica et Biophysica Acta 979(2):166-176. 1989
7. Johnson, W. Sub-Cellular Biochemistry 28:235-276. 1997
8. Leonard, A. Biochimie 73(10):1295-1302. 1991

9. Mason, R. Annals of the New York Academy of Sciences 777:368-373. 1996
10. Mukherjee, S. Biochemistry 35(4):1311-1322. 1996
11. Reyes, M. Biophysical J. 68(3):978-987. 1995
12. Sakanishi, A. Biochemistry 18(12):2636-2642. 1979
13. Schroeder, F. Molecular Membrane Biology 12(1):113-119. 1995
14. Spink, C. Biochimica et Biophysica Acta 1279(2):190-196. 1996
15. Taylor, K. Biochemistry 34(11):3841-3850. 1995
16. Tirosh, O. Chemistry & Physics of Lipids 87(1):17-22. 1997

3-4

1. Bonte, F. Archives of Dermatological Research 289(2):78-82. 1997
2. Downing, D. J. Investigative Dermatology 88(3 Suppl):2s-6s. 1987
3. Feingold, K. J. Clinical Investigation 86(5):1738-1745. 1990
4. Ghadially, R. J. Investigative Dermatology 106(5)1064-1069. 1996
5. Mao-Qiang, M. J. Investigative Dermatology 101(2):185-190. 1993
6. Pharmaceutical Skin Penetration Enhancement(eds Walters, K. & Hadgraft, J.)(Marcel Dekker, Inc. 1993
7. Ponec, M. J. Investigative Dermatology 109(3):348-355. 1997
8. Proksch, E. J. Investigative Dermatology 99(2):216-220. 1992
9. Proksch, E. British J. Dermatology 128(5):473-482. 1993
10. Suetake, T. Archives of Dermatology 132(12):1453-1458. 1996
11. Wertz, P. Seminars in Dermatology 11(2):106-113. 1992

3-5

1. Gower, D. in Biochemistry of Steroid Hormones (ed Makin, H.)47-49,77-79(Blackwell Scientific Publications, 1975)

3-6

1. Aigueperse, J. Biochimie 64(3):185-193. 1982
2. Betteridge, D. European J. Clinical Investigation 10(3):227-230. 1980
3. Cella, L. American J. Physiology 269(3 Pt 1):E489-498. 1995
4. Cella, L. American J. Physiology 269(5 Pt 1):E878-883. 1995
5. Ho, K. Proceedings of the Society for Experimental Biology & Medicine 150(2):271-277. 1975
6. Ho, K. International J. Chronobiology 6(1):39-50. 1979
7. Jones, P. J. Lipid Research 31(4):667-673. 1990
8. Kandutsch, A. in Lipoprotein and Cholesterol Metabolism in Steroidogenic Tissues(eds Strauss, J. & Menon, K.) l-7(George Stickley Company, 1985)
9. Kempen, H. Biochimica et Biophysica Acta 876(3):494-499. 1986
10. Parker, T. Proceedings/America 79(9):3037-3041. 1982
11. Parker, T. J. Clinical Investigation 74(3):795-804. 1984
12. Sato, R. Cell Structure & Function 20(6):421-427. 1995
13. Tilvia, R. European J. Clinical Investigation 9(2 Pt 1):155-160. 1979

3-7

1. Mahley, R. Science 240(4852):622-630. 1988
2. Olson, R. J. Nutrition 128(2 Suppl):439S-443S. 1998

3-8

1. Brown, M. Science 232(4746):34-47. 1986
2. Fagan, A. J. Biological Chemistry 271(47):30121-30125. 1996
3. Igbavboa, U. J. Neurochemistry 69(4):1661-1667. 1997
4. Lange, Y. J. Biological Chemistry 272(27):17018-17022. 1997
5. Lestavel, S. Cellular & Molecular Biology 40(4);461-481. 1994
6. Myant,N. in Cholesterol Metabolism, LDL, and the LDL Receptor. Publ. By Academic Press, 1990
7. Osono, Y. J. Clinical Investigation 95(3):1124-1132. 1995
8. Poirier, J. Trends in Neurosciences 17(12):525-530. 1994

3-9

1. Anderson, D. Central Nervous System Trauma 2(4):257-267. 1985
2. Baranowski, A. Atherosclerosis 41(2-3):255-266. 1982
3. Davies, K. Biochemical Society Symposia 61:1-31. 1995
4. Guardiola, F. Food & Chemical Toxicology 34(2):193-211. 1996
5. Joseph, J. Free Radical Biology & Medicine 22(3):455-462. 1997
6. Lomnitski, L. Pharmacology, Biochemistry & Behavior 56(4):669-673. 1997
7. Mason, R. Free Radical Biology & Medicine 23(3):419-425. 1997
8. Metcalfe, T. Neurochemical Research 14(12):1209-1212. 1989
9. Slotte, J. J. Lipid Research 31(12):2235-2242. 1990
10. Traber, M. Annual Review of Nutrition 16:321-347. 1996
11. Vandewoude, M. J. American College of Nutrition 6(4):307-311. 1987
12. Vatassery, G. Lipids 32(8):879-886. 1997
13. Weight, M. International J. Vitamin & Nutrition Research 52(3):298-306. 1982

3-10   —None

3-11

1. Faix, D. J. Lipid Research 34(12):2063-2075. 1993
2. Pagana, K. in Mosby's Manual of Diagnostic and Laboratory Tests. Publ. By Mosby 1998

3-12

1. Bonte, F. Archives of Dermatological Research 289(2):78-82. 1997
2. Caughman, G. In Vitro Cellular & Developmental Biology. Animal. 29a(9):693-698. 1993
3. Cox, P. J. Investigative Dermatology 87(6):741-744. 1986
4. Denning, M. Cell Growth & Differentiation 6(12):1619-1626. 1995
5. Jetten, A. J. Investigative Dermatology 92(2):203-209. 1989
6. Lampe, M. J. Lipid Research 24(2):131-140. 1983
7. Ponec,M. Archives of Dermatological Research 279(1):32-36. 1986
8. Ponec, M. J. Investigative Dermatology 109(3):348-355. 1997
9. Rodrigueza, W. Biochemistry 34(18):6208-6217. 1995

10. Serizawa, S. Clinical & Experimental Dermatology 15(1):13-15. 1990
11. Serizawa, S. J. Investigative Dermatology 99(2):232-236. 1992
12. Wertz,P. Lipids 23(9):878-881. 1988
13. Wertz, P. Comparative Biochemistry & Physiology-B: Comparative Biochemistry 92(4):759-761. 1989
14. Williams, M. Biochimica et Biophysica Acta 845(3):349-357. 1985
15. Williams, M. J. Lipid Research 28(8):955-967. 1987

Chapter 4

4-1

1. Alivisatos, S. Biochimica et Biophysica Acta 643(3):642-649. 1981
2. De Chaves, E. J. Biological Chemistry 272(49):30766-30773. 1997
3. Deliconstantinos, G. Experientia 39(7):748-750. 1983
4. Kabara, J. Progress in Brain Research 40(0):363-382. 1973
5. Ramsey, R. Advances in Lipid Research 10:143-232. 1972

4-2

1. Chia, L. Biochimica et Biophysica Acta 775(3):308-312. 1984
2. Connor, J. Glia 17(2):83-93. 1996
3. Jurevics, H. J. Neurochemistry 64(2):895-901. 1995
4. Koenig, S. Magnetic Resonance in Medicine 20(2):285-291. 1991
5. Lowry, N. Canadian J. Neurological Sciences 11(1):60-63. 1984
6. Malone, M. J. Gerontology 37(3):262-267. 1982
7. Martenson, R. in Myelin: Biology and Chemistry. Publ. By CRC Press. 1992
8. Morell, P. Neurochemical Research 21(4):463-470. 1996
9. Myelin, Second Edition (edited by Morell, P.). Publ. By Plenum Press. 1984
10. Smith, M. Lipids 5:665-671. 1970
11. Yeh, Y. J. Neuroscience Research 19(3):357-363. 1988

4-3

1. Banati, R. Glia 14(3):209-215. 1995
2. Benkovic, S. J. Comparative Neurology 338(1):97-113. 1993
3. Connor, J. J. Comparative Neurology 355(1):111-123. 1995
4. Connor, J. Glia 17(2):83-93. 1996
5. Koper, J. Biochimica et Biophysica Acta 796(1):20-26. 1984
6. Kreutzberg, G. Arzneimittel-Forschung 45(3a):357-360. 1995
7. Lopes-Cardozo, M. J. Neurochemistry 46(3):773-778. 1986
8. Ludwin, S. J. Neuropathology and Experimental Neurology 56(2):111-124. 1997
9. McRae, A. Gerontology 43(1-2):95-108. 1997
10. Poduslo, S. J. Biological Chemistry 253(5):1592-1597. 1978
11. Stoll, G. Glia 2(3):170-176. 1989

4-4

1. Balint, Z. Neoplasma 25(1):25-29. 1978
2. Binder, L. J. Cell Biology 101(4):1371-1378. 1985

3. Butner, K. J. Cell Biology 115(3):717-730. 1991

4. Conrad, P. J. Cell Biology 131(6 Pt 1):1421-1433. 1995

5. Drechsel, D. Molecular Biology of the Cell 3(10):1141-1154. 1992

6. Erickson, S. Biochimica et Biophysica Acta 409(1):59-67. 1975

7. Fielding, P. Biochemistry 35(47):14932-14938. 1996

8. Garcia-Perez, J. J. Neuroscience Research 52(4):445-452. 1998

9. Hanger, D. Neuroscience Letters 147(1):58-62. 1992

10. Hyman, B. Neurobiology of Aging 18(4 Suppl):s27-32. 1997

11. Latimer, D. FEBS Letters 365(1):42-46. 1995

12. Lee, G. J. Cell Science 102(Pt 2):227-237. 1992

13. Lovestone, S. Current Biology 4(12):1077-1086. 1994

14. Lovestone, S. Neuroscience 73(4):1145-1157. 1996

15. Mandelkow, E. FEBS Letters 314(3):315-321. 1992

16. Markesberry, W. Neurobiology of Aging 18(4 Suppl):s13-19.1997

17. Naves, F. Anatomical Record 244(2):246-256. 1996

18. Pei, J. J. Neuropathology & Experimental Neurology 56(1):70-78. 1997

19. Pelech, S. Neurobiology of Aging 16(3):247-256. 1995

20. Price, J. Neurobiology of Aging 18(4 Suppl):s67-70. 1997

21. Rajan, V. Endocrinology 117(6):2408-2416. 1985

22. Regenass-Klotz, M. Canadian J. Biochemistry & Cell Biology 62(2-3):94-99. 1984

23. Shiurba, R. Brain Research 737(1-2):119-132. 1996

24. Singh, T. Molecular & Cellular Biochemistry 131(2):181-189. 1994

25. Sperber, B. Neuroscience Letters 197(2):149-153. 1995

26. Weingarten, M. Proceedings/America 72(5):1858-1862. 1975

4-5

1. Dehouck, B. J. Cell Biology 138(4):877-889. 1997

2. Kito, A. No to Shinkei-Brain & Nerve 39(8):783-788. 1987

3. Lucarelli, M. FEBS Letters 401(1):53-58. 1997

4. Meresse, S. J. Neurochemistry 53(2):340-345. 1989

5. Osanai, T. Neurochemical Research 9(10):1407-1416. 1984

6. Shibata, S. Neurologia Medico-Chirurgica 30(4):242-245. 1990

7. Wahler, J. Hepatology 17(6):1103-1108. 1993

4-6

1. Beffert, U. J. Neurochemistry 70(4):1458-1466. 1998

2. Boyles, J. J. Clinical Investigation 83(3):1015-1031. 1989

3. Dickson, T. Neuropathology & Applied Neurobiology 23(6):483-491. 1997

4. Fagan, A. J. Biological Chemistry 271(47):30121-30125. 1996

5. Handelmann, G. J. Lipid Research 33(11):1677-1688. 1992

6. Hass, S. J. Biological Chemistry 273(22):13892-13897. 1998

7. Ignatius, M. Proceedings/America 83(4):1125-1129. 1986

8. Ignatius, M. Science 236(4804):959-962. 1987

9. Laskowitz, D. J. Cerebral Blood Flow & Metabolism 18(5):465-471. 1998

10. Lomnitski, L. Pharmacology, Biochemistry & Behavior 56(4):669-673. 1997
11. Mahley, R. Science 240(4852):622-630. 1988
12. Martel, C. J. Neurochemistry 69:1995-2004. 1997
13. Masliah,E. Experimental Neurology 136(2):107-122. 1995
14. Metzger, R. J. Neuropathology & Experimental Neurology 55(3):372-380. 1996
15. Oitzl, M. Brain Research 752(1-2):189-196. 1997
16. Pitas, R. Biochimica et Biophysica Acta 917(1):148-161. 1987
17. Pitas,R. J. Biological Chemistry 262(29):14352-14360. 1987
18. Poirier, J. Neuroscience 55(1):81-90. 1993
19. Poirier, J. Annals of Medicine 27:663-670. 1995
20. Stewart, J. International J. Biochemistry & Cell Biology 30(3):407-415. 1998
21. Strittmatter, W. Proceedings/America 90(5):1977-1981. 1993
22. Strittmatter, W. Proceedings/America 90(17):8098-8102. 1993

4-7

1. Fleming, L. Experimental Neurology 138(2):252-260. 1996
2. Han, S. J. Neuropathology & Experimental Neurology 53(5):535-544. 1994
3. Masliah, E. Experimental Neurology 136(2):107-122. 1995
4. Masliah, E. Progress in Neurobiology 50(5-6):493-503. 1996
5. Roses, A. Annals of the New York Academy of Sciences 777:146-157. 1996

4-8

1. Crawford, M. Upsala J. Medical Science, Suppl 48:43-78. 1990
2. Cunnane, S. Nutrition & Health 9(3):219-235. 1993
3. Foley, R. Philosophical Transactions of the Royal Society of London-Series B: Biological Sciences 334(1270):223-231. 1991

4-9

1. Hyman, B. Annals of the New York Academy of Sciences 640:14-19. 1991
2. Mesholam, R. Archives of Neurology 55(1):84-90. 1998
3. Ninfali, P. Brain Research 744:138-142. 1997

4-10

1. Balazs, L. Neurochemical Research 19(9):1131-1137. 1994
2. Behl, C. Biochemical & Biophysical Research Communications 186(2):944-950. 1992
3. Binkova, B. General Physiology & Biophysics 9(3):311-318. 1990
4. Choi, B. Yonsei Medical J. 34(1):1-10. 1993
5. Davies, K. Biochemical Society Symposia 61:1-31. 1995
6. Kabara, J. Advances in Lipid Research 5:279-327. 1967
7. Lo, W. J. Neurochemistry 46(2):394-398. 1986
8. Lovell, M. Neurology 45(8):1594-1601. 1995
9. Lyras, L. J. Neurochemistry 68(5):2061-2069. 1997
10. Mecocci, P. Annals of Neurology 36(5):747-751. 1994
11. Palmer, A. Brain Research 645(1-2):338-342. 1994
12. Perrig, W. J. American Geriatrics Society 45(6):718-724. 1997
13. Palladini, G. Experimental Cell Research 223(1):72-82. 1996

14. Schroeder, F. Molecular Membrane Biology 12(1):113-119. 1995

15. Subbarao, K. J. Neurochemistry 55(1):342-345. 1990

16. Sugawa, M. Brain Research 761:165-172. 1997

17. Tayarani, I. J. Neurochemistry 48(5):1399-1402. 1987

18. Urano, S. Biofactors 7(1-2):103-112. 1998

19. Vatassery, G. Lipids 32(8):879-886. 1997

20. Wood, W. Brain Research 683(1):36-42. 1995

4-11

1. Kondo, T. Neuroscience Letters 215(2):103-106. 1996

2. Leestma, J. Archives of Neurology 41(2):147-152. 1984

3. Moseley, J. Archives of Pathology & Laboratory Medicine 100(2):61-64. 1976

4. Towbin, A. Human Pathology 4(4):583-594. 1973

5. Walker, A. J. Neuropathology & Experimental Neurology 34(4):295-323. 1975

4-12

1. Andersson, M. Mechanisms of Ageing & Development 85(1):1-14. 1995

2. Barness, L. American J. Medical Genetics 50(4):353-354. 1994

3. Darmady, J. British Medical J. 2(815):685-688. 1972

4. Dehouck, B. J. Cell Biology 126(2):465-473. 1994

5. Dehouck, B. J. Cell Biology 138(4):877-889. 1997

6. Duhamel-Clerin, E. Glia 11(1):35-46. 1994

7. Edmond, J. J. Nutrition 121(9):1323-1330. 1991

8. Fabrizi, C. Brain Research 776(1-2):154-161. 1997

9. Horrocks, L. in Handbook of Neurochemistry, Second Edition, pgs 1-12. (ed by Lajtha, A.). Publ by Plenum Press. 1983

10. Jung-Testas, I. J. Steroid Biochemistry & Molecular Biology 42(6):597-605. 1992

11. Jurevics, H. J. Neurochemistry 64:895-901. 1995

12. Jurevics, H. J. Lipid Research 38(4):723-733. 1997

13. Kabara, J. J. American Oil Chemists' Society 42(12):1003-1008. 1965

14. Kabara, J. Progress in Brain Research 40(0):363-382. 1973

15. Kim, S. Laboratory Investigation 32(6):720-728. 1975

16. Kobayashi, K. Acta Medica Okayama 50(2):67-72. 1996

17. Koper, J. Biochimica et Biophysica Acta 796(1):20-26. 1984

18. Lucarelli, M. FEBS Letters 401(1):53-58. 1997

19. Meresse, S. J. Neurochemistry 53(2):340-345. 1989

20. Morell, P. Neurochemical Research 21(4):463-470. 1996

21. Ness, G. Lipids 14(5):447-450. 1979

22. Ness, G. American J. Medical Genetics 50(4):355-357. 1994

23. Nygren, C. British J. Neurosurgery 11(3):216-220. 1997

24. Osanai, T. Neurochemical Research 9(10):1407-1416. 1984

25. Pardridge, W. J. Neurochemistry 34(2):463-466. 1980

26. Plotz, E. American J. Obstetrics & Gynecology 101(4):534-538. 1968

27. Poirier, J. Neuroscience 55(1):81-90. 1993

28. Potter, J. Australian & New Zealand J. Medicine 7(2):155-160. 1977

29. Ramsey, R. Advances in Lipid Research 10:143-232. 1972

30. Roeder, L. J. Neuroscience Research 8(4):671-682. 1982

31. Roux, F. J. Neuropathology & Experimental Neurology 48(4):437-447. 1989

32. Schoknecht, P. J. Nutrition 124(2):305-314. 1994

33. Serougne-Gautheron, C. Biochimica et Biophysica Acta 316(2):244-250. 1973

34. Serougne, C. Experimental Neurology 44(1):1-9. 1974

35. Serougne, C. Experimental Neurology 51(1):229-240. 1976

36. Shah, S. J. Neurochemistry 50(5):1529-1536. 1988

37. Shibata, S. Neurologia Medico-Chirurgica 30(4):242-245. 1990

38. Smith, M. J. American Oil Chemists' Society 42:1013-1018. 1965

39. Sparks, D. Neuroscience Letters 187(2):142-144. 1995

40. Spohn, M. J. Lipid Research 13(5):563-570. 1972

41. Turley, S. J. Lipid Research 37(9):1953-1961. 1996

42. Van Biervliet, J. J. Pediatrics 120(4 Pt 2):s101-108. 1992

4-13

1. Bergstresser, P. British J. Dermatology 96(5):503-509. 1977

2. Bjorkhem, I. J. Biological Chemistry 272(48):30178-30184. 1997

3. Dell, R. J. Lipid Research 26(3):327-337. 1985

4. Dhopeshwarkar, G. Lipids 16(5):389-392. 1981

5. Diczfalusy, U. Scandinavian J. Clinical & Laboratory Investigation-Suppl 226:9-17. 1996

6. Iizuka, H. J. Dermatological Science 8(3):215-217. 1994

7. Lutiohann, D. Proceedings/America 93(18):9799-9804. 1996

8. Nicholas, H. Lipids 29(9):611-617. 1994

9. Ramsey, R. Lipids 17(3):263-267. 1982

4-14

1. Goldstein, S. J. American Geriatrics Society 33(9):579-584. 1985

2. Ito, M. British J. Radiology 54(641):384-390. 1981

3. McEwen, B. Molecular Psychiatry 2(3):255-262. 1997

4. Takeda, S. J. American Geriatrics Society 32(7):520-524. 1984

5. Takeda, S. Tohoku J. Experimental Medicine 144(4):361-367. 1984

Chapter 5

5-1

1. Akama, K. Proceedings of the National Academy of Sciences of the United States of America 95(10):5795-5800. 1998

2. Akiyama, H. Tohoku J. Experimental Medicine 174(3):295-303. 1994

3. Arispe, N. Molecular & Cellular Biochemistry 140(2):119-125. 1994

4. Avdulov, N. J. Neurochemistry 68(5):2086-2091. 1997

5. Behl, C. Brain Research 645(1-2):253-264. 1994

6. Behl, C. J. Neural Transmission. Suppl 49:125-134. 1997

7.   Blanc, E. J. Neurochemistry 68(5):1870-1881. 1997

8.   Blanchard, B. Brain Research 776(1-2):40-50. 1997

9.   Busciglio, J. Neuron 14(4):879-888. 1995

10. Dickson, D. J. Neuropathology & Experimental Neurology 56(4):321-339. 1997

11. Garcia-Garcia, M. Nephrology, Dialysis, Transplantation 12(6):1192-1198. 1997

12. Good, T. Biochemical & Biophysical Research Communications 201(1):209-215. 1995

13. Gouin-Charnet, A. Biochemical & Biophysical Research Communications 231(1):48-51. 1997

14. Hoshi, M. Proceedings/America 93(7):2719-2723. 1996

15. Hu, J. Brain Research 785(2):195-206. 1998

16. Iwamoto, N. Acta Neuropathologie 93:334-340. 1997

17. Hartmann, H. Biochemical & Biophysical Research Communications 194(3):1216-1220. 1993

18. Hartmann, H. Life Sciences 55(25-26):2011-2018. 1994

19. Klegeris, A. Biochemical & Biophysical Research Communications 199(2):984-991. 1994

20. Lassmann, H. Annals of the New York Academy of Sciences 695:59-64. 1993

21. Lorenzo, A. Annals of the New York Academy of Sciences 777:89-95. 1996

22. Mark, R. J. Neuroscience 15(9):6239-6249. 1995

23. Mark, R. Molecular Neurobiology 12(3):211-224. 1996

24. Mark, R. J. Neuroscience 17(3):1046-1054. 1997

25. Mattson, M. J, Neuroscience 12(2):376-389. 1992

26. Mattson, M. Brain Research 676(1):219-224. 1995

27. Meier-Ruge, W. Annals of the New York Academy of Sciences 826:229-241. 1997

28. Miyakawa, T. Annals of Medicine 21(2):99-102. 1989

29. Parpura-Gill, A. Brain Research 754:65-71. 1997

30. Perlmutter, L. Microscopy Research & Technique 28(3):204-215. 1994

31. Pike, C. J. Neuroscience 13(4):1676-1687. 1993

32. Pike, C. J. Neurochemistry 69:1601-1611. 1997

33. Qiu, W. J. Biological Chemistry 272(10):6641-6646. 1997

34. Rhee, S. J. Biological Chemistry 273(22):13379-13382. 1998

35. Sanderson, K. Brain Research 744(1):7-14. 1997

36. Schultz, J. Neuroscience Letters 175(1-2):99-102. 1994

37. Sheng, J. J. Neuropathology & Experimental Neurology 57(7):714-717. 1998

38. Smith, M. J. Neurochemistry 70(5):2212-2215. 1998

39. Tan, S. Histopathology 25(5):403-414. 1994

40. Ueda, K. J. Neurochemistry 68(1):265-271. 1997

41. Wu, A. Neuroscience 80(3):675-684. 1997

42. Ye, C. J. Neuroscience Research 47(5):547-554. 1997

43. Zhou, Y. J. Neurochemistry 67(4):1419-1425. 1996

5-2

1.   Banati, R. Glia 9(3):199-210. 1993

2. Bellotti, V. Nephrology, Dialysis, Transplantation. 11 Suppl 9:53-62. 1996
3. Garcia-Ladona, F. J. Neuroscience Research 50(1):50-61. 1997
4. LeBlanc, A. J. Neurochemistry 66:2300-2310. 1996
5. Mark, R. Molecular Neurobiology 12(3):211-224. 1996
6. Schubert, W. Brain Research 563(1-2):184-194. 1991
7. Shinkai, Y. Annals of Neurology 42(6):899-908. 1997

5-3

1. Bush, A. J. Biological Chemistry 265(26):15977-15983. 1990
2. Chen, M. Biochemical & Biophysical Research Communications 213(1):96-103. 1995
3. Chugh, K. Postgraduate Medical J. 57(663):31-35. 1981
4. Davies, T. J. Laboratory & Clinical Medicine 130(1):21-32. 1997
5. Gardella, J. Biochemical & Biophysical Research Communications 173(3):1292-1298. 1990
6. Gardella, J. Laboratory Investigation 67(3):303-313. 1992
7. Li, Q. Blood 84(1):133-142. 1994
8. Li, Q. Laboratory Investigation 78(4):461-469. 1998
9. Maness,L. Life Sciences 55(21):1643-1650. 1994
10. Miyakawa, T. Annals of the New York Academy of Sciences 826:25-34. 1997
11. Rosenberg, R. Archives of Neurology 54(2):139-144. 1997
12. Rosenthal, C. J. Clinical Investigation 55(4):746-753. 1975
13. Schlossmacher, M. Neurobiology of Aging 13(3):421-434. 1992
14. Smith, C. Neuroscience Letters 235(3):157-159. 1997
15. Van Nostrand, W. Science 248(4956):745-748. 1990
16. Whyte, S. Annals of Neurology 41(1):121-124. 1997

5-4

1. Alonso, A. Nature Medicine 2(7):783-787. 1996
2. Braak, E. Acta Neuropathologica 87(6):554-567. 1994
3. Arai, H. J. American Geriatrics Society 45:1228-1231. 1997
4. Holzer, M. Neuroscience 63(2):499-516. 1994
5. Hoshi, M. Proceedings/America 93(7):2719-2723. 1996
6. Igbal, K. International Psychogeriatrics. 9 Suppl 1:289-296. 1997
7. Imahori, K. J. Biochemistry 121(2):179-188. 1997
8. Latimer, D. FEBS Letters 365(1):42-46. 1995
9. Morishima, M. Dementia 5(5):282-288. 1994
10. Pei, J. J. Neuropathology & Experimental Neurology 56(1):70-78. 1997

5-5

1. Arriagada, P. Neurology 42(3 Pt 1):631-639. 1992
2. Bancher, C. J. Neural Transmission. Suppl 50:141-152. 1997
3. Berg, L. Archives of Neurology 55:326-335. 1998
4. Bierer,L. Archives of Neurology 52(1):81-88. 1995
5. Blennow, K. J. Neural Transmission 103:603-618. 1996
6. Bobinski, M. Neurobiology of Aging 17(6):909-919. 1996

7. Braak, H. Neurobiology of Aging 18(4 Suppl):s85-88. 1997

8. Cras, P. Proceedings/America 88(17):7552-7556. 1991

9. Cummings, B. Neurobiology of Aging 17(6):921-933. 1996

10. Fowler, C. Gerontology 43:132-142. 1997

11. Geula, C. J. Neuropathology & Experimental Neurology 57(1):63-75. 1998

12. Giannakopoulos, P. Acta Neuropathologica 85(6):602-610. 1993

13. Giannakopoulos, P. Dementia 5(6):348-356. 1994

14. Giannakopoulos, P. Progress in Neuro-Psychopharmacology & Biological Psychiatry 19(4):577-592. 1995

15. Giannakopoulos P. Archives of Neurology 52(12):1150-1159. 1995

16. Gomez-Isla, T. Annals of Neurology 41(1):17-24. 1997

17. Hansen, L. Neurobiology of Aging 18(4 Suppl):s71-73. 1997

18. Hatanpaa, K. Annals of Neurology 40:411-420. 1996

19. Hardy, J. Trends in Pharmacological Sciences 12(10):383-388. 1991

20. Hyman, B. Neurobiology of Aging 18(4 Suppl):s27-32. 1997

21. Lue, L. J. Neuropathology & Experimental Neurology 55(10):1083-1088. 1996

22. Mackenzie, I. Neurology 46(2):425-429. 1996

23. Markesbery, W. Neurobiology of Aging 18(4 Suppl):s13-19. 1997

24. Martin, L. American J. Pathology 145(6):1358-1381. 1994

25. Masliah, E. American J. Pathology 137(6):1293-1297. 1990

26. Mirra, S. Neurobiology of Aging 18(4 Suppl):s91-94. 1997

27. Mukaetova-Ladinska, E. Dementia and Geriatric Cognitive Disorders 8(5):288-295. 1997

28. Onorato, M. Progress in Clinical & Biological Research 317:781-789. 1989

29. Price, J. Neurobiology of Aging 18(4 Suppl):s67-70. 1997

30. Rosenblum, W. J. Neuropathology & Experimental Neurology 56:213. 1997

31. Roses, A. J. Neuropathology & Experimental Neurology 53(5):429-437. 1994

32. Selkoe, D. J. Neuropathology & Experimental Neurology 53(5):438-447. 1994

33. Shinkai, Y. Annals of Neurology 42(6):899-908. 1997

34. Snowdon, D. Gerontologist 37(2):150-156. 1997

35. Spillantini, M. Acta Neuropathologica 92(1):42-48. 1996

36. Tabaton, M. Annals of Neurology 26(6):771-778. 1989

37. Terry, R. J. Neuropathology & Experimental Neurology 55(10):1023-1025. 1996

38. Terry, R. Annals of Neurology 41:7. 1997

39. Troncoso, J. J. Neuropathology & Experimental Neurology 55(11):1134-1142. 1996

5-6

1. Citron, M. Nature Medicine 3(1):67-72. 1997

2. Clark, R. Cold Spring Harbor Symposia on Quantitative Biology 61:551-558. 1996

3. De Strooper, B. J. Biological Chemistry 272(6):3590-3598. 1997

4. De Strooper, B. Nature 391(6665):387-390. 1998

5. Frangione, B. Ciba Foundation Symposium 199:132-141. 1996

6. Iwatsubo, T. Neurobiology of Aging 19(1 Suppl):s11-13. 1998

7. Lippa, C. Neurology 46(2):406-412. 1996
8. Mann, D. Annals of Neurology 40:149-156. 1996
9. Mattson, M. J. Neurochemistry 70(1):1-14. 1998
10. Pericak-Vance, M. JAMA 278(15):1237-1241. 1997
11. Podlisny, M. Science 238(4827):669-671. 1987
12. Rosenberg, R. JAMA 278(15):1282-1283. 1997
13. St. George-Hyslop, P. Science 238(4827):664-666. 1987
14. Scheuner, D. Nature Medicine 2(8):864-869. 1996
15. Tanzi, R. Nature 329(6135):156-157. 1987
16. Tanzi, R. Neurobiology of Disease 3(3):159-168. 1996
17. Van Broeckhoven, C. Nature 329(6135):153-155. 1987
18. Walter, J. Molecular Medicine 2(6):673-691. 1996
19. Wasco, W. Annals of the New York Academy of Sciences 695:203-208. 1993
20. Xia, W. Proceedings/America 94(15):8208-8213. 1997

5-7

1. Bouras, C. Neuroscience Letters 153(2):131-135. 1993
2. Bouras, C. Cerebral Cortex 4(2):138-150. 1994
3. Delaere, P. Neurobiology of Aging 14(2):191-194. 1993
4. Giannakopoulos, P. Acta Neuropathologica 87(5):456-468. 1994
5. Giannakopoulos, P. Archives of Neurology 52(12):1150-1159. 1995
6. Giannakopoulos, P. J. Neuropathology & Experimental Neurology 55(12):1210-1220. 1996
7. Hauw, J. Revue Neurologique 142(2):107-115. 1986
8. Hof, P. J. American Geriatrics Society 44(7):857-864. 1996
9. Hof, P. Histology & Histopathology 11(4):1075-1088. 1996
10. Kyle, R. Medicine 54(4):271-299. 1975
11. Mizutani, T. J. Neurological Sciences 108(2):168-177. 1992
12. Morris, J. Neurology 46:707-719. 1996
13. Terry, R. Annals of Neurology 10(2):184-192. 1981
14. Yasha, T. Indian J. Medical Research 105:141-150. 1997

5-8

1. Bornebroek, M. Brain Pathology 6(2):111-114. 1996
2. Cohen, D. Annals of the New York Academy of Sciences 826:390-395. 1997
3. Feldmann, E. Clinics in Geriatric Medicine 7(3):617-630. 1991
4. Ferreiro, J. J. Neurology 236(5):267-272. 1989
5. Gilles, C. Neurology 34(6):730-735. 1984
6. Greenberg, S. Neurology 43(10):2073-2079. 1993
7. Greenberg, S. Annals of Neurology 38(3):254-259. 1995
8. Itoh, Y. Stroke 27(2):216-218. 1996
9. Iwamoto, N. Acta Neuropathologica 86(5):418-421. 1993
10. Kalaria, R. Annals of the New York Academy of Sciences 826:263-271. 1997
11. Leblanc, R. Neurosurgery 29(5):712-718. 1991

12. Levy, E. Science 248(4959):1124-1126. 1990
13. Maat-Schieman, M. Acta Neuropathologica 88(4):371-378. 1994
14. Maat-Schieman, M. J. Neuropathology & Experimental Neurology 56(3):273-284. 1997
15. Mandybur, T. Neurology 29(10):1336-1340. 1979
16. Premkumar, D. American J. Pathology 148(6):2083-2095. 1996
17. Roos, R. Annals of the New York Academy of Sciences 640:155-160. 1991
18. Tagliavini,F. Acta Neuropathologica 85(3):267-271. 1993
19. Thomas, R. Archives of Internal Medicine 157(6):605-617. 1997
20. Urmoneit, B. Laboratory Investigation 77(2):157-166. 1997
21. Van Duinen, S. Proceedings/America 84(16):5991-5994. 1987
22. Wattendorff, A. J. Neurological Sciences 55(2):121-135. 1982
23. Wisniewski, H. Annals of the New York Academy of Sciences 826:161-172. 1997

5-9

1. Biere, A. J. Biological Chemistry 271(51):32916-32922. 1996
2. Koudinov, A. Biochemical & Biophysical Research Communications 205(2):1164-1171. 1994
3. Koudinov, A. Clinica Chimica Acta 270(2):75-84. 1998
4. Mackic, J. J. Clinical Investigation 102(4):734-743. 1998.
5. Poduslo, J. Neurobiology of Disease 4(1):27-34. 1997

5-10

1. Alafuzoff, I. Acta Neuropathologica 73(2):160-166. 1987
2. Burns, E. Advances in Neurology 30:301-306. 1981
3. Caserta, M. J. Neuropsychiatry & Clinical Neurosciences 10(1):78-84. 1998
4. Claudio, L. Acta Neuropathologica 91(1):6-14. 1996
5. Elovaara, I. J. Neurological Sciences 70(1):73-80. 1985
6. Kalaria, R. Brain Research 516(2):349-353. 1990
7. Kalaria, R. Cerebrovascular & Brain Metabolism Reviews 4(3):226-260. 1992
8. Kalaria,R. Annals of the New York Academy of Sciences 826:263-271. 1997
9. Maness, L. Life Sciences 55(21):1643-1650. 1994
10. Mooradian, A. Neurobiology of Aging 9(1):31-39. 1988
11. Mooradian, A. Brain Research 609(1-2):41-44. 1993
12. Munoz, D. Annals of the New York Academy of Sciences 826:173-189. 1997
13. Perlmutter, L. J. Comparative Neurology 352(1):92-105. 1995
14. Pluta, R. Neuroreport 7(7):1261-1265. 1996
15. Stewart, P. Microvascular Research 33(2):270-282. 1987
16. Stewart, P. Laboratory Investigation 67(6):734-742. 1992
17. Saito, Y. Proceedings/America 92(22):10227-10231. 1995
18. Vinters, H. Ultrastructural Pathology 18(3):333-348. 1994
19. Wahler, J. Hepatology 17(6):1103-1108. 1993
20. Wisniewski, H. Annals of the New York Academy of Sciences 826:161-172. 1997

21. Zlokovic, B. Biochemical & Biophysical Research Communications 197(3):1034-1040. 1993

Chapter 6

6-1

1. Barrett- Connor, E. J. American Geriatrics Society 44(10):1147-1152. 1996
2. Cronin-Stubbs, D. BMJ 314:178-179. 1997
3. Donaldson, K. J. American Geriatrics Society 44(10):1232-1234. 1996
4. Du, W. J. Geriatric Psychiatry & Neurology 6(1):34-38. 1993
5. Ferrara, A. Circulation 96(1):37-43. 1997
6. Franklin, C. J. American Dietetic Association 89(6):790-792. 1989
7. Gray, G. J. American Dietetic Association 89(12):1795-1802. 1989
8. Grundman, M. Neurology 46(6):1585-1591. 1996
9. Gustafson, D. Archives Internal Medicine 163(13):1524-1528. 2003
10. Knittweis, J. J. American Geriatrics Society 46(4):540-541. 1998
11. Kyle, R. Medicine 54(4):271-299. 1975
12. Paganini-Hill, A. American J. Epidemiology 140(3):256-261. 1994
13. Poehlman, E. Neurology 48(4):997-1002. 1997
14. Potter, J. J. Gerontology 43(3):m59-63. 1988
15. Priefer, B. Dysphagia 12(4):212-221. 1997
16. Renvall, M. J. American Dietetic Association 93(1):47-52. 1993
17. Sandman, P. J. American Geriatrics Society 35(1):31-38. 1987
18. Scobie, I. BMJ 316:707. 1998
19. Singh, S. Age & Ageing 17(1):21-28. 1988
20. Skullerud, K. Acta Neurologica Scandinavica. Suppl 102:1-94. 1985
21. Smith, G. Neuropsychiatry, Neuropsychology, & Behavioral Neurology 11(2):97-102. 1998
22. Tavares, A. Zeitschrift Fur Alternsforschung 42(3):165-167. 1987
23. Tully, C. J. American Geriatrics Society 43(12):1394-1397. 1995
24. White, H. J. American Geriatrics Society 44(3):265-272. 1996
25. White, H. J. American Geriatrics Society 46(10):1223-1227. 1998
26. Winograd, C. Alzheimer Disease & Associated Disorders 5(3):173-180. 1991
27. Wolf-Klein, G. International Psychogeriatrics 4(1):103-118. 1992
28. Wolf-Klein, G. International Psychogeriatrics 6(2):135-142. 1994

6-2

1. Doty, R. Science 226(4681):1441-1443. 1984
2. Hyman, B. Annals of the New York Academy of Sciences 640:14-19. 1991
3. Schiffman, S. JAMA 278(16):1357-1362. 1997
4. Ship, J. J. Gerontology 51a(2):m86-91. 1996
5. Yamagishi, M. Annals of Otology, Rhinology & Laryngology 103(6):421-427. 1994
6. Yamagishi, M. Annals of Otology, Rhinology & Laryngology 107(5 Pt 1):421-426. 1998

6-3

1. Abbasi, A. J. American Geriatrics Society 41(2):117-121. 1993
2. Baumgartner, R. J. Gerontology 50a(6):m307-316. 1995
3. Bernard, M. J. Nutrition for the Elderly 14(2-3):55-67. 1995
4. Bianchetti, A. J. American Geriatrics Society 38(5):521-526. 1990
5. Brownell, K. Archives of Internal Medicine 141(9):1142-1146. 1981
6. Buckler, D. J. American Geriatrics Society 42(10):1100-1102. 1994
7. Cefalu, C. American Family Physician, issue Sept 15,1995, pg 1105
8. Chandra, V. Neurology 36(2):209-211. 1986
9. Clevidence, B. American J. Clinical Nutrition 55(3):689-694. 1992
10. Curb, J. J. American Geriatrics Society 34(11):773-780. 1986
11. Ettinger, W. Circulation 86(3):858-869. 1992
12. Ettinger, W. Coronary Artery Disease 4(10):854-859. 1993
13. Ferrara, A. Circulation 96(1):37-43. 1997
14. Fischer, J. J. American Dietetic Association 90(12):1697-1706. 1990
15. Frishman, W. Annals of Epidemiology 2(1-2):43-50. 1992
16. Garry, P. American J. Clinical Nutrition 55(3):682-688. 1992
17. Grant, M. J. American Geriatrics Society 44(1):31-36. 1996
18. Groom, D. J. Gerontological Nursing 19(6):12-16. 1993
19. Heiss, G. Circulation 61(2):302-315. 1980
20. Kannel, W. American J. Cardiology 76(9):69c-77c. 1995
21. Kayser-Jones, J. American J. Alzheimer's Disease, Mar/Apr 1997 issue, pg 67-71
22. Keller, H. J. American Geriatrics Society 43:165-169. 1995
23. Lamon-Fava, S. American J. Clinical Nutrition 59(1):32-41. 1994
24. Lipschitz, D. Seminars in Dermatology 10(4):273-281. 1991
25. Lowik, M. J. American College of Nutrition 11(6):673-681. 1992
26. Maaravi, Y. Israel J. Medical Sciences 32(8):620-625. 1996
27. Mattila, K. Scandinavian J. Clinical & Laboratory Investigation 46(2):131-136. 1986
28. Miller, D. J. American Geriatrics Society 39(5):462-466. 1991
29. Mitchell, C. American J. Clinical Nutrition 35(2):398-406. 1982
30. Mookhoek, E. Tijdschrift voor Gerontologie en Geriatrie 23(4):127-131. 1992
31. Morgan, D. Human Nutrition-Clinical Nutrition 36(6):439-448. 1982
32. Morley, J. Annals of Internal Medicine 109(11):890-904. 1988
33. Morley, J. J. American Geriatrics Society 42(6):583-585. 1994
34. Morley, J. Annals of Internal Medicine 123(11):850-859. 1995
35. Morley, J. Drugs & Aging 8(2):134-155. 1996
36. Morley, J. American J, Clinical Nutrition 66(4):760-773. 1997
37. Mowe, M. American J. Clinical Nutrition 59(2):317-324. 1994
38. Mowe, M. Nutrition Reviews 54(1 Pt 2):s22-24. 1996
39. Muls, E. International J. Obesity & Related Metabolic Disorders 17(12):711-716. 1993
40. Newschaffer,C. American J. Epidemiology 136(1):23-34. 1992
41. Nguyen, P. Blood Pressure Suppl 3:26-30. 1995

42. Ritchie, C. American J. Clinical Nutrition 66:815-818. 1997
43. Shay, K. J. American Geriatrics Society 43:1414-1422. 1995
44. Sullivan D. J. Parenteral & Enteral Nutrition 13(3):249-254. 1989
45. Sullivan D. American J. Clinical Nutrition 53:599-605. 1991
46. Sullivan, D. J. American Geriatrics Society 43:507-512. 1995
47. Tayback, M. Archives of Internal Medicine 150(5):1065-1072. 1990
48. Thompson, M. J. American Geriatrics Society 39:497-500. 1991
49. Tully, C. J. American Geriatrics Society 43:1394-1397. 1995
50. Vellas, B. Nutrition 13(6):515-519. 1997
51. Wallace, J. J. American Geriatrics Society 43:329-337. 1995
52. Wallace, R. Annals of Epidemiology 2(1-2):15-21. 1992
53. Weijenberg, M. American J. Public Health 86(6):798-803. 1996
54. Willard, M. JAMA 243(17):1720-1722. 1980
55. Wilson, P. J. Gerontology 49(6):m252-257. 1994
56. Wing, R. American J. Clinical Nutrition 55(6):1086-1092. 1992
57. Woo, J. J. Clinical Pathology 42(12):1241-1245. 1989
58. Zimmerman, J. Arteriosclerosis 4(2):115-123. 1984

6-4

1. Anderson, K. JAMA 257(16):2176-2180. 1987
2. Baggio, G. FASEB J. 12(6):433-437. 1998
3. Casiglia, E. European J. Epidemiology 9(6):577-586. 1993
4. Chan, Y. J. American College of Nutrition 16(3):229-235. 1997
5. Dontas, A. J. Aging and Health 8(2):220-237. 1996
6. Emond, M. J. Womens Health 6(3):295-307. 1997
7. Forette, B. Lancet 1(8643):868-870. 1989
8. Grant, M. J. American Geriatrics Society 44:31-36. 1996
9. Harris, T. J. Clinical Epidemiology 45(6):595-601. 1992
10. Higgins, M. Annals of Epidemiology 2(1-2):69-76. 1992
11. Hirose, N. Japanese J. Geriatrics 34(4):324-330. 1997
12. Hulley, S. JAMA 272(17):1372-1374. 1994
13. Ives, D. J. Gerontology 48(3):m103-107. 1993
14. Jacobsen, S. J. Clinical Epidemiology 45(10):1053-1059. 1992
15. Kronmal, R. Archives of Internal Medicine 153(9):1065-1073. 1993
16. Krumholz,H. JAMA 272(17):1335-1340. 1994
17. Krumholz, H. JAMA 275(2):110-111. 1996
18. Lammi, U. Acta Psychiatrica Scandinavica 80(5):459-468. 1989
19. Morgan, R. Lancet 341(8837):75-79. 1993
20. Osterlind, P. Gerontology 30(4):247-252. 1984
21. Paolisso, G. American J. Clinical Nutrition 62(4):746-750. 1995
22. Rudman, D. J. American Geriatrics Society 35(6):496-502. 1987
23. Schaefer, E. Metabolism: Clinical & Experimental 38(4):293-296. 1989
24. Tietz, N. Clinical Chemistry 38(6):1167-1185. 1992

25. Yoshimura, A. J. Cardiology 25(3):113-118. 1995

6-5 —None

6-6

1. Albini, A. Collagen & Related Research 8(1):23-37. 1988
2. Ashcroft, G. J. Pathology 183(2):169-176. 1997
3. Gerstein, A. Dermatologic Clinics 11(4):749-757. 1993
4. Holt, D. Surgery 112(2):293-297. 1992
5. Katzman, R. Archives of Neurology 54:1201-1205. 1997
6. Mo, J. Mechanisms of Ageing & Development 81(2-3):73-82. 1995
7. Ravindranath, V. Neuroscience Letters 101(2):187-190. 1989
8. Uitto, J. Dermatologic Clinics 4(3):433-446. 1986

Chapter 7

7-1

1. Andersson, B. Acta Medica Scandinavica 223(6):485-490. 1988
2. Bajaj, J. Metabolism: Clinical & Experimental 28(5):594-598. 1979
3. Beer, S. J. Endocrinology 120(2):337-350. 1989
4. Behl, C. Endocrinology 138(1):101-106. 1997
5. Beitins, I. J. Clinical Endocrinology & Metabolism 60(6):1120-1126. 1985
6. Bergendahl, M. J. Clinical Endocrinology & Metabolism 81(2):692-699. 1996
7. Bondareff, W. Alzheimer Disease & Associated Disorders 1(4):256-262. 1987
8. Boyd, G. J. Steroid Biochemistry 19(1c):1017-1027. 1983
9. Boyle, P. American J. Physiology 256(5 Pt 1):e651-661. 1989
10. Broocks, A. J. Neural Transmission-General Section 79(1-2):113-124. 1990
11. Cella, L. American J. Physiology 269(5 Pt 1):e878-883. 1995
12. Davis, B. J. American Geriatrics Society 33(11):741-748. 1985
13. Davis, K. American J. Psychiatry 143(3):300-305. 1986
14. De Leon, M. Lancet 2(8607):391-392. 1988
15. Drott, C. Annals of Surgery 208(5):645-650. 1988
16. Elrod, R. American J. Psychiatry 154(1):25-30. 1997
17. Endo, Y. Neuroscience 79(3):745-752. 1997
18. Engelborghs, S. Acta Neurologica Belgica 97(2):67-84. 1997
19. Fichter, M. Psychiatry Research 17(1):61-72. 1986
20. Franceschi, M. J. Neurology, Neurosurgery & Psychiatry 54(9):836-837. 1991
21. Garruti, G. International J. Obesity & Related Metabolic Disorders 19(1):46-49. 1995
22. Gotoh, M. Brain Research 706(2):351-354. 1996
23. Gross, H. J. Clinical Endocrinology & Metabolism 49(6):805-809. 1979
24. Gurevich, D. Progress in Neuro-Psychopharmacology & Biological Psychiatry 14(3):297-308. 1990
25. Hartmann, A. Neurobiology of Aging 18(3):285-289. 1997
26. Hatzinger, M. Neurobiology of Aging 16(2):205-209. 1995
27. Ho, K. International J. Chronobiology 6(1):39-50. 1979

28. Ichimiya, Y. Acta Neuropathologica 70(2):112-116. 1986

29. Jones, P. American J. Clinical Nutrition 66:438-446. 1997

30. Lambeth, J. in Lipoprotein and Cholesterol Metabolism in Steroidogenic Tissues (ed by Strauss,J. and Menon, K.). Pgs beginning 237. Publ by George Stickley Company, 1985

31. Lawlor, B. American J. Psychiatry 149(4):546-548. 1992

32. Leiter, L. American J, Physiology 247(2 Pt 1):e190-197. 1984

33. Lupien, S. J. Neuroscience 14(5 Pt 1):2893-2903. 1994

34. Malozowski, S. Clinical Endocrinology 32(4):461-465. 1990

35. Mandal, S. Indian J. Physiology & Pharmacology 29(4):255-258. 1985

36. Marniemi, J. European J. Applied Physiology & Occupational Physiology 53(2):121-127. 1984

37. Martignoni, E. Acta Neurologica Scandinavica 81(5):452-456. 1990

38. Masugi, F. Methods & Findings in Experimental & Clinical Pharmacology 11(11):707-710. 1989

39. Miller, H. American J. Psychiatry 151(2):267-270. 1994

40. Mortaud, S. Behavior Genetics 26(4):367-372. 1996

41. Nasman, B. Biological Psychiatry 39(5):311-318. 1996

42. Nieman, D. J. Applied Physiology 63(6):2502-2509. 1987

43. O'Brien, J. Psychological Medicine 26(1):7-14. 1996

44. O'Brien, J. British J. Psychiatry 168(6):679-687. 1996

45. Olusi, S. Clinica Chimica Acta 74(3):261-269. 1977

46. Peskind, E. Biological Psychiatry 40(1):61-68. 1996

47. Pirke, K. Acta Endocrinologica 100(2):168-176. 1982

48. Pirke, K. Neuroscience & Biobehavioral Reviews 17(3):287-294. 1993

49. Pirke, K. Psychiatry Research 62(1):43-49. 1996

50. Raskind, M. Archives of General Psychiatry 41(4):343-346. 1984

51. Reinikainen, K. J. Neuroscience Research 27(4):576-586. 1990

52. Sapolsky, R. J. Neuroscience 6(8):2240-2244. 1986

53. Seckl, J. Brain Research. Molecular Brain Research 18(3):239-245. 1993

54. Smith, S. J. Clinical Endocrinology & Metabolism 40(1):43-52. 1975

55. Storga, D. Neuroscience Letters 203(1):29-32. 1996

56. Swanwick, G. Biological Psychiatry 39(11):976-978. 1996

57. Swanwick, G. American J. Psychiatry 155(2):286-289. 1998

58. Tejani-Butt, S. Brain Research 631(1):147-150. 1993

59. Titov, V. Voprosy Meditsinskoi Khimii 28(4):38-42. 1982

60. Van Binsbergen, C.Psychosomatic Medicine 53(4):440-452. 1991

61. Van Cauter, E. J. Clinical Endocrinology & Metabolism 81(7):2468-2473. 1996

62. Webber, J. British J. Nutrition 71(3):437-447. 1994

63. Weiner, M. Biological Psychiatry 42(11):1030-1038. 1997

7-2

1. Adolfsson, R. Acta Medica Scandinavica 208(5):387-388. 1980

2. Bajaj, J. Metabolism: Clinical & Experimental 28(5):594-598. 1979

3. Blanc, E. J. Neurochemistry 68(5):1870-1881. 1997

4. Blesa, R. Dementia 7(5):239-245. 1996

5. Boyle, P. American J, Physiology 256(5 Pt 1):e651-661. 1989

6. Bucht, G. Acta Medica Scandinavica 213(5):387-392. 1983

7. Cheng, B. Experimental Neurology 117(2):114-123. 1992

8. Clotet, J. European J. Biochemistry 229(1):207-214. 1995

9. Cohen, P. Biochimica et Biophysica Acta 1094(3):292-299. 1991

10. Copani, A. Neuroreport 2(12):763-765. 1991

11. Craft, S. Neurobiology of Aging 17(1):123-130. 1996

12. Cryer, P. J. Internal Medicine. Suppl 735:31-39. 1991

13. Delvenne, V. J. Affective Disorders 44(1):69-77. 1997

14. Ferrigno, P. Molecular Biology of the Cell 4(7):669-677. 1993

15. Hasselbalch, S. J. Cerebral Blood Flow & Metabolism 14(1):125-131. 1994

16. Horner, H. Neuroendocrinology 52(1):57-64. 1990

17. Hoyer, S. J. Neurology 235(3):143-148. 1988

18. Hoyer, S. Annals of the New York Academy of Sciences 777:374-379. 1996

19. Ibanez, V. Neurology 50(6):1585-1593. 1998

20. Itagaki, T. Japanese J. Geriatrics 33(8):569-572. 1996

21. Jagust, W. J. Neuroimaging 6(3):156-160. 1996

22. Kalaria, R. J. Neurochemistry 53(4):1083-1088. 1989

23. Krakower, G. J. Biological Chemistry 256(5):2408-2413. 1981

24. Korol, D. American J. Clinical Nutrition 67(4):764s-771s. 1998

25. Landin, K. J. Internal Medicine 233(4):357-363. 1993

26. Lau, K. Molecular & Cellular Biochemistry 44(3):149-159. 1982

27. Manning, C. Neurobiology of Aging 14(6):523-528. 1993

28. Marcus, D. Annals of Neurology 26(1):91-94. 1989

29. Marcus, D. Annals of the New York Academy of Sciences 826:248-253. 1997

30. Mark, R. J. Neuroscience 17(3):1046-1054. 1997

31. Meier-Ruge, W. Gerontology 40(5):246-252. 1994

32. Peppard, R. J. Neuroscience Research 27(4):561-568. 1990

33. Piert, M. J. Nuclear Medicine 37(2):201-208. 1996

34. Redies, C. American J. Physiology 256(6 Pt 1):e805-810. 1989

35. Serra, D. J. Lipid Research 31(5):919-926. 1990

36. Shi, J. Brain Research 772(1-2):247-251. 1997

37. Smith, M. Lipids 5:665-671. 1970

38. Sorbi, S. Alzheimer Disease & Associated Disorders 9(2):73-77. 1995

39. Sugden, M. Advances in Enzyme Regulation 33:71-95. 1993

40. Swerdlow, R. American J. Medical Sciences 308(3):141-144. 1994

41. Webber, J. British J. Nutrition 71(3):437-447. 1994

42. Welsh, G. Biochemical J. 294(Pt 3):625-629. 1993

43. Winograd, C. Biological Psychiatry 30(5):507-511. 1991

44. Yamaguchi, S. J. Neurology, Neurosurgery & Psychiatry 62(6):596-600. 1997
45. Yasuno, F. Dementia and Geriatric Cognitive Disorders 9(2):63-67. 1998

7-3

1. Borjigin, J. Nature 378(6559):783-785. 1995
2. Cacabelos, R. Methods & Findings in Experimental & Clinical Pharmacology 18(10):693-706. 1996
3. Cooper, J. Aging 4(2):165-169. 1992
4. Corey-Bloom, J. Drugs & Aging 7(2):79-87. 1995
5. D'Amato, R. Annals of Neurology 22(2):229-236. 1987
6. Daniels, W. J. Pineal Research 24(2):78-82. 1998
7. Hasegawa, H. Archives of Histology & Cytology 52 Suppl:69-74. 1989
8. Holmes, M. J. Neuroscience 17(11):4056-4065. 1997
9. Huether, G. European J. Pharmacology 238(2-3):249-254. 1993
10. Joshi, B. Life Sciences 38(17):1573-1580. 1986
11. Kaplan, J. Psychosomatic Medicine 56(6):479-484. 1994
12. Kumar, A. Neuropsychobiology 32(1):9-12. 1995
13. Lawlor, B. Biological Psychiatry 37(12):895-896. 1995
14. Leibowitz, S. Drugs 39 Suppl 3:33-48. 1990
15. Maurizi, C. Medical Hypotheses 45(4):339-340. 1995
16. McEntee, W. Psychopharmacology 103(2):143-149. 1991
17. Pappolla, M. J. Neuroscience 17(5):1683-1690. 1997
18. Reiter, R. J. Neural Transmission. Suppl 21:35-54. 1986
19. Shor-Posner, G. Brain Research Bulletin 17(5):663-671. 1986
20. Skene, D. Brain Research 528(1):170-174. 1990
21. Song, W. J. Molecular Neuroscience 9(2):75-92. 1997
22. Steegmans, P. BMJ 312(7025):221. 1996
23. Tohgi, H. Neuroscience Letters 141(1):9-12. 1992
24. Uchida, K. Brain Research 717(1-2):154-159. 1996
25. Wurtman, R. Obesity Research 3 Suppl 4:477s-480s. 1995

7-4

1. Aisen, P. Gerontology 43(1-2):143-149. 1997
2. Anderson, D. Central Nervous System Trauma 2(4):257-267. 1985
3. Dzenko, K. J. Neuroimmunology 80(1-2):6-12. 1997
4. Ettinger, W. J. American Geriatrics Society 43:264-266. 1995
5. Garbagnati, E. Acta Paediatrica 82(11):948-952. 1993
6. Gordon, B. Critical Care Medicine 24(4):584-589. 1996
7. Jacobs, D. American J. Epidemiology 146(7):558-564. 1997
8. Kunitomo,M. Japanese J. Pharmacology 44(1):15-22. 1987
9. Lindhorst, E. Biochimica et Biophysica Acta 1339(1):143-154. 1997
10. Lopez Martinez, J. Nutricion Hospitalaria 10(1):24-31. 1995
11. McGeer, P. Neurology 47(2):425-432. 1996
12. Nanji, A. Hepatology 26(1):90-97. 1997

13. Read, T. European Heart J. 14 Suppl K:125-129. 1993

14. Reynolds, C. J. Neurochemistry 68(4):1736-1744. 1997

15. Rogers, J. Neurobiology of Aging 17(5):681-686. 1996

16. Stephenson, D. Neurobiology of Disease 3(1):51-63. 1996

7-5

1. Blommaart, E. Histochemical J. 29(5):365-385. 1997

2. Bondareff, W. American J. Pathology 137(3):711-723. 1990

3. Cochran, E. American J. Pathology 139(3):485-489. 1991

4. Dickson, D. Acta Neuropathologica 79(5): 486-493. 1990

5. Dickson, D. Neurobiology of Aging 13(1):179-189. 1992

6. Ding, X. Mineral & Electrolyte Metabolism 23(3-6):194-197. 1997

7. Hampton, R. Proceedings/America 94(24):12944-12948. 1997

8. Igbal, K. International Psychogeriatrics 9 Suppl 1:289-296. 1997

9. Ii, K. J. Neuropathology & Experimental Neurology 56(2):125-131. 1997

10. Master, E. Neuroreport 8(12):2781-2786. 1997

11. Migheli, A. Neuropathology & Applied Neurobiology 18(1):3-11. 1992

12. Morishima, M. Dementia 5(5):282-288. 1994

13. Muller, S. Bioessays 17(8):677-684. 1995

14. Skoog, I. Neurodegeneration 4(4):433-442. 1995

15. Tabaton, M. Neurology 41(3):391-394. 1991

16. Takada, K. Clinical Chemistry 43(7):1188-1195. 1997

17. Wang, G. Brain Research 566(1-2):146-151. 1991

18. Wilkinson, K. Annual Review of Nutrition 15:161-189. 1995

19. Wing, S. Biochemical J. 307(Pt 3):639-645. 1995

7-6

1. Bruhwyler, J. Neuroscience & Biobehavioral Reviews 17(4):373-384. 1993

2. Casino, P. Circulation 88(6):2541-2547. 1993

3. Dorheim, M. Biochemical & Biophysical Research Communications 205(1):659-665. 1994

4. Good, P. American J. Pathology 149(1):21-28. 1996

5. Grammas, P. Annals of the New York Academy of Sciences 826:47-55. 1997

6. John, S. Circulation 98(3):211-216. 1998

7. Knudsen, H. American J. Physiology 273(1 Pt 2):h347-355. 1997

8. Laufs, U. Circulation 97(12):1129-1135. 1998

9. Molina, J. Drugs & Aging 12(4):251-259. 1998

10. Nicotera, P. Advances in Neuroimmunology 5(4):411-420. 1995

11. O'Driscoll, G. Circulation 95(5):1126-1131. 1997

12. Preik, M. J. Cardiovascular Risk 3(5):465-471. 1996

13. Quyyumi, A. Circulation 92(3):320-326. 1995

14. Rossi, F. Biochemical & Biophysical Research Communications 225(2):474-478. 1996

15. Smith, M. J. Neuroscience 17(8):2653-2657. 1997

16. Stroes, E. Cardiovascular Research 36(3):445-452. 1997

17. Tanaka, S. Clinical Cardiology 20(4):361-365. 1997

18. Vodovotz, Y. J. Experimental Medicine 184(4):1425-1433. 1996

19. Weldon, D. Geriatrics 52 Suppl 2:s13-16. 1997

7-7

1. Altstiel, L. Progress in Neuro-Psychopharmacology & Biological Psychiatry 15(4):481-495. 1991

2. Barger, S. Proceedings/America 92(20):9328-9332. 1995

3. Blumberg, D. J. Surgical Oncology 59(4):220-224. 1995

4. Bongioanni, P. J. Neurology 244(7):418-425. 1997

5. Cue, J. Archives of Surgery 129(2):193-197. 1994

6. DeRijk, R. J. Clinical Endocrinology & Metabolism 82(7):2182-2191. 1997

7. Ershler, W. Drugs & Aging 5(5):358-365. 1994

8. Evans, D. American J. Physiology 257(5 Pt 2):r1182-1189. 1989

9. Feingold, K. J. Clinical Investigation 80(1):184-190. 1987

10. Feingold, K. Endocrinology 125(1):267-274. 1989

11. Fillit, H. Neuroscience Letters 129(2):318-320. 1991

12. Forloni, G. Brain Research. Molecular Brain Research 16(1-2):128-134. 1992

13. Gadient, R. Progress in Neurobiology 52(5):379-390. 1997

14. Gershenwald, J. Proceedings/America 87(13):4966-4970. 1990

15. Gordon, B. Critical Care Medicine 24(4):584-589. 1996

16. Griffin, W. Neuroscience Letters 176(2):133-136. 1994

17. Gruol, D. Molecular Neurobiology 15(3):307-339. 1997

18. Hall-Angeras, M. Surgery 108(2):460-466. 1990

19. Hardardottir, I. Lymphokine & Cytokine Research 13(3):161-166. 1994

20. Hermus, A. Arteriosclerosis& Thrombosis 12(9):1036-1043. 1992

21. Holden, R. Medical Hypotheses 47(6):423-438. 1996

22. Hull, M. Neurobiology of Aging 17(5):795-800. 1996

23. Ikeda, T. Acta Psychiatrica Scandinavica 84(3):262-265. 1991

24. Kalman, J. Acta Neurologica Scandinavica 96:236-240. 1997

25. Kato, M. J. Clinical Anesthesia 9(4):293-298. 1997

26. Knapp, M. Annals of Clinical Biochemistry 28(Pt 5):480-486. 1991

27. Laskowitz, D. J. Neuroimmunology 76(1-2):70-74. 1997

28. Leblhuber, F. Deutsche Medizinische Wochenschrift 123(25-26):787-791. 1998

29. Mattson, M. Brain Research-Brain Research Reviews 23(1-2):47-61. 1997

30. Mealy, K. Archives of Surgery 125(1):42-47. 1990

31. Memon, R. Endocrinology 132(5):2246-2253. 1993

32. Moss, M. J. Neuroimmunology 72(2):127-129. 1997

33. Nanji, A. Hepatology 26(1):90-97. 1997

34. Neese, R. American J. Physiology 264(1 Pt 1):e136-147. 1993

35. Rosenzweig, I. Biotherapy 2(3):193-198. 1990

36. Schattner, A. J. Clinical & Laboratory Immunology 32(4):183-184. 1990

37. Shalit, F. Neuroscience Letters 174(2):130-132. 1994

38. Sheng, J. Neurobiology of Aging 17(5):761-766. 1996

39. Steer, J. British J. Clinical Pharmacology 43(4):383-389. 1997

40. Stopeck, A. J. Biological Chemistry 268(23):17489-17494. 1993

41. Swaminathan, N. Biochemical Medicine & Metabolic Biology 49(2):212-216. 1993

42. Vaisman, N. Metabolism: Clinical & Experimental 40(7):720-723. 1991

43. Vasilakos, J. FEBS Letters 354(3):289-292. 1994

44. Waage, A. Immunology 63(2):299-302. 1988

45. Wood, J. Brain Research 629(2):245-252. 1993

46. Xia, M. American J. Pathology 150(4):1267-1274. 1997

47. Yasuhara, O. Acta Neuropathologica 93(4):414-420. 1997

7-8

1. Anderson, I. Psychological Medicine 20(4):785-791. 1990

2. Arneric, S. J. Pharmacology & Experimental Therapeutics 228(3):551-559. 1984

3. Christie, J. British J. Psychiatry 150:674-681. 1987

4. Cincotta, A. Annals of Nutrition & Metabolism 33(6):305-314. 1989

5. Cincotta, A. Life Sciences 45(23):2247-2254. 1989

6. Cincotta, A. American J. Physiology 264(2 Pt 1):e285-293. 1993

7. Cooper, J. Aging 4(2):165-169. 1992

8. Cowen, P. Psychological Medicine 26(6):1155-1159. 1996

9. Culebras, A. Epilepsia 28(5):564-570. 1987

10. Dewey, K. J. Nutrition 128(2 Suppl):386s-389s. 1998

11. El-Shazly, M. Biological Psychiatry 22(5):661-663. 1987

12. El Sobky, A. Acta Psychiatrica Scandinavica 74(1):13-17. 1986

13. Gianoulakis, C. Annales de la Nutrition et l Alimentation 33(1):91-112. 1979

14. Gonzalez, C. J. Endocrinological Investigation 4(1):65-69. 1981

15. Goodwin, G. Archives in General Psychiatry 44(11):952-957. 1987

16. Heuser, I. Neurobiology of Aging 13(2):255-260. 1992

17. Mazzocchi, G. Cell & Tissue Research 262(1):41-46. 1990

18. McLoughlin, D. American J. Psychiatry 151(11):1701-1703. 1994

19. Merimee, T. J. Clinical Endocrinology & Metabolism 62(5):931-937. 1976

20. Middleton, B. J. Biological Chemistry 256(10):4827-4831. 1981

21. Mori, M. Neuropeptides 16(2):57-61. 1990

22. Nemeroff, C. Neuroendocrinology 50(6):663-666. 1989

23. Olusi, S. Clinica Chimica Acta 74(3):261-269. 1977

24. Oscarsson, J. J. Endocrinology 128(3):433-438. 1991

25. Pelkonen, R. Clinical Endocrinology 16(4):383-390. 1982

26. Pouplard, A. Revue Neurologique 139(3):187-191. 1983

27. Reber, P. American J. Medicine 95(6):637-644. 1993

28. Schmidt, M. European J. Pharmacology 90(2-3):169-177. 1983

29. Shand, J. J. Endocrinology 152(3):447-454. 1997

30. Smith, S. J. Clinical Endocrinology & Metabolism 39(1):53-62. 1974

31. Takeshita, H. Japanese J. Psychiatry & Neurology 40(4):617-623. 1986

32. Thomas, D. Acta Psychiatrica Scandinavica 76(2):158-163. 1987

33. Walsh, A. J. Affective Disorders 33(2):89-97. 1995

7-9

1. Fillit, H. Psychoneuroendocrinology 11(3):337-345. 1986

2. Hanyu, H. Japanese J. Geriatrics 30(10):857-863. 1993

3. Melton, L. J. American Geriatrics Society 42(6):614-619. 1994

7-10

1. Barbir, M. International J. Cardiology 32(1):51-56. 1991

2. Becker, D. American J. Medicine 85(5):632-638. 1988

3. Bentson, J. J. Computer Assisted Tomography 2(1):16-23. 1978

4. Ettinger, W. Atherosclerosis 63(2-3):167-172. 1987

5. Fredrikson, M. Biological Psychology 34(1):45-58. 1992

6. Gogia, P. Archives of Physical Medicine & Rehabilitation 74(5):463-467. 1993

7. Jover, E. J. Medicine 7(2):131-142. 1976

8. Keenan, P. Neurology 47(6):1396-1402. 1996

9. Kobashigawa, J. J. Heart & Lung Transplantation 14(5):963-967. 1995

10. Lieu, F. J. Applied Physiology 75(2):763-771. 1993

11. Lopez-Miranda, J. Clinical Biochemistry 25(5):379-386. 1992

12. Magarinos, A. Neuroscience 69(1):89-98. 1995

13. Mandal, S. Indian J. Physiology & Pharmacology 29(4):255-258. 1985

14. Maxwell, S. Postgraduate Medical J. 70(830):863-870. 1994

15. McCaughan, G. J. Gastroenterology & Hepatology 8(6):569-573. 1993

16. McDiarmid, S. Transplantation 60(12):1443-1450. 1995

17. Nanjee, M. Clinica Chimica Acta 180(2):113-120. 1989

18. Nashel, D. American J. Medicine 80(5):925-929. 1986

19. Nelson, A. Mayo Clinic Proceedings 55(12):758-769. 1980

20. Ong, C. Medicine 73(4):215-223. 1994

21. Petri, M. American J. Medicine 93(5):513-519. 1992

22. Raine, A. Nephrology, Dialysis, Transplantation 3(4):458-463. 1988

23. Renlund, D. J. Heart Transplantation 8(3):214-219. 1989

24. Romano, M. Pediatric Research 11(10 Pt 1):1042-1045. 1977

25. Schwertner, H. Atherosclerosis 67(2-3):237-244. 1987

26. Seene, T. J. Steroid Biochemistry & Molecular Biology 50(1-2):1-4. 1994

27. Solveborn, S. Clinical Orthopaedics & Related Research (316):99-105. 1995

28. Stamler, J. American J. Cardiology 62(17):1268-1272. 1988

29. Takacs, O. Acta Physiologica Academiae Scientiarum Hungaricae 55(2):121-128. 1980

30. Taylor, D. J. Heart Transplantation 8(3):209-213. 1989

31. Titov, V. Biokhimiia 43(11):2002-2010. 1978

32. Titov, V. Voprosy Meditsinskoi Khimii 28(4):38-42. 1982

33. Troxler, R. Atherosclerosis 26(2):151-162. 1977

7-11

1. Arden, M. J. Adolescent Health Care 11(3):199-202. 1990

2. Bannai, C. Endocrinologia Japonica 35(3):455-462. 1988
3. Fichter, M. Psychiatry Research 17(1):61-72. 1986
4. Frankel, R. Acta Endocrinologica 78(2):209-221. 1975
5. Gold, P. New England J. Medicine 314(21):1335-1342. 1986
6. Kennedy, S. Biological Psychiatry 30(3):216-224. 1991
7. Laessle, R. Psychoneuroendocrinology 17(5):475-484. 1992
8. McClain, C. J. American College of Nutrition 12(4):466-474. 1993
9. Mira, M. Pediatrician 12(2-3):148-156. 1983-85
10. Mordasini, R. Metabolism: Clinical & Experimental 27(1):71-79. 1978
11. Phinney, S. American J. Clinical Nutrition 53(6):1404-1410. 1991
12. Sanchez-Muniz, F. European J. Clinical Nutrition 45(1):33-36. 1991
13. Savendahl, L. American J. Clinical Nutrition 66(3):622-625. 1997
14. Stone, N. Medical Clinics of North America 78(1):117-141. 1994
15. Thibault, L. International J. Vitamin & Nutrition Research 57(4):447-452. 1987
16. Walsh, B. J. Clinical Endocrinology & Metabolism 53(1):203-205. 1981
17. Walsh, B. Psychoneuroendocrinology 12(2):131-140. 1987
18. Umeki, S. J. Nervous & Mental Disease 176(8):503-506. 1988

7-12

1. Abo-Hussein, S. J. Tropical Medicine & Hygiene 87(6):237-240. 1984
2. Codina, J. Revista Espanola de Fisiologia 35(4):457-460. 1979
3. Fisman, M. American J. Psychiatry 142(1):71-73. 1985
4. Giesecke, K. Metabolism: Clinical & Experimental 38(12):1196-1200. 1989
5. Hoyer, S. J. Neurology 235(3):143-148. 1988
6. Hoyer, S. Neuroscience Letters 117(3):358-362. 1990
7. Kilroe-Smith, T. South African Medical J. 71(11):723-724. 1987
8. Nowacka, M. Acta Physiologica Polonica 39(5-6):427-434. 1988
9. Seiler, N. Neurochemical Research 18(3):235-245. 1993

Chapter 8

8-1

1. Andersson, M. J. Neurochemistry 49(3):685-691. 1987
2. Aronica, E. Neuroscience 82(4):979-991. 1998
3. Arriagada, P. Neurology 42(9):1681-1688. 1992
4. Blennow, K. Neuroreport 5(118):2534-2536. 1994
5. Blennow, K. J. Neural Transmission-General Section 103(5):603-618. 1996
6. Buee, L. Annals of the New York Academy of Sciences 826:7-24. 1997
7. Chia, L. Biochimica et Biophysica Acta 775(3):308-312. 1984
8. Detoledo-Morrell, L. Neurobiology of Aging 18(5):463-468. 1997
9. Draczynska-Lusiak, B. Molecular & Chemical Neuropathology 33(2):139-148. 1998
10. Erkinjuntti, T. Comprehensive Gerontology 2(1):1-6. 1988
11. Ferrara, A. Circulation 96(1):37-43. 1997
12. Gomez-Isla, T. Annals of Neurology 41(1):17-24. 1997

13. Goodwin, J. JAMA 249(21):2917-2921. 1983
14. Gottfries, C. Alzheimer Disease and Associated Disorders 10(2):77-81. 1996
15. Gottfries, C. International Psychogeriatrics 8(3):365-372. 1996
16. Ginsberg, L. Molecular & Chemical Neuropathology 19(1-2):37-46. 1993
17. Ginsberg, L. Brain Research 615(2):355-357. 1993
18. Hanyu, H. Gerontology 43(6):343-351. 1997
19. Henderson, A. Psychological Medicine 22(2):429-436. 1992
20. Herishanu, Y. J. Neurological Sciences 26(4):583-586. 1975
21. Heun, R. Dementia and Geriatric Cognitive Disorders 8(6):329-336. 1997
22. Hyman, B. J. Neuropathology & Experimental Neurology 53(5):427-428. 1994
23. Igbavboa, U. J. Neurochemistry 69(4):1661-1667. 1997
24. Jarvik, G. Neurology 45(6):1092-1096. 1995
25. Joseph, J. Molecular & Chemical Neuropathology 28(1-3):35-40. 1996
26. Joseph, J. Free Radical Biology & Medicine 22(3):455-462. 1997
27. Kalaria, R. Annals of the New York Academy of Sciences 826:263-271. 1997
28. Kaplan, J. Psychosomatic Medicine 56(6):479-484. 1994
29. Katyal, S. Biochemical Pharmacology 21(5):747-751. 1972
30. Katz, A. J. Molecular & Cellular Cardiology 23(11):1343-1344. 1991
31. Knebl, J. Mechanisms of Aging & Development 73(1):69-77. 1994
32. Kuo, Y. Biochemical & Biophysical Research Communications 252(3):711-715. 1998
33. Lehtonen, A. Age & Ageing 15(5):267-270. 1986
34. Mark, R. J. Neuroscience 17(3):1046-1054. 1997
35. Masliah, E. Experimental Neurology 136(2):107-122. 1995
36. Mason, R. J. Molecular & Cellular Cardiology 23(11):1339-1342. 1991
37. Mason, R. Neurobiology of Aging 13(3):413-419. 1992
38. Mason, R. Annals of the New York Academy of Sciences 695:54-58. 1993
39. Mason, R. Annals of the New York Academy of Sciences 747:125-139. 1994
40. Mason, R. Neurobiology of Aging 16(4):531-539. 1995
41. Mason, R. Annals of the New York Academy of Sciences 777:368-373. 1996
42. Matthies, H. Neuroscience 79(2):341-346. 1997
43. McEwen B. Molecular Psychiatry 2(3):255-262. 1997
44. Miyakawa, T. Annals of the New York Academy of Sciences 826:25-34. 1997
45. Montine, T. American J. Pathology 151(6):1571-1575. 1997
46. Mulder, M. Alzheimer Disease & Associated Disorders 12(3):198-203. 1998
47. Oliver, M. Lancet 337(8756):1529-1531. 1991
48. Oliver, M. J. Molecular & Cellular Cardiology 23(11):1335-1337. 1991
49. Oliver, M. Cardiovascular Drugs & Therapy 7(5):785-788. 1993
50. Paresce, D. J. Biological Chemistry 272(46):29390-29397. 1997
51. Park, I. Neurobiology Aging 24(5):637-643. 2003
52. Pavlov, O. Neurotoxicology & Teratology 17(1):31-39. 1995
53. Pfrieger, F. Cellular Molecular Life Sciences 60(6):1158-1171. 2003
54. Praprotnik, D. Acta Neuropathologica 91(1):1-5. 1996

55. Roth, G. Trends in Neurosciences 18(5):203-206. 1995
56. Ruggiero, F. J. Neurochemistry 59(2):487-491. 1992
57. Scacchi, R. Dementia & Geriatric Cognitive Disorders 9(4):186-190. 1998
58. Scheffel, A. Psychiatria Polska 30(1):159-170. 1996
59. Soderberg, M. J. Neurochemistry 54(2):415-423. 1990
60. Soderberg, M. J. Neurochemistry 59(9):1646-1653. 1992
61. Stommel, A. Mechanisms of Ageing & Development 48(1):1-14. 1989
62. Svennerholm, L. J. Neurochemistry 62(3):1039-1047. 1994
63. Svennerholm, L. J. Neurochemistry 63(5):1802-1811. 1994
64. Svennerholm L. Acta Neuropathologica 94(4):345-352. 1997
65. Tacconi, M. Neurobiology of Aging 12(1):55-59. 1991
66. Takeda, S. Japanese J. Geriatrics 24:348-353. 1987
67. Torello, L. Neurobiology of Aging 7(5):337-346. 1986
68. Uchihara, T. Stroke 28(10):1948-1950. 1997
69. Upadhyay, S. Indian J. Medical Research 90:430-441. 1989
70. Van Rensburg, S. Neuroreport 5(17):2221-2224. 1994
71. Wada, T. J. American Geriatrics Society 45(1):122-123. 1997
72. Wada, T. J. American Geriatrics Society 45(11):1411-1412. 1997
73. Wender, M. Folia Neuropathologica 32(2):75-79. 1994
74. Wood, W. Brain Research 683(1):36-42. 1995

8-2

1. Araki, W. Biochemical & Biophysical Research Communications 181(1):265-271. 1991
2. Askanas, V. Neuroreport 6(7):1045-1049. 1995
3. Avdulov, N. J. Neurochemistry 69(4):1746-1752. 1997
4. Badolato, R. J. Experimental Medicine 180(1):203-209. 1994
5. Banati, R. Glia 14(3):209-215. 1995
6. Beer, J. Neurodegeneration 4(1):51-59. 1995
7. Beffert, U. J. Neurochemistry 70(4):1458-1466. 1998
8. Benson, M. Arthritis & Rheumatism 22(1):36-42. 1979
9. Beyreuther, K. Annals of the New York Academy of Sciences 640:129-139. 1991
10. Bohl, J. Progress in Clinical & Biological Research 317:1007-1019. 1989
11. Brachova, L. Brain Research. Molecular Brain Research 18(4):329-334. 1993
12. Bramlett, H. J. Neuropathology & Experimental Neurology 56(10:1132-1141. 1997
13. Breen, K. Molecular & Chemical Neuropathology 16(1-2):109-121. 1992
14. Brown, M. Cell 89(3):331-340. 1997
15. Cohen, A. Current Opinion in Rheumatology 5(1):62-76. 1993
16. Cole, G. Biochemical & Biophysical Research Communications 170(1):288-295. 1990
17. Cook, D. Nature Medicine 3(9):1021-1023. 1997
18. Cotman, C. Neurobiology of Aging 17(5):723-731. 1996
19. Dickson, D. Neurobiology of Aging 13(1):179-189. 1992
20. Dickson, T. Neuropathology & Applied Neurobiology 23(6):483-491. 1997
21. De Strooper, B. Nature 391(6665):387-390. 1998

22. Eikelenboom, P. Virchows Archiv 424(4):421-427. 1994
23. Eikelenboom, P. Neurobiology of Aging 17(5):673-680. 1996
24. Elovaara, I. Acta Neurologica Scandinavica 74(3):245-250. 1986
25. Frackowiak, J. Acta Neuropathologica 84(3):225-233. 1992
26. Gentleman, S. Neuroscience Letters 160(2):139-144. 1993
27. Ghiso, J. Biochemical J. 288(Pt 3):1053-1059. 1992
28. Ghiso, J. FEBS Letters 408(1):105-108. 1997
29. Gillmore, J. British J. Haematology 99(2):245-256. 1997
30. Gondo, T. Virchows Archiv-A, Path Anat & Histo 422(3):225-231. 1993
31. Gruys, E. Baillieres Clinical Rheumatology 8(3):599-611. 1994
32. Haas, C. Biochemical J. 325(Pt 1):169-175. 1997
33. Hartmann, T. Nature Medicine 3(9):1016-1020. 1997
34. Hoshii, Y. American J. Pathology 151(4):911-917. 1997
35. Hyman, B. J. Neuropathology & Experimental Neurology 52(6):594-600. 1993
36. Ikeda, K. Brain Research 527(1):140-144. 1990
37. Islam, K. American J. Pathology 151(1):265-271. 1997
38. Joachim, C. Nature 341(6239):226-230. 1989
39. King, C. Neuroreport 8(7):1663-1665. 1997
40. Kisilevsky, R. Annals of the New York Academy of Sciences 826:117-127. 1997
41. Knauer, M. Proceedings/America 89(16):7437-7441. 1992
42. Koo, E. J. Cell Science 109(Pt 5):991-998. 1996
43. Korotzer, A. Experimental Neurology 134(2):214-221. 1995
44. Koudinov, A. Cell Biology International 21(5):265-271. 1997
45. Kounnas, M. Cell 82(2):331-340. 1995
46. Kumon, Y. Clinical Biochemistry 26(6):505-511. 1993
47. LeBlanc, A. J. Neuroscience 15(12):7837-7846. 1995
48. Lee, S. Nature Medicine 4(6):730-734. 1998
49. Li, Q. Blood 84(1):133-142. 1994
50. Li, Q. Laboratory Investigation 78(4):461-469. 1998
51. Liang, J. J. Lipid Research 36(1):37-46. 1995
52. Liang,J. J. Lipid Research 37(10):2109-2116. 1996
53. Lindhorst, E. Biochimica et Biophysica Acta 1339(1):143-154. 1997
54. Linke, R. Clinical Neuropathology 1(4):172-182. 1982
55. Liu, Y. Proceedings/America 95(22):13266-13271. 1998
56. Maness, L. Life Sciences 55(21):1643-1650. 1994
57. Marhaug, G. Baillieres Clinical Rheumatology 8(3):553-573. 1994
58. Mason, R. Neurobiology of Aging 13:413-419. 1992
59. Mason, R. Annals of the New York Academy of Sciences 695:54-58. 1993
60. Mason, R. Biochemical & Biophysical Research Communications 222(1):78-82. 1996
61. Mattson, M. Neuron 10(2):243-254. 1003
62. Mazur-Kolecka, B. Brain Research 760(1-2):255-260. 1997
63. Meier-Ruge, W. Annals of the New York Academy of Sciences 826:229-241. 1997

64. Mirzabekov, T. Biochemical & Biophysical Research Communications 202(2):1142-1148. 1994

65. Miwata, H. Archives of Disease in Childhood 68(2):210-214. 1993

66. Mozes, G. J. Trauma 29(1):71-74. 1989

67. Paresce, D. J. Biological Chemistry 272(46):29390-29397. 1997

68. Puttfarcken, P. J. Neurochemistry 68:760-769. 1997

69. Praprotnik, D. Acta Neuropathologica 91(1):1-5. 1996

70. Qiu, W. J. Biological Chemistry 272(1):6641-6646. 1997

71. Schubert, W. Brain Research 563(1-2):184-194. 1991

72. Schwartz, P. Fortschritte der Medizin 94(15):890-896. 1976

73. Selkoe, D. Trends in Neurosciences 16(10):403-409. 1993

74. Skodras, G. Annals of Clinical & Laboratory Science 23(4):275-280. 1993

75. Smith, M. J. Neurochemistry 70(5):2212-2215. 1998

76. Smith, R. Science 248(4959):1126-1128. 1990

77. Soreghan, B. J. Biological Chemistry 269(46):28551-28554. 1994

78. Tan, S. Histopathology 25(5):403-414. 1994

79. Tennent, G. Proceedings/America 92(10):4299-4303. 1995

80. Terzi, E. J. Molecular Biology 252(5):633-642. 1995

81. Terzi, E. Biochemistry 36(48):14845-14852. 1997

82. Urban, B. Radiographics 13(6):1295-1308. 1993

83. Walter, M. Biochemical & Biophysical Research Communications 233(3):760-764. 1997

84. Whitson, J. Science 243(4897):1488-1490

85. Yam, P. Brain Research 760:150-157. 1997

86. Yamazaki, T. J. Cell Science 109(Pt 5):999-1008. 1996

87. Zhang, M. Clinical Neuropathology 15(2):74-78. 1996

88. Zunarelli, E. Neuroreport 8(1):45-48. 1996

8-3

1. Bodovitz, S. J. Biological Chemistry 271(8):4436-4440. 1996

2. Clemens, J. Neurobiology of Aging 13(5):581-586. 1992

3. Dzenko K. J. Neuroimmunology 80(1-2):6-12. 1997

4. Farhangrazi, Z. Neuroreport 8(5):1127-1130. 1997

5. Hartmann, H. Biochemical & Biophysical Research Communications 200(3):1185-1192. 1994

6. Howland, D. J. Biological Chemistry 273(26):16576-16582. 1998

7. Kim, S. J. Neurochemistry 67(3):1172-1182. 1996

8. LaFerla, F. J. Clinical Investigation 100(2):310-320. 1997

9. Liao, F. Arteriosclerosis& Thrombosis 14(9):1475-1479. 1994

10. Mark, R. Neurobiology of Aging 16(2):187-198. 1995

11. Mason, R. Neurobiology of Aging 13(3):413-419. 1992

12. Mason, R. Annals of the New York Academy of Sciences 695:54-58. 1993

13. Mason, R. Annals of the New York Academy of Sciences 747:125-139. 1994

14. Puttfarcken, P. J. Neurochemistry 68(2):760-769. 1997
15. Racchi, M. Biochemical J. 322(Pt 3):893-898. 1997
16. Simons, M. Proceedings/America 95(11):6460-6464. 1998
17. Sparks, D. Neurobiology Aging 17(2):291-299. 1996
18. Whitson, J. Biochemical & Biophysical Research Communications 199(1):163-170. 1994
19. Zhou, Y. Neuroreport 7(15-17):2487-2490. 1996

<u>8-4</u>

1. Aviram, M. Progress in Cardiovascular Diseases 30(1):61-72. 1987
2. Bastiaanse, E. Cardiovascular Research 33(2):272-283. 1997
3. Berlin, E. Atherosclerosis 63(1):85-96. 1987
4. Bodovitz, S. J. Biological Chemistry 271(8):4436-4440. 1996
5. Bosman, G. Neurobiology of Aging 13(6):711-716. 1992
6. Cataliotti, R. Research in Experimental Medicine 180(2):117-125. 1982
7. Cohen, B. Life Sciences 40(25):2445-2451. 1987
8. Corvera, E. Biochimica et Biophysica Acta 1107(2):261-270. 1992
9. Davi, G. Atherosclerosis 79(1):79-83. 1989
10. Davies, T. Biochemical & Biophysical Research Communications 194(1):537-543. 1993
11. Di Luca, M. Archives of Neurology 53(11):1162-1166. 1996
12. Ghosh, C. Neurochemistry International 23(5):479-484. 1993
13. Hajimohammadreza, I. Biochimica et Biophysica Acta 1025(2):208-214. 1990
14. Hassall, D. Arteriosclerosis 3(4):332-338. 1983
15. Heemskerk, J. Biochimica et Biophysica Acta 1255(1):87-97. 1995
16. Hicks, N. Alzheimer Disease and Associated Disorders 1(2):90-97. 1987
17. Kaczmarek, D. European J. Clinical Pharmacology 45(5):451-457. 1993
18. Kalman, J. Biological Psychiatry 35(3):190-194. 1994
19. Latta, E. Arteriosclerosis & Thrombosis 14(8):1372-1377. 1994
20. Le Quan Sang, K. Thrombosis & Haemostasis 69(1):70-76. 1993
21. Li, Q. Blood 84(1):133-142. 1004
22. Lijnen, P. Methods & Findings in Experimental & Clinical Pharmacology 18(2):123-136. 1996
23. Piletz, J. Neurobiology of Aging 12(5):401-406. 1991
24. Rao, G. Indian J. of Physiology & Pharmacology 40(1):5-14. 1996
25. Rosenberg, R. Archives of Neurology 54(2):139-144. 1997
26. Schror, K. Eicosanoids 2(1):39-45. 1989
27. Shattil, S. Biochemistry 15(22):4832-4837. 1976
28. Smith, C. Neuroscience Letters 235(3):157-159. 1997
29. Spink, C. Biochimica et Biophysica Acta 1279(2):190-196. 1996
30. Srivastava, S. Thrombosis Research 76(5):451-461. 1994
31. Surya, I. Thrombosis & Haemostasis 65(3):306-311. 1991
32. Van Rensburg, S. Neuroreport 5(17):2221-2224. 1994
33. Winocour, P. Diabetes 39(2):241-244. 1990

34. Zubenko, G. Annals of Neurology 22(2):237-244. 1987
35. Zubenko, G. Psychopharmacology 94(3):347-349. 1988
36. Zubenko, G. Biological Psychiatry 24(8):925-936. 1988
37. Zubenko, G. American J. Psychiatry 153(3):420-423. 1996
38. Zubenko, G. American J. Psychiatry 156(1):50-57. 1999

<u>8-5</u>   —None

<u>8-6</u>

1. Alonso, A. Nature Medicine 2(7):783-787. 1996
2. Arebalo, R. J. Biological Chemistry 256(2):571-574. 1981
3. Arendt, T. Neurobiology of Aging 19(1):3-13. 1998
4. Asins, G. J. Lipid Research 32(9):1391-1401. 1991
5. Auer, I. Acta Neuropathologica 90(6):547-551. 1995
6. Benzing, W. Experimental Neurology 132(2):162-171. 1995
7. Bifulco, M. J. Cellular Physiology 155(2):340-348. 1993
8. Cohen, P. Biochimica et Biophysica Acta 1094(3):292-299. 1991
9. Conrad, P. J. Cell Biology 131(6 Pt 1):1421-1433. 1995
10. De Mattos, A. Developmental Neuroscience 16(1-2):38-43. 1994
11. Fielding, P. Biochemistry 35(47):14932-14938. 1996
12. Genis, I. Neuroscience Letters 199(1):5-8. 1995
13. Goedert, M. Neurobiology of Aging 16(3):325-334. 1995
14. Goedert, M. J. Neurochemistry 65(6):2804-2807. 1995
15. Gordon, I. Molecular & Chemical Neuropathology 28(1-3):97-103. 1996
16. Ingebritsen, T. European J. Biochemistry 132(2):255-261. 1983
17. Ingebritsen T. European J. Biochemistry 132(2):297-307. 1983
18. Krakower, G. J. Biological Chemistry 256(5):2408-2413. 1981
19. Marcus, D. Annals of the New York Academy of Sciences 826:248-253. 1997
20. Merrick, S. J. Biological Chemistry 271(10):5589-5594. 1996
21. ONO, T. Neurochemistry International 26(3):205-215. 1995
22. Pei, J. J. Neuropathology & Experimental Neurology 56(1):70-78. 1997
23. Pei, J. J. Neural Transmission 105(1):69-83. 1998
24. Pipeleers, D. Science 191(4222):88-90. 1976
25. Redies, C. American J. Physiology 256(6 Pt 1):e805-810. 1989
26. Sauk, J. J. Oral Pathology 16(2):69-74. 1987
27. Serra, D. J. Lipid Research 31(5):919-926. 1990
28. Volpe, J. J. Neurochemistry 33(1):97-106. 1979
29. Wang, J. Brain Research. Molecular Brain Research 38(2):200-208. 1996
30. Welsh, G. Biochemical J. 294(Pt 3):625-629. 1993

<u>8-7</u>

1. Beg, Z. J. Biological Chemistry 260(3):1682-1687. 1985
2. Chang, H. J. Membrane Biology 143(1):51-63. 1995
3. Mason, R. Biochemical Pharmacology 45(11):2173-2183. 1993
4. Mason, R. Annals of the New York Academy of Sciences 747:125-139. 1994

5. Nakahara, K. Biochemical & Biophysical Research Communications 202(3):1579-1585. 1994
6. Roitelman, J. J. Biological Chemistry 266(24):16085-16091. 1991
7. Zammit, V. Biochemical J. 269(2):373-379. 1990
8. Zammit, V. Biochemical J. 279(Pt 2):377-383. 1991

8-8

1. Crino, P. Annals of Otology, Rhinology & Laryngology 104(8):655661. 1995
2. Doty, R. in Smell and Taste in Health and Disease (ed by Getchell, T. et al), pgs 735-751. Publ by Raven Press, 1991
3. Taste and Smell Disorders(ed by Seiden, A.), publ by Thieme, 1997
4. Solomon, G. J. Neuropsychiatry & Clinical Neurosciences 10(1):64-67. 1998
5. Thompson, M. Neuropsychology Review 8(1):11-23. 1998
6. Yamagishi, M. Annals of Otology, Rhinology & Laryngology 107(5 Pt 1):421-426. 1998
7. Zucco, G. Perceptual & Motor Skills 78(2):627-631. 1994

8-9

1. Abushov, B. Arkhiv Anatomii, Gistologii i Embriologii 86(1):40-45. 1984
2. Andrade, J. J. Anatomy 187(Pt 2):379-393. 1995
3. Andrade, J. Experimental Brain Research 109(3):419-433. 1996
4. Andrade, J. Hippocampus 8(1):33-47. 1998
5. Barrett-Connor, E. J. American Geriatrics Society 44(10):1147-1152. 1996
6. Beard, C. Annals of Epidemiology 7(3):219-224. 1997
7. Bjornsson, O. Archives of Biochemistry & Biophysics 238(1):135-145. 1985
8. Dahl, N. Acta Neuropathologica 57(2-3):111-120. 1982
9. Dickson, D. Neurobiology of Aging 13(1):179-189. 1992
10. Donaldson, K. J. American Geriatrics Society 44(10):1232-1234. 1996
11. Easom, R. Biochemical J. 241(1):183-188. 1987
12. Efendiev, A. Voprosy Meditsinskoi Khimii 40(2):34-37. 1994
13. Franklin, C. J. American Dietetic Association 89(6):790-792. 1989
14. Garcia-Ruiz, M. Brain Research 625(2):203-212. 1993
15. Haupt, M. Acta Neurologica Scandinavica 88(5):349-353. 1993
16. Heller, D. New England J. Medicine 328(16):1150-1156. 1993
17. Henderson, A. Psychological Medicine 22(2):429-436. 1992
18. Hoyer, S. Aging 2(3):245-258. 1990
19. Jarvik, G. Neurology 45(1092-1096. 1995
20. Jeandel, C. Gerontology 35(5-6):275-282. 1989
21. Jones, P. American J. Clinical Nutrition 57(6):868-874. 1993
22. Jungmann, H. Klinische Wochenschrift 59(18):1061-1064. 1981
23. Kannel, W. American J. Cardiology 76(9):69c-77c. 1995
24. Kaur, K. Neuroscience Letters 145(2):168-170. 1992
25. Kempen, H. Biochimica et Biophysica Acta 876(3):494-499. 1986
26. Mozes, S. Physiology & Behavior 43(3):287-291. 1988

27. Mulder, M. Alzheimer Disease & Associated Disorders 12(3):198-203. 1998

28. Redies, C. American J. Physiology 256(6 Pt 1):e805-810. 1989

29. Roth, G. Trends in Neurosciences 18(5):203-206. 1995

30. Tacconi, M. Neurobiology of Aging 12:55-59. 1991

31. Valenta, L. Postgraduate Medicine 79(4):263-267. 1986

32. Volicer, L. Alzheimer Disease & Associated Disorders 11 Suppl 6:60-65. 1997

33. White, H. J. American Geriatrics Society 46(10):1223-1227. 1998

34. Wolf-Klein, G. International Psychogeriatrics 4(1):103-118. 1992

35. Wolf-Klein, G International Psychogeriatrics 6(2):135-142. 1994

8-10

1. Avdulov, N. J. Neurochemistry 68(5):2086-2091. 1997

2. Gwebu, E. In Vitro Cellular & Developmental Biology. Animal 33(9):672-673. 1997

3. Mattson, M. Brain Research 676(1):219-224. 1995

4. Sano, M. New England J. Medicine 336(17):1216-1222. 1997

5. Ueda, K. J. Neurochemistry 68(1):265-271. 1997

6. Zhou, Y. J. Neurochemistry 67(4):1419-1425. 1996

8-11

1. Bretscher, M. Science 261(5126):1280-1281. 1993

2. Conrad, P. J. Cell Biology 131(6 Pt 1):1421-1433. 1995

3. Dal Canto, M. American J. Pathology 148(2):355-360. 1996

4. Deshmukh, D. Neurochemical Research 13(6):571-582. 1988

5. Fielding, P. Biochemistry 35(47):14932-14938. 1996

6. Gabuzda, D. J. Biological Chemistry 269(18):13623-13628. 1994

7. Higgins, J. J. Lipid Research 25(12):1295-1305. 1984

8. Hutton, M. Human Molecular Genetics 6(10):1639-1646. 1997

9. Kovacs, D. Nature Medicine 2(2):224-229. 1996

10. Lahiri, D. Cellular & Molecular Neurobiology 14(4):297-313. 1994

11. Lee, S. Nature Medicine 4(6):730-734. 1998

12. Lehmann, S. J. Biological Chemistry 272(18):12047-12051. 1997

13. Mendez, A. J. Lipid Research 37(12):2510-2524. 1996

14. Mok, S. Biochemistry 36(1):156-163. 1997

15. Moreau, P. J. Biological Chemistry 266(7):4322-4328. 1991

16. Neufeld, E. J. Biological Chemistry 271(21604-21613. 1996

17. Pitas, R. Biochimica et Biophysica Acta 917(1):148-161. 1987

18. Robakis, N. Annals of the New York Academy of Sciences 695:132-138. 1993

19. Rusinol, A. J. Biological Chemistry 268(5):3555-3562. 1993

20. Salehi, A. Neuroscience 59(4):871-880. 1994

21. Salehi, A. J. Neuropathology & Experimental Neurology 54(5):704-709. 1995

22. Salehi, A. Neuroscience Letters 193(1):29-32. 1995

23. Stephens, D. J. Neuroscience Research 46(2):211-225. 1996

24. Stieber, A. American J. Pathology 148(2):415-426. 1996

25. Swift, L. J. Clinical Investigation 66(3):415-425. 1980

26. Thinakaran, G. J. Biological Chemistry 271(16):9390-9397. 1996
27. Walter, J. Molecular Medicine 2(6):673-691. 1996
28. Wild-Bode, C. J. Biological Chemistry 272(26):16085-16088. 1997

8-12

1. Brunk, U. Free Radical Biology & Medicine 19(6):813-822. 1995
2. Dowson, J. Neurobiology of Aging 134(4):493-500. 1992
3. Lange, Y. J. Biological Chemistry 272(27):17018-17022. 1997
4. Nilsson, E. Histochemical J. 29(11-12):857-865. 1997
5. Nixon, R. Annals of the New York Academy of Sciences 674:65-88. 1992
6. Nixon, R. Annals of the New York Academy of Sciences 679:87-109. 1993

Chapter 9

9-1

1. Breteler, M. American J. Epidemiology 142(12):1300-1305. 1995
2. Gentlemen, S. Neuroreport 8(6):1519-1522. 1997
3. Graham, D. Neuropathology & Applied Neurobiology 21(1):27-34. 1995
4. Henderson, A. Psychological Medicine 22(2):429-436. 1992
5. Meier-Ruge, W. Annals of the New York Academy of Sciences 826:229-241. 1997
6. Nemetz, P. American J. Epidemiology 149(1):32-40. 1999
7. O'Meara, E. American J. Epidemiology 146(5):373-384. 1997
8. Poduri, A. Neuroscience Letters 197(1):1-4. 1995
9. Rasmusson, D. Brain Injury 9(3):213-219. 1995
10. Roberts, G. J. Neurology, Neurosurgery & Psychiatry 57(4):419-425. 1994
11. Rudelli, R. Archives of Neurology 39(9):570-575. 1982
12. Schofield, P. J. Neurology, Neurosurgery & Psychiatry 62(2):119-124. 1997
13. Smith, D. American J. Pathology 153(3):1005-1010. 1998
14. Tang, M. Annals of the New York Academy of Sciences 802:6-15. 1996
15. Van Duijn, C. American J. Epidemiology 135(7):775-782. 1992

9-2

1. Davie, C. J. Neurology, Neurosurgery & Psychiatry 58(6):688-691. 1995
2. Hof, P. Acta Neuropathologica 85(1):23-30. 1992
3. Jordan, B. JAMA 278(2):136-140. 1997
4. Roberts, G. J. Neurology, Neurosurgery & Psychiatry 53(5):373-378. 1990
5. Unterharnscheidt, F. Revista de Neurologia 23(123):1027-1032. 1995

Chapter 10

10-1 —None
10-2 —None
10-3

1. Andersson, B. Acta Medica Scandinavica 223(6):485-490. 1988
2. Burke, W. J. Autonomic Nervous System 48(1):65-71. 1994
3. Elmstahl, S. Age & Ageing 21(4):301-307. 1992

4. Franke, H. Aktuelle Gerontologie 10(3):137-147. 1980
5. Garbarino, K. American J. Medicine 86:734-735. 1989
6. Gilles, C. Neurology 34(6):730-735. 1984
7. Goldstein, S. J. American Geriatrics Society 33(9):579-584. 1985
8. Goode, G. Circulation 91(12):2898-2903. 1995
9. Guo, Z. BMJ 312(7034):805-808. 1996
10. Itoh, Y. J. Neurological Sciences 116(2):135-141. 1993
11. Ives, D. J. Gerontology 48(3):m103-107. 1993
12. Kyle, R. Medicine 54(4):271-299. 1975
13. Landin, K. J. Internal Medicine 233(357-363. 1993
14. Langer, R. American J. Epidemiology 134(1):29-38. 1991
15. Leiter, L. American J. Physiology 247(2 Pt 1):e190-197. 1984
16. Melby, C. American J. Clinical Nutrition 59(1):103-109. 1994
17. Menotti, A. European J. Epidemiology 13(4):379-386. 1997
18. Morrison, R. Hypertension 28(4):569-575. 1996
19. Murdoch, J. British Medical J. 2:226-228. 1977
20. Rouse, I. Lancet 1(8314-5):5-10. 1983
21. St. Clair, D. British J. Psychiatry 143:274-276. 1983
22. Skoog, I. Neurology Research 25(6):675-680. 2003
23. Takeda, S. Japanese J. Geriatrics 24:348-353. 1987
24. Tresch, D. J. American Geriatrics Society 33(8):530-537. 1985
25. Wang, S. Age & Ageing 23(5):400-404. 1994
26. Zaninelli, A. Giornale Italiano di Cardiologia 23(2):153-158. 1993

10-4

1. Anwaar, I. International Angiology 15(3):201-206. 1996
2. Brorson, J. J. Neurochemistry 69(5):1882-1889. 1997
3. Busse, R. J. Vascular Research 33:181-194. 1996
4. Candipan, R. Arteriosclerosis, Thrombosis & Vascular biology 16(1):44-50. 1996
5. Casino, P. Circulation 88(6):2541-2547. 1993
6. Gilligan, D. J. American College of Cardiology 24(7):1611-1617. 1994
7. Goodwin, J. Brain Research 768(279-286. 1997
8. Hu, J. J. Neurochemistry 69(6):2294-2301. 1997
9. Hu, J. Brain Research 785(2):195-206. 1998
10. Kingwell, B. American J. Physiology 270(6 Pt 2):h2008-2013. 1996
11. Knudsen, H. American J. Physiology 273(1 Pt 2):h347-355. 1997
12. Laight, D. British J. Pharmacology 117(7):1471-1474. 1996
13. Mathew, V. Circulation 96(6):1930-1936. 1997
14. Middlemas, D. Biochemistry 26(5):1219-1223. 1987
15. O'Driscoll, G. Circulation 95(5):1126-1131. 1997
16. Preik, M. J. Cardiovascular Risk 3(5):465-471. 1996
17. Quyyumi, A. Circulation 92(3):320-326. 1995
18. Shiode, N. Internal Medicine 35(2):89-93. 1996

19. Tanaka, S. Clinical Cardiology 20(4):361-365. 1997

20. Wallace, M. Experimental Neurology 144:266-272. 1997

21. Weisbrod, R. Arteriosclerosis, Thrombosis & Vascular Biology 17(2):394-402. 1997

10-5

1. Abbott, R. J. Neurology, Neurosurgery & Psychiatry 43(2):163-167. 1980

2. Anderson, C. J. Nervous and Mental Disease 109:210-219. 1949

3. Anderson, R. International J. Hyperthermia 1(4):337-347. 1985

4. Ashton, H. Drugs 48(1):25-40. 1994

5. Bagaev, V. Neuroreport 5(14):1705-1708. 1994

6. Bauer, J. J. Neurology 241(4):242-245. 1994

7. Bauer, J. Epilepsy Research 24(1):1-7. 1996

8. Bekkelund, S. Acta Neurologica Scandinavica 94(6):378-382. 1996

9. Bell, F. Atherosclerosis 50(3):345-352. 1984

10. Bell, F. Lipids 20(2):75-79. 1985

11. Bierkamper, G. Epilepsia 19(2):155-167. 1978

12. Bierkamper, G. Brain Research 150(2):343-351. 1978

13. Botez, M. Canadian J. Neurological Sciences 15(3):299-303. 1988

14. Breteler, M. International J. Epidemiology 20 Suppl 2:s36-42. 1991

15. Breteler, M. American J. Epidemiology 142(12):1300-1305. 1995

16. Brodtkorb, E. Seizure 3(4):277-285. 1994

17. Brown, D. J. Clinical Psychopharmacology 12(6):431-437. 1992

18. Calandre, E. Acta Neurologica Scandinavica 83(4):250-253. 1991

19. Cascino, G. Mayo Clinic Proceedings 71(8):787-792. 1996

20. Cenedella, R. Epilepsia 23(3):257-268. 1982

21. Chandra, V. Neurology 36(2):209-211. 1986

22. Cheng, K. Cancer Research 47(5):1255-1262. 1987

23. Colannino, N. Epilepsia 24(5):597-603. 1983

24. Cress, A. Cancer Research 42(5):1716-1721. 1982

25. Culebras, A. Epilepsia 28(5):564-570. 1987

26. Cuparencu, B. Clinical & Experimental Pharmacology & Physiology 12(6):593-602. 1985

27. Dastur, D. Epilepsia 28(2):147-159. 1987

28. Davis, J. Biochimica et Biophysica Acta 597(3):477-491. 1980

29. De Bock, F. Neuroreport 7(6):1125-1129. 1996

30. De la Court, A. Epilepsia 37(2):141-147. 1996

31. Despland, P. Schweizerische Rundschau fur Medizin Praxis 86(37):1414-1417. 1997

32. Dessi, S. Research Communications in Chemical Pathology & Pharmacology 31(2):375-378. 1981

33. Dirik, E. Acta Paediatrica Japonica 38(2):118-120. 1996

34. Eiris, J. Neurology 45(6):1155-1157. 1995

35. Franzoni, E. Epilepsia, 33(5):932-935. 1992

36. Garbagnati, E. Acta Paediatrica 82(11):948-952. 1993

37. Garcia-Cairasco, N. Pharmacology, Biochemistry & Behavior 53(3):503-510. 1996

38. Gouras, G. Annals of Neurology 41(3):402-404. 1997

39. Goerdt, C. J. Clinical Pharmacology 35(8):767-775. 1995

40. Hallowitz, R. Brain Research 130(2):271-286. 1977

41. Hatazawa, J. Japanese J. Clinical Radiology 34(11):1343-1348. 1989

42. Healy, B. Epilepsy Research 28(2):101-104. 1997

43. Heldenberg, D. Neurology 33(4):510-513. 1983

44. Hendricks, H. Neurology 40(8):1308-1310. 1990

45. Henry, T. Epilepsia 39(9):983-990. 1998

46. Hesdorffer, D. Neurology 46:727-730. 1996

47. Hirvasniemi, A. Acta Neurologica Scandinavica 90(3):388-393. 1994

48. Honghan, G. Nippon Igaku Hoshasen Gakkai Zasshi- Nippon Acta Radiologica 54(2):122-128. 1994

49. Inui, T. Brain Research 517(1-2):123-133. 1990

50. Iontov, A. Zhurnal Nevropatologii i Psikhiatrii Imeni s-s-Korsakova 81(6):891-895. 1981

51. Isojarvi, J. Archives of Neurology 50(6):590-593. 1993

52. Jacobs, D. American J. Epidemiology 146(7):558-564. 1997

53. Jallon, P. Revue Neurologique 153(3):173-184. 1997

54. Johannsen, P. Seizure 5(2):121-125. 1996

55. Johnson, E. Neurology 42(4):811-815, 1992

56. Jurgelski, W. Brain Research 64:466-471. 1973

57. Kao, F. Genomics 23(3):700-703. 1994

58. Kaste, M. Stroke 14(4):525-530. 1983

59. Kaukola, S. J. Cardiovascular Pharmacology 3(1):207-214. 1981

60. Kenneback, G. Seizure 6(5):369-375. 1997

61. Lannon, S. J. Neuroscience Nursing 25(5):273-282. 1993

62. Lin, Y. Neurology 49(2):528-532. 1997

63. Luoma, P. European Neurology 19(1):67-72. 1980

64. Luoma, P. J. Cardiovascular Pharmacology 4(6):1024-1027. 1982

65. Luoma,P. European J. Clinical Pharmacology 28(6):615-618. 1985

66. Luoma, P. Research Communications in Chemical Pathology & Pharmacology 62(1):125-128. 1988

67. Mackenzie, I. Acta Neuropathologica 87(5):504-510. 1994

68. Mackenzie, I. Neurology 46(2):425-429. 1996

69. Mark, R. Neurobiology of Aging 16(2):187-198. 1995

70. Masada, T. Neuroreport 7(2):446-448. 1996

71. Massetani, R. Epilepsia 38(3):363-369. 1997

72. Mathern, G. J. Neuropathology & Experimental Neurology 56(2):199-212. 1997

73. McVicker, R. British J. Psychiatry 164(4):528-532. 1994

74. Melanson, M. Neurology 49(6):1732-1733. 1997

75. Mendez, M. J. Geriatric & Neurology 7(4):230-233. 1994

76. Mudher, A. Neuroscience 89(2):329-333. 1999

77. Natelson, S. Clinical Chemistry 25(6):889-897. 1979

78. Nikkila, E. Acta Medica Scandinavica 204(6):517-520

79. O'Neill, B. Acta Neurologica Scandinavica 65(2):104-109. 1982

80. Patel, D. Artery 10(4):237-249. 1982

81. Pitkanen, A. Neurology 46(6):1724-1730. 1996

82. Pohlmann-Eden, B. Fortschritte der Neurologie-Psychiatrie 61(11):363-368. 1993

83. Prasher, V. Seizure 4(1):53-56. 1995

84. Pritchard, P. Epilepsia 32 Suppl 6:s46-50. 1991

85. Rausch, R. Archives of Neurology 51(2):139-144. 1994

86. Reddy, M. Proceedings of the Society for Experimental Biology & Medicine 180(2):359-363. 1985

87. Rigaud-Monnet, A. Brain Research 673(2):297-303. 1995

88. Romanelli, M. Archives of Neurology 47(8):847-850. 1990

89. Rundfeldt, C. J. Pharmacology & Experimental Therapeutics 275(2):693-702. 1995

90. Rutecki, P. Epilepsia 31 Suppl 2:s1-6. 1990

91. Sadzot, B. Epilepsy Research 12(2):121-129. 1992

92. Saija, A. Experimental Brain Research 88(1):151-157. 1992

93. Sarkar, C. Epilepsia 23(3):243-255. 1982

94. Sawchenko, P. J. Autonomic Nervous System 9(1):13-26. 1983

95. Schoch, P. Biochemical Society Symposia 59:121-134. 1993

96. Sheng, J. J. Neurochemistry 63(5):1872-1879. 1994

97. Shoham, S. Experimental Neurology 147(2):361-376. 1997

98. Singh, U. Indian Pediatrics 31(6):667-669. 1994

99. Smith, K. European J. Pharmacology 176(1):45-55. 1990

100. Smith, K. Brain Research 729(2):147-150. 1996

101. Soejima, S. Cancer Letters 60(2):159-167. 1991

102. Takeshita, H. Japanese J. Psychiatry & Neurology 40(4):617-623. 1986

103. Thomas, R. Archives of Internal Medicine 157(6):605-617. 1997

104. Tomson, T. Epilepsy Research 30(1):77-83. 1998

105. Verrotti, A. J. Paediatrics & Child Health 33(3):242-245. 1997

106. Volicer, L. Dementia 6(5):258-263. 1995

107. Wallace, R. Circulation 62(4 Pt 2):IV77-82. 1980

108. Yamamoto, T. International J. Clinical Pharmacology, Therapy, & Toxicology 27(9):463-466. 1989

109. Zelnik, N. Pediatrics 88(3):486-489. 1991

10-6

1. Berry, P. American J. Pathology 132(3):427-443. 1988

2. Blaker, W. J. Neurobiology 11(3):243-250. 1980

3. Bron, A. Cornea 8(2):135-140. 1989

4. Brosnahan, D. Ophthalmology 101(1):38-45. 1994

5. Brown, N. Eye 12(Pt 1):127-133. 1998

6. Cenedella, R. Experimental Eye Research 37(1):33-43. 1983

7. Cenedella, R. J. Lipid Research 30(7):1079-1084. 1989

8. Cenedella, R. Survey of Ophthalmology 40(4):320-337. 1996

9. Chambless, L. American J. Public Health 80(10):1200-1204. 1990

10. Chandra, V. Neurology 36(2):209-211. 1986

11. Christen, W. Annals of Epidemiology 6(1):60-66. 1996

12. Das, B. Eye 4(Pt 5):723-726. 1990

13. Donnelly, C. British J. Ophthalmology 79(11):1036-1041. 1995

14. Donnelly C. Ophthalmic Research 29(4):207-217. 1997

15. Dreyfus H. Investigative Ophthalmology & Visual Science 37(4):574-585. 1996

16. Frederikse, P. J. Biological Chemistry 271(17):10169-10174. 1996

17. Gaynor, P. J. Lipid Research 37(9):1849-1861. 1996

18. Gerson, R. Experimental Eye Research 50(1):65-78. 1990

19. Gerson, R. Fundamental & Applied Toxicology 16(2):320-329. 1991

20. Green, K. Ophthalmic Research 27 Suppl 1:143-149. 1995

21. Guo, J. Investigative Ophthalmology & Visual Science 39(2):292-300. 1998

22. Harding, J. Alzheimer Disease & Associated Disorders 11(3):123. 1997

23. Hill R. Archives d Ophthalmologie 36(2):155-160. 1976

24. Hiller, R. Annals of Epidemiology 5(6):490-496. 1995

25. Hockwin, O. Fortschritte der Ophthalmologie 88(4):393-395. 1991

26. Jacques, P. American J. Clinical Nutrition 66:911-916. 1997

27. Jahn, C. Ophthalmic Research 15(4):220-224. 1983

28. Keller, R. J. Biological Chemistry 263(5):2250-2254. 1988

29. Kivela, T. Progress in Retinal & Eye Research 17(3):385-428. 1998

30. Klaver, C. American J. Human Genetics 63(1):200-206. 1998

31. Klein, R. Ophthalmology 100(3):406-414. 1993

32. Konishi, M. Cornea 16(6):635-638. 1997

33. Kuszak, J. Investigative Ophthalmology & Visual Science 29(2):261-267. 1988

34. Loffler, K. Investigative Ophthalmology & Visual Science 36(1):24-31. 1995

35. Li, D. Molecular & Cellular Biochemistry 173(1-2):59-69. 1997

36. Liu, I. American J. Public Health 79(6):765-769. 1989

37. Marks, R. J Cataract & Refractive Surgery 14(1):58-63. 1988

38. Morley, J. Annals of Internal Medicine 109(11):890-904. 1988

39. Mosley, S. J. Lipid Research 30(9):1411-1420. 1989

40. Murdoch, I. British J. Ophthalmology 80(12):1083-1086. 1996

41. Nishimoto, J. J. American Optometric Association 61(1):44-49. 1990

42. Pollack, A. Ophthalmic Surgery & Lasers 29(4):286-294. 1998

43. Rouhiainen, P. Cornea 12(2):142-145. 1993

44. Sakuragawa, M. Investigative Ophthalmology 15(12):1022-1027. 1976

45. Shanmugaratnam, J. Brain Research. Molecular Brain Research 50(1-2):113-120. 1997

46. Shimazaki, J. Ophthalmology 102(1):139-144. 1995

47. Smith, W. Archives of Ophthalmology 116(5):583-587. 1998

48. Spector, A. FASEB J. 9(12):1173-1182. 1995
49. Sperduto, R. Archives of Ophthalmology 108(10):1403-1405. 1990
50. Tielsch, J. New England J. Medicine 332(18):1205-1209. 1995
51. Van Haeringen, N. Experimental Eye Research 20(3):271-274. 1975
52. Van Setten, G. Investigative Ophthalmology & Visual Science 37(13):2585-2593. 1996
53. Young, R. J. National Medical Association 84(4):353-358. 1992
54. Yu, F. Investigative Ophthalmology & Visual Science 36(10):1997-2007. 1995
55. Zelenka, P. Current Eye Research 3(11):1337-1359. 1984

10-7

1. Askanas, V. Current Opinion in Rheumatology 5(6):732-741. 1993
2. Chou, S. Baillieres Clinical Neurology 2(3):557-577. 1993
3. Dalakas, M. Current Opinion in Neurology & Neurosurgery 5(5):645-654. 1992
4. Garlepp, M. Annals of Neurology 38(6):957-959. 1995
5. Harrington, C. Neuroscience Letters 183(1-2):35-38. 1995
6. London, S. Neurology 41(7):1159-1160. 1991
7. Manoukian, A. Clinical Chemistry 36(12):2145-2147. 1990
8. Pierno, S. J. Pharmacology & Experimental Therapeutics 275(3):1490-1496. 1995
9. Querfurth, H. J. Neurochemistry 69(4):1580-1591. 1997
10. Robertson, T. American J. Pathology 150(2):417-427. 1997
11. Sarkozi, E. Neuroreport 4(6):815-818. 1993
12. Veerkamp, J. Biochimica et Biophysica Acta 1315(3):217-222. 1996

10-8

1. Benson, M. New England J. Medicine 336(7):502-504. 1997
2. Bergfeldt, B. American J. Cardiology 56(10):647-652. 1985
3. Dubrey, S. American J. Cardiology 76(10):739-741. 1995
4. Gertz, M. American J. Cardiology 80(1):93-95. 1997
5. Goffin, Y. J. Clinical Pathology 3393):262-268. 1980
6. Hosenpud, J. Circulation 84(5 Suppl):III 338-343. 1991
7. Ikeda, S. J. Neurological Sciences 79(1-2):129-139. 1987
8. Ishii, T. J. American Geriatrics Society 26(3):108-115. 1978
9. Johansson, B. International J. Cardiology 32(1):83-92. 1991
10. Kyle, R. American J. Medicine 101(4):395-400. 1996
11. Ott, A. Stroke 28(2):316-321. 1997
12. Pelosi, F. American J. Cardiology 79(4):532-535. 1997
13. Psaty, B. Circulation 96)7):2455-2461. 1997
14. Shimamoto, T. J. Epidemiology 6(3 Suppl):s43-47. 1996

10-9

1. Aho, K. J. Rheumatology 13(5):899-902. 1986
2. Akatsuka, H. Microbiology & Immunology 41(4):367-370. 1997
3. Akiyama, H. Japanese J. Clinical Medicine 52(11):2990-2994. 1994
4. Athanasou, N. Histopathology 20(1):41-46. 1992
5. Badolato, R. Seminars in Arthritis & Rheumatism 26(2):526-538. 1996

6. Beard, C. Lancet 337(8754):1426. 1991

7. Bekkelund, S. American J. Neuroradiology 16(4):767-772. 1995

8. Bely, M. Acta Morphologica Hungarica 40(1-4):49-69. 1992

9. Blackburn, W. American J. Medicine 100(2a):24s-30s. 1996

10. Bondeson, J. General Pharmacology 29(2):127-150. 1997

11. Breitner, J. Neurology 44(2):227-232. 1994

12. Chikanza, I. Arthritis & Rheumatism 35(11):1281-1288. 1992

13. Chikanza, I. British J, Rheumatology 32(6):445-448. 1993

14. Comstock, G. Annals of the Rheumatic Diseases 56:323-325. 1997

15. Crofford, L. J. Clinical Endocrinology & Metabolism 82(4):1279-1283. 1997

16. Dawes, P. Annals of the Rheumatic Diseases 45(11):945-949. 1986

17. De Beer, F. Lancet 2(8292):231-234. 1982

18. Dennison, E. BMJ 316:789-790. 1998

19. Duff, G. Scandinavian J. Rheumatology- suppl 100:9-19. 1994

20. Ettinger, W. Atherosclerosis 63(2-3):167-172. 1987

21. Fairburn, K. Clinical Science 83(6):657-664. 1992

22. Farrell, A. Annals of the Rheumatic Diseases 51(11):1219-1222. 1992

23. Gogia, P. Archives of Physical Medicine & Rehabilitation 74(5):463-467. 1993

24. Grabowski, P. British J. Rheumatology 35(3):207-212. 1996

25. Gudbjornsson, B. J. Rheumatology 23(4):596-602. 1996

26. Hall, J. Arthritis & Rheumatism 37(8):1132-1137. 1994

27. Henderson, N. Current Opinion in Rheumatology 8(4):365-369. 1996

28. Hilliquin, P. Arthritis & Rheumatism 40(8):1512-1517. 1997

29. Honkanen, V. Clinical & Experimental Rheumatology 8(2):187-191. 1990

30. Horrobin, D. Medical Hypotheses 22(4):421-428. 1987

31. Husby, G. Clinical & Experimental Rheumatology 3(2):173-180. 1985

32. Jacobsson, L. Arthritis & Rheumatism 37(8):1158-1165. 1994

33. Jarvinen, P. Seminars in Arthitis & Rheumatism 24(1):19-28. 1994

34. Jenkinson, M. British J. Rheumatology 28(1):86-88. 1989

35. Jongen-Lavrencic, M. J. Rheumatology 24(8):1504-1509. 1997

36. Jorgensen, C. Clinical & Experimental Rheumatology 13(6):705-709. 1995

37. Kaur, H. FEBS Letters 350(1):9-12. 1994

38. Kobayashi, H. British J. Rheumatology 35(1):44-49. 1996

39. Kunitomo, M. Japanese J. Pharmacology 44(1):15-22. 1987

40. Kyle, R. Medicine 54(4):271-299. 1975

41. Lazarevic, M. Seminars in Arthritis & Rheumatism 22(3):172-178. 1992

42. Lee, C. J. Formosan Medical Association 96(8):573-578. 1997

43. Liew, F. Ciba Foundation Symposium 195-234-239. 1995

44. Lorber, M. British J. Rheumatology 24(3):250-255. 1985

45. Maini, R. Clinical & Experimental Rheumatology 11 Suppl 8:s173-175. 1993

46. Mandi, B. Acta Biologica Academiae Scientiarum Hungaricae 26(3-4):115-133. 1975

47. Mandybur, T. Neurology 29(10):1336-1340. 1979

48. Masoom-Yasinzai, M. Zeitschrift fur Naturforschung. Section C. J. Biosciences 51(5-6):401-403. 1996

49. Maury, C. Rheumatology International 8(3):107-111. 1988

50. Mazanec, K. Ceskoslovenska Patologie 28(3):136-141. 1992

51. McGeer, P. Lancet 335(8696):1037. 1990

52. McGeer, P. Neurology 47(2):425-432. 1996

53. McMurray, R. J. Rheumatology 22(8):1577-1580. 1995

54. Migita, K. Laboratory Investigation 75(3):371-375. 1996

55. Mohr, W. Virchows Archiv. B, Cell Pathology Including Molecular Pathology 60(4):259-262. 1991

56. Munro, R. Annals of the Rheumatic Diseases 56:326-329. 1997

57. Myllykangas-Luosujarvi, R. British J. Rheumatology 33(5):501-502. 1994

58. Nashel, D. American J. Medicine 80(5):925-929. 1986

59. Noseda, G. Schweizerische Medizinische Wochenschrift. J. Suisse de Medecine 105(31 Suppl):1-58. 1975

60. Okuda, Y. Ryumachi 34(6):939-946. 1994

61. Partsch, G. J. Rheumatology 24(3):518-523. 1997

62. Rantapaa-Dahlqvist, S. Annals of the Rheumatic Diseases 50(6):366-368. 1991

63. Ravussin, E. Diabetes Care 19(9):1067-1074. 1994

64. Rosenthal, C. J. Clinical Investigation 55(4):746-753. 1975

65. Rossner, S. Atherosclerosis 28(1):41-52. 1977

66. Saitou, H. J. Japanese Orthopaedic Association 68(7):534-544. 1994

67. Senturk, T. Rheumatology International 16(4):141-144. 1996

68. Setton, L. Agents & Actions- Suppl 39):27-48. 1993

69. Silman, A. British J. Rheumatology 32(10):903-907. 1993

70. Silman, A. APMIS 102(10):721-728. 1994

71. Situnayake, R. Annals of the Rheumatic Diseases 56:341-342. 1997

72. Solveborn, S. Clinical Orthopaedics & Related Research 316:99-105. 1995

73. Spector, T. Current Opinion in Rheumatology 3(2):266-271. 1991

74. Svenson, K. Archives of Internal Medicine 147(11):1912-1916. 1987

75. Svenson K. Archives of Internal Medicine 147(11):1917-1920. 1987

76. Takada, K. Clinical Chemistry 43(7):1188-1195. 1997

77. Ueki, Y. J. Rheumatology 23(2):230-236. 1996

78. Urban, B. Radiographics 13(6):1295-1308. 1993

79. Wigand, R. Annals of the Rheumatic Diseases 56(5):330-332. 1997

80. Wuthier, R. Biochimica et Biophysica Acta 409(1):128-143. 1975

81. Yamaguchi, Y. Japanese J. Pharmacology 50(4):377-386. 1989

82. Ylinen, K. Nephrology, Dialysis, Transplantation 7(9):908-912. 1992

83. Youssef, P. Arthritis & Rheumatism 40(8):1400-1408. 1997

10-10

1. Ahmed, Q. J. Rheumatology 23(6):1107-1110. 1996

2. Ameglio, F. Dermatology 189(4):359-363. 1994

3. Bergstresser, P. British J. Dermatology 96(5):503-509. 1977
4. Bonifati, C. Clinical & Experimental Dermatology 19(5):383-387. 1994
5. Bonte, F. Archives of Dermatological Research 289(2):78-82. 1997
6. Brandrup, F. Acta Dermato-Venereologica 62(3):229-236. 1982
7. Brazzelli, V. Dermatology 192(3):214-216. 1996
8. Brenner, S. Dermatologica 150(2):96-102. 1975
9. Bruch-Gerharz, D. J. Experimental Medicine 184(5):2007-2012. 1996
10. Christophers, E. International Archives of Allergy & Immunology 110(3):199-206. 1996
11. Cox, P. J. Investigative Dermatology 87(6):741-744. 1986
12. Deiana, L. Bollettino- Societa Italiana Biologia Sperimentale 68(12):755-759. 1992
13. Duffy, D. J. American Academy of Dermatology 29(3):428-434. 1993
14. Edwards, B. QJM 88(2):109-113. 1995
15. Ellis, C. Archives of Dermatology 118(8):559-562. 1982
16. Feingold, K. J. Investigative Dermatology 96(2):201-209. 1991
17. FitzGerald, O. Current Opinion in Rheumatology 9(4):295-301. 1997
18. Guilhou, J. Presse Medicale 26(24):1168-1172. 1997
19. Gupta, A. J. American Academy of Dermatology 20(6):1088-1093. 1989
20. Heenen, M. Cell & Tissue Kinetics 20(6):561-570. 1987
21. Hohler, T. J. Investigative Dermatology 109(4):562-565. 1997
22. Horrobin, D. Medical Hypotheses 22(4):421-428. 1987
23. Iizuka, H. J. Dermatological Science 8(3):215-217. 1994
24. Imamura, T. Japanese J. Dermatology 100(10):1023-1028. 1990
25. Jackson, S. J. Lipid Research 33(9):1307-1314. 1992
26. Jackson, S. Western J. Medicine 158(3):279-285. 1993
27. Kadunce, D. Dermatologic Clinics 13(4):723-737. 1995
28. Kolb-Bachofen, V. Lancet 344(8915):139. 1994
29. Krasovec, M. Dermatology 186(4):248-252. 1993
30. Krueger, G. J. Investigative Dermatology 102(6):14s-18s. 1994
31. Krupp, P. British J. Dermatology 122 Suppl 36:47-56. 1990
32. Lampe, M. J. Lipid Research 24(2):131-140. 1983
33. Lazarevic, M. Seminars in Arthritis & Rheumatism 22(3):172-178. 1992
34. Leren, T. Clinical Genetics 25(3):230-241. 1984
35. Lu, I. J. Cutaneous Pathology 23(5):419-430. 1996
36. Man, M. J. Investigative Dermatology 106(5):1096-1101. 1996
37. Mizushima, H. J. Lipid Research 37(2):361-367. 1996
38. Mizutani, H. J. Dermatological Science 14(2):145-153. 1997
39. Morimoto, S. Archives of Dermatology 125(2):231-234. 1989
40. Morimoto, S. J. Dermatological Science 1(4):277-282. 1990
41. Oxholm, A. APMIS. Suppl 24:1-32. 1992
42. Partsch, G. J. Rheumatology 24(3):518-523. 1997
43. Paus, R. Medical Hypotheses 36(1):33-42. 1991

44. Pilgram, G. J. Microscopy 189(Pt 1):71-78. 1998
45. Ponec, M. J. Investigative Dermatology 98(6 Suppl):50s-56s. 1992
46. Proksch, E. Hautarzt 43(6):331-338. 1992
47. Proksch, E. British J. Dermatology 128(5):473-482. 1993
48. Proksch, E. Hautarzt 46(2):76-80. 1995
49. Prystowsky, J. J. American Academy of Dermatology 35(Pt 1)690-695. 1996
50. Quiec, D. Biochemical J. 310(Pt 1):305-309. 1995
51. Rowe, A. Lancet 344(8933):1371. 1994
52. Serizawa, S. J. Investigative Dermatology 99(2):232-236. 1992
53. Sirsjo, A. British J. Dermatology 134(4):643-468. 1996
54. Stiller, M. J. American Academy of Dermatology 27(3):434-438. 1992
55. Tsuda, S. Clinical & Experimental Dermatology 21(2):141-144. 1996
56. Veys, E. Dermatology 189 Suppl 2:35-41. 1994
57. Weinstein, G. J. Investigative Dermatology 82(6):623-628. 1984
58. Wen, G. Acta Neuropathologica 88(3):201-206. 1994
59. Wertz, P. J. Investigative Dermatology 87(5):582-584. 1986
60. Williams, M. Archives of Dermatology 123(11):1535-1538. 1987
61. Wittenberg, G. J. American Academy of Dermatology 32(3):465-468. 1995
62. Wang, R. J. Investigative Dermatology 106(3):419-427. 1996
63. Wu-Pong, S. J. Investigative Dermatology 102(5):799-802. 1994
64. Zettersten, E. J. American Academy of Dermatology 37(3 Pt 1):403-408. 1997

10-11

1. Abe-Hashimoto, J. Cancer Research 53(11):2534-2537. 1993
2. Ainsleigh, H. Preventive Medicine 22(1):132-140. 1993
3. Ashton, R. J. Investigative Dermatology 79(4):229-232. 1982
4. Belleli, A. Carcinogenesis 13(12):2293-2298. 1992
5. Boutron, M. British J. Cancer 74(1):145-151. 1996
6. Brenner, R. Cancer Letters 92(1):77-82. 1995
7. Chel, V. J Bone & Mineral Research 13(8):1238-1242. 1998
8. Christakos, S. Advances in Experimental Medicine & Biology 364:115-118. 1994
9. Chuang, T. J. American Academy of Dermatology 26(2 Pt 1):173-177. 1992
10. Colston, K. Lancet 1(8631)188-191. 1989
11. Colston, K. Biochemical Pharmacology 44(4):693-702. 1992
12. Colston, K. British J. Cancer 76(8):1017-1020. 1997
13. Crivello, J. Archives Biochemical Biophysics 262(2):471-480. 1988
14. Emerson, J. Cancer Causes & Control 3(1):95-99. 1992
15. Feldman, D. Advances in Experimental Medicine & Biology 375:53-63. 1995
16. Garland, F. Archives of Environmental Health 45(5):261-267. 1990
17. Garland, F. Preventive Medicine 19(6):614-622. 1990
18. Getzenberg, R. Urology 50(6):999-1006. 1997
19. Glinghammar, B. American J. Clinical Nutrition 66(5):1277-1282. 1997
20. Halprin, K. J. American Academy of Dermatology 7(5):633-638. 1982

21. Hanchette, C. Cancer 70(12):2861-2869. 1992

22. Harkonen, M. J. Steroid Biochemistry 11(3):1205-1208. 1979

23. He, R. J. Pharmacology & Experimental Therapeutics 281(1):464-469. 1997

24. Higashimoto, Y. Anticancer Research 16(5a):2653-2659. 1996

25. Holick, M. Bone 17(2 Suppl):107s-111s. 1995

26. Kaiser, U. J. Cancer Research & Clinical Oncology 122(6):356-359. 1996

27. Kawa, S. Gastroenterology 110(5):1605-1613. 1996

28. Klaui, H. Proceedings Nutrition Society 38(1):135-141. 1979

29. Kornfehl, J. European Archives of Oto-Rhino-Laryngology 253(6):341-344. 1996

30. Kragballe, K. Archives of Dermatological Research 284 Suppl 1:s30-36. 1992

31. Lefkowitz, E. International J. Epidemiology 23(6):1133-1136. 1994

32. Light, B. Cancer Research 57(17):3759-3764. 1997

33. Lointier, P. Anticancer Research 9(6):1921-1924. 1989

34. Martinez, M. J. National Cancer Institute 88(19):1375-1382. 1996

35. Martinez, M. Cancer Epidemiology, Biomarkers & Prevention 7(2):163-168. 1998

36. Mercier, T. Biochemical Pharmacology 52(3):505-510. 1996

37. Naveilhan, P. J. Neuroscience 37(2):271-277. 1994

38. Newman, M. Archives of Dermatology 125(9):1218-1224. 1989

39. Newmark, H. Advances in Experimental Medicine & Biology 364:109-114. 1994

40. Numahara, T. Dermatologica 178(2):73-74. 1989

41. Peehl, D. Cancer Research 54(3):805-810. 1994

42. Pritchard, R. Cancer Epidemiology, Biomarkers & Prevention 5(11):897-900. 1996

43. Sadava, D. Biology of the Cell 87(1-2):113-115. 1996

44. Saunders, D. Gynecologic Oncology 51(2):155-159. 1993

45. Saunders, D. Anti-Cancer Drugs 6(4):562-569. 1995

46. Schmidt, J. Ugeskrift for Laeger 160(30):4411-4414. 1998

47. Schwartz, G. Anticancer Research 14(3a):1077-1081. 1994

48. Schwartz, G. Cancer Epidemiology, Biomarkers & Prevention 6(9):727-732. 1997

49. Shabahang, M. Cancer Research 54(15):4057-4064. 1994

50. Simboli-Campbell, M. J. Steroid Biochemistry & Molecular Biology 58(4):367-376. 1996

51. Simboli-Campbell, M. Breast Cancer Research & Treatment 42(1):31-41. 1997

52. Skowronski, R. Endrocrinology 132(5):1952-1960. 1993

53. Skowronski, R. Endocrinology 136(1):20-26. 1995

54. Stern, R. J. Investigative Dermatology 108(6):897-900. 1997

55. Stern, R. J. National Cancer Institute 90(17):1278-1284. 1998

56. Tangrea, J. Cancer Causes & Control 8(4):615-625. 1997

57. Themido, R. Acta Dermato-Venereologica 72(5):361-364. 1992

58. Thomas, M. Gut 33(12):1660-1663. 1992

59. Tong, W. International J. Cancer 75(3):467-472. 1998

60. Van Dooren-Greebe, R. British J. Dermatology 130(2):204-210. 1994

61. Verstuyf, A. Current Opinion in Nephrology & Hypertension 7(4):397-403. 1998

62. Vink-Van Wijngaarden, T. Cancer Research 54(21):5711-5717. 1994

63. Wang, X. British J. Urology 80(2):260-262. 1997

64. Yabushita, H. J. Obstetrics & Gynaecology Research 22(6):529-539. 1996

65. Zheng, W. Cancer Epidemiology, Biomarkers & Prevention 7(3):221-225. 1998

Chapter 11

1. Armstrong, R. Neurodegeneration 5(1):35-41. 1996

2. Banik, N. Brain 98(2):213-218. 1975

3. Becker, L. APMIS Suppl 40:57-70. 1993

4. Ben-Yoseph, O. Neurochemical Research 21(9):1005-1012. 1996

5. Berk, A. Ophthalmic Genetics 17(1):15-19. 1996

6. Beyreuther, K. Annals of the New York Academy of Sciences 640:129-139. 1991

7. Beyreuther, K. Annals of the New York Academy of Sciences 695:91-102. 1993

8. Brodtkorb, E. Seizure 3(4):277-285. 1994

9. Brooksbank, B. Brain Research 318(1):37-44. 1984

10. Brunk, U. Free Radical Biology & Medicine 19(6):813-822. 1995

11. Busciglio, J. Nature 378(6559);776-779. 1995

12. Carmeliet, G. Mutation Research 256(2-6):221-231. 1991

13. Ceballos-Picot, I. Brain Research 552(2):198-214. 1991

14. Ceballos-Picot, I. EXS 62:89-98. 1992

15. Ceballos-Picot, I. Comptes Rendus des Seances de la Societe de Biologie et de Ses Filiales 187(3):308-323. 1993

16. Chada, S. Genomics 6(2):268-271. 1990

17. Chu, F. Cytogenetics & Cell Genetics 66(2):96-98. 1994

18. Clemens, M. Free Radical Research Communications 3(1-5):265-271. 1987

19. Crino, P. Annals of Otology, Rhinology & Laryngology 104(8):655-661. 1995

20. Da Cunha, R. American J. Ophthalmology 122(2):236-244. 1996

21. De Haan, J. Brain Research. Molecular Brain Research 13(3):179-187. 1992

22. De Haan, J. Biochemistry & Molecular Biology International 35(6):1281-1297. 1995

23. De Haan, J. Human Molecular Genetics 5(2):283-292. 1996

24. De La Torre, R. Experientia 52(9):871-873. 1996

25. Denisova, N. J. Neurochemistry 69(3):1259-1266. 1997

26. Diamond, A. Gene 122(2):377-380. 1992

27. Dorner, K. Clinica Chimica Acta 142(3):307-311. 1984

28. Eberhard, Y. Pathologie Biologie 41(5):482-486. 1993

29. Emerson, J. Progress in Clinical & Biological Research 393:123-138. 1995

30. Feaster, W. American J. Human Genetics 29(6):563-570. 1977

31. Finney, J. Angiology 17(4):223-228. 1966

32. Furuta, A. American J. Pathology 146(2):357-367. 1995

33. Hemdal, P. Neuropsychologia 31(9):977-984. 1993

34. Hof, P. Archives of Neurology 52(4):379-391. 1995

35. Holland, A. J. Neurology, Neurosurgery & Psychiatry 59(2):111-114. 1995

36. Hughes, W. British Medical J. dated Sept 10, 1977, page 702.
37. Hyman, B. Proceedings/America 92(8):3586-3590. 1995
38. Johannsen, P. Seizure 5(2):121-125. 1996
39. Joseph, J. Free Radical Biology & Medicine 22(3):455-462. 1997
40. Kallen, B. American J. Medical Genetics 65(2):160-166. 1996
41. Kalman, J. Acta Neurologica Scandinavica 96(4):236-240. 1997
42. Kao, F. Genomics 23(3):700-703. 1994
43. Korenberg, J. Genomics 5(1):124-127. 1989
44. Kyle, M. Biochemical Pharmacology 38(21):3797-3805. 1989
45. Lee, J. International J. Food Sciences & Nutrition 48(2):151-159. 1997
46. Lemere, C. Neurobiology of Disease 3(1):16-32. 1996
47. Leverenz, J. Experimental Neurology 150(2):296-304. 1998
48. Lott, I. Annals of the New York Academy of Sciences 396:15-27. 1982
49. Mann, D. J. Neurological Sciences 80(1):79-89. 1987
50. Mann, D. J. Neurological Sciences 89(2-3):169-179. 1989
51. Mann, D. Neuroscience Letters 196(1-2):105-108. 1995
52. Mattiace, L. J. Neuropathology & Experimental Neurology 50(5):547-559. 1991
53. McBride, O. Biofactors 1(4):285-292. 1988
54. McCoy, E. J. Mental Deficiency Research 15(1):1-12. 1971
55. McVicker, R. British J. Psychiatry 164(4):528-532. 1994
56. Mickel, H. Lipids 7(2):121-124. 1972
57. Morrison, R. Hypertension 28(4):569-575. 1996
58. Murdoch, J. British Medical J. 2(6081):226-228. 1977
59. Murphy, C. Neurobiology of Aging 17(4):631-637. 1996
60. Murphy, G. Brain Research 537(1-2):102-108. 1990
61. Murphy, M. J. Immunology 149(7):2506-2512. 1992
62. Nishida, Y. Atherosclerosis 26(3):369-372. 1977
63. Pearlson, G. American J. Neuroradiology 11(4):811-816. 1990
64. Pearlson, G. Developmental Medicine & Child Neurology 40(5):326-334. 1998
65. Pouplard, A. Revue Neurologique 139(3):187-191. 1983
66. Prasher, V. Seizure 4(1):53-56. 1995
67. Pueschel, S. Archives of Neurology 48(3):318-320. 1991
68. Pueschel, S. J. Intellectual Disability Research 36(Pt 4):365-369. 1992
69. Richards, B. J. Mental Deficiency Research 23(2):123-135. 1979
70. Roth, G. American J. Neuroradiology 17(7):1283-1289. 1996
71. Rumble, B. New England J. Medicine 320(22):1446-1452. 1989
72. Salo, M. Scandinavian J. Clinical & Laboratory Investigation 39(5):485-490. 1979
73. Schapiro, M. American J. Ophthalmology 99(6):659-663. 1985
74. Schapiro, M. Neurology 38(6):938-942. 1988
75. Schapiro, M. Neurology 39(10):1349-1353. 1989
76. Schapiro, M. J. Cerebral Blood Flow & Metabolism 10(2):199-206. 1990
77. Shireman, R. Biochimica et Biophysica Acta 958(3):352-360. 1988

78. Sinet, P. Life Sciences 24(1):29-33. 1979
79. Sinet, P. Annals of the New York Academy of Sciences 396:83-94. 1982
80. Speller, C. British J. Psychiatry 165(2):270. 1994
81. Tayarani, I. J. Neurochemistry 48(5):1399-1402. 1987
82. Teller, J. Nature Medicine 2(1):93-95. 1996
83. Tokuda, T. Annals of Neurology 41:271-273. 1997
84. Tolksdorf, M. Human Genetics- Suppl 2:3-31. 1981
85. Urakami, K. Dementia 7(2):82-85. 1996
86. Vallfors, B. Acta Neurochirurgica 64(3-4):225-232. 1982
87. Van Gool, W. Annals of Neurology 38(2):225-230. 1995
88. Van Leeuwen, F. Science 279(5348):242-247. 1998
89. Walsh, S. J. Mental Deficiency Research 25 Pt 4:243-251. 1981
90. Wisniewski, K. Annals of Neurology 17(3):278-282. 1985
91. Wisniewski, K. American J. Medical Genetics- Suppl 7:274-281. 1990
92. Wisniewski, T. Annals of Neurology 37(1):136-138. 1995
93. Yla-Herttuala, S. Atherosclerosis 76(2-3):269-272. 1989
94. Yoshimura, N. Acta Pathologica Japonica 40(10):735-743. 1990
95. Zamorano, A. Archivos de Biologia y Medicina Experimentales 24(1):49-55. 1991
96. Zubenko, G. J. Geriatric Psychiatry & Neurology 1(4):218-219. 1988
97. Zucco, G. Perceptual & Motor Skills 78(2):627-631. 1994

Chapter 12
12-1

1. Araki, W. J. Internal Medicine 229(2):197-199. 1991
2. Bawle, E. Pediatric Neurology 13(1):14-18. 1995

12-2

1. Arlazoroff, A. Epilepsia 32(5):657-661. 1991
2. Ballantyne C. Metabolism: Clinical & Experimental 36(3):270-276. 1987
3. Bencze, K. J. Neurology, Neurosurgery & Psychiatry 53(2):166-167. 1990
4. Berginer, V. J. Neurological Sciences 122(1):102-108. 1994
5. Dotti, M. American J. Neuroradiology 15(9):1721-1726. 1992
6. Fujiyama, J. Japanese J. Medicine 30(2):189-192. 1991
7. Fujiyama, J. Clinica Chimica Acta 299(1):1-11. 1991
8. Katz, D. Archives of Neurology 42(10):1008-1010. 1985
9. Leitersdorf, E. American J. Human Genetics 55(5):907-915. 1994
10. Ohnishi, A. Acta Neuropathologica 45(1):43-45. 1979
11. Salen, G. Metabolism: Clinical & Experimental 43(8):1018-1022. 1994
12. Shibata, N. Rinsho Shinkeigaku- Clinical Neurology 30(9):978-984. 1990

12-3

1. Acosta, P. American J. Medical Genetics 50(4):358-363. 1994
2. Chambers, C. American J. Medical Genetics 68(3):322-327. 1997
3. Elias, E. American J. Medical Genetics 68(3):305-310. 1997

4. Irons, M. American J. Medical Genetics 68(3):311-314. 1997
5. Llirbat, B. J. Lipid Research 38(1):22-34. 1997
6. Ness, G. American J. Medical Genetics 68(3):294-299. 1997
7. Nwokoro, N. American J. Medical Genetics 68(3):315-321. 1997
8. Opitz, J. American J. Medical Genetics 50(4):326-338. 1994
9. Pauli, R. American J. Medical Genetics 68(3):260-262. 1997
10. Salen, G. J. Lipid Research 37(6):1169-1180. 1996
11. Tint, G. New England J. Medicine 330:107-113. 1994
12. Tzouvelekis, g. Clinical Genetics 40(3):229-232. 1991
13. Van Rooij, A. J. Inherited Metabolic Disease 20(4):578-580. 1997

12-4

1. Gibson, K. European J. Pediatrics 148(3):250-252. 1988
2. Hoffman, G. New England J. Medicine 314(25):1610-1614. 1986
3. Hoffman, G. Pediatrics 91(5):915-921. 1993
4. Hoffman, G. Pediatric Research 41(4 Pt 1):541-546. 1997
5. Mancini, J. Pediatric Neurology 9(3):243-246. 1993

12-5

1. Auer, I. Acta Neuropathologica 90(6):547-551. 1995
2. Blanchette-Mackie, E. Proceedings/America 85(21):8022-8026. 1988
3. Brown, D. J. Inherited Metabolic Disease 19(3):319-330. 1996
4. Coxey, R. J. Lipid Research 34(7):1165-1176. 1993
5. Hulette, C. Clinical Neuropathology 11(6):293-297. 1992
6. Litvan, I. Neurology 49(1):62-69. 1997
7. Love, S. Brain 118(Pt 1):119-129. 1995
8. Suzuki, K. Acta Neuropathologica 89(3):227-238. 1995
9. Turpin, J. Developmental Neuroscience 13(4-5):304-306. 1991

12-6

1. Lancaster, F. Alcohol 9(1):9-15. 1992
2. Landers, D. American Family Physician 28(4):219-222. 1983
3. Lundsberg, L. Annals of Epidemiology 7:498-508. 1997
4. Pierce, J. Southern Medical J. 75(4):463-469. 1982
5. Pirovino, M. Schweizerische Medizinische Wochenschrift. J. Suisse de Medecine 123(17):873-880. 1993
6. Plotz, E. American J. Obstetrics & Gynecology 101(4):534-538. 1968
7. Potter, J. Australian & New Zealand J. of Medicine 7(2):155-160. 1977

Chapter 13

13-1

1. El-Tatawy,S. American J. Neuroradiology 4(3):434-436. 1983
2. Gunston, G. Archives of Diseases in Childhood 67(8):1030-1032. 1992
3. Househam, K. Archives of Diseases in Childhood 62(6):589-592. 1987
4. Kessel, A. Israel J. Medical Sciences 32(5):306-308. 1996

13-2

1. Ainley, C. Gastroenterology 100(6):1616-1625. 1991
2. Arden, M. J. Adolescent Health Care 11(3):199-202. 1990
3. Argente, J. J. Clinical Endocrinology & Metabolism 82(7):2084-2092. 1997
4. Artmann, H. Neuroradiology 27(4):304-312. 1985
5. Ball, W. J. Pediatrics 129(6):779-781. 1996
6. Beumont, P. J. Clinical Endocrinology & Metabolism 51(6):1283-1285. 1980
7. Blickle, J. Hormone & Metabolic Research 16(7):336-340. 1984
8. Bradley, S. J. Clinical & Experimental Neuropsychology 19(1):20-33. 1997
9. Bridgers, S. Archives of Neurology 44(3):312-316. 1987
10. Broocks, A. J. Neural Transmission- General Section 79(1-2):113-124. 1990
11. Counts, D. J. Clinical Endocrinology & Metabolism 75(3):762-767. 1992
12. Croner, S. Acta Paediatrica Scandinavica 74(2):230-236. 1985
13. Delvenne, V. Biological Psychiatry 40(8):761-768. 1996
14. Delvenne, V. J. Affective Disorders 44(1):69-77. 1997
15. De Marinis, L. Psychoneuroendocrinology 16(6):499-504. 1991
16. Divertie, G. Diabetes 40(10):1228-1232. 1991
17. Dolan, R. Psychological Medicine 18(2):349-353. 1988
18. Esca, S. Acta Dermato-Venereologica 59(4):361-364. 1979
19. Fenley, J. General Hospital Psychiatry 12(4):264-270; 1990
20. Fichter, M. Acta Psychiatrica Scandinavica 66(6):429-444. 1982
21. Fichter, M. Psychiatry Research 17(1):61-72. 1986
22. Fohlin, L. Acta Medica Scandinavica 204(1-2):61-65. 1978
23. Frankel, R. Acta Endocrinologica 78(2):209-221. 1975
24. Garfinkel, P. Archives of General Psychiatry 32(6):739-744. 1975
25. Gold, P. New England J. Medicine 314(21):1335-1342. 1986
26. Golden, N. J. Pediatrics 128(2):296-301. 1996
27. Golden, N. Archives of Pediatrics & Adolescent Medicine 151(1):16-21. 1997
28. Gupta, M. Archives of Dermatology 123(10):1386-1390. 1987
29. Gwirtsman, H. Archives of General Psychiatry 46(1):61-69. 1989
30. Heinz, E. J. Computer Assisted Tomography 1(4):415-418. 1977
31. Hertlova, M. Casopis Lekaru Ceskych 133(24):759-761. 1994
32. Holden, R. Medical Hypotheses 47(6):423-438. 1996
33. Jornod, P. Revue Medicale de la Suisse Romande 117(6):485-494. 1997
34. Joyce, J. J. Nuclear Medicine 31(3):325-331. 1990
35. Katzman, D. J. Pediatrics 129(6):794-803. 1996
36. Kingston, K. Psychological Medicine 26(1):15-28. 1996
37. Krieg, J. Biological Psychiatry 23(4):377-387. 1988
38. LaBan, M. Archives of Physical Medicine & Rehabilitation 76(9):884-887. 1995
39. Laessle, R. Psychoneuroendocrinology 17(5):475-484. 1992
40. Lambe, E. Archives of General Psychiatry 54(6):537-542. 1997
41. Lankenau, H. Comprehensive Psychiatry 26(2):136-147. 1985

42. Leibowitz, S. Drugs 39 Suppl 3:33-48. 1990
43. Lesem, M. Biological Psychiatry 25(4):509-512. 1989
44. Licinio, J. Psychiatry Research 62(1):75-83. 1996
45. Maugars, Y. Presse Medicale 23(4):156-158. 1994
46. Maugars, Y. European J. Endocrinology 135(5):591-597. 1996
47. McClain, C. J. American College Nutrition 12(4):466-474. 1993
48. Mira, M. Annals of Clinical Biochemistry 24(Pt 1):29-35. 1987
49. Mordasini, R. Metabolism: Clinical & Experimental 27(1):71-79. 1978
50. Muuss, R. Adolescence 20(79):525-536. 1985
51. Newman, M. Psychiatry Research 29(1):105-112. 1989
52. Pirke, K. Neuroscience & Biobehavioral Reviews 17(3):287-294. 1993
53. Pirke, K. Psychiatry Research 62(1):43-49. 1996
54. Pomeroy, C. Biological Psychiatry 36(12):836-839. 1994
55. Rencken, M. JAMA 276:238-240. 1996
56. Rich, L. Archives of Internal Medicine 150(4):894-895. 1990
57. Roberts, W. Medicine & Science in Sports & Exercise 23(5):513-516. 1991
58. Rock, C. International J. Eating Disorders 18(3):257-262. 1995
59. Salisbury, J. American J. Psychiatry 148(768):774. 1991
60. Sanchez-Muniz, F. European J. Clinical Nutrition 45(1):33-36. 1991
61. Scacchi, M. J. Clinical Endocrinology & Metabolism 82(10):3225-3229. 1997
62. Schattner, A. J. Clinical & Laboratory Immunology 32(4):183-184. 1990
63. Signer, S. American J. Psychiatry 147(2):235-238. 1990
64. Sirinathsinghji, D. Acta Endocrinologica 108(2):255-260. 1985
65. Stephan, F. Nouvelle Presse Medicale 11(14):1055-1058. 1982
66. Tachibana, N. Japanese J. Psychiatry & Neurology 43(1):77-84. 1989
67. Thibault, L. International J. for Vitamin & Nutrition Research 57(4):447-452. 1987
68. Umeki, S. J. Nervous & Mental Disease 176(8):503-506. 1988
69. Vaisman, N. Metabolism: Clinical & Experimental 40(7):720-723. 1991
70. Van Binsbergen, C. Psychosomatic Medicine 53(4):440-452. 1991
71. Vierhapper, H. Acta Endocrinologica 122(6):753-758. 1990
72. Walsh, B. J. Clinical Endocrinology & Metabolism 53(1):203-205. 1981
73. Walsh, B. Psychoneuroendocrinology 12(2):131-140. 1987
74. Yamada, Y. Internal Medicine 35(7):560-563. 1996

13-3
1. Abe, S. American Heart J. 131(6):1137-1144. 1996
2. Allieu, Y. Annales de Chirurgie de la Main et du Membre Superieur 13(2):113-121. 1994
3. Aguilera, A. Nephrology, Dialysis, Transplantation 13(6):1476-1483. 1998
4. Avram,M. American J. Kidney Diseases 26(1):209-219. 1995
5. Avram, M. American J. Kidney Diseases 28(6):910-917. 1996
6. Bailey, J. Mineral & Electrolyte Metabolism 24(1):13-19. 1998
7. Balaskas, E. Clinical Nephrology 42(1):54-62. 1994

8. Bergstrom, J. J. American Society of Nephrology 6(5):1329-1341. 1995
9. Besbas, N. Nephrology, Dialysis, Transplantation 13(6):1484-1488. 1998
10. Brauner, A. American J. Kidney Diseases 27(3):402-408. 1996
11. Brem, A. Archives of Internal Medicine 149(11):2541-2544. 1989
12. Candy, J. J. Neurological Sciences 107(2):210-218. 1992
13. Carbone, V. Anna J. 22(5):452-455. 1995
14. Cianciaruso, B. American J. Kidney Diseases 26(3):475-486. 1995
15. Cohen, A. Current Opinion in Rheumatology 5(1):62-76. 1993
16. Cohen, G. Mineral & Electrolyte Metabolism 23(3-6):210-213. 1997
17. Davison, A. Lancet 2(8302):785-787. 1982
18. Degoulet, P. Nephron 31(2):103-110. 1982
19. De Precigout, V. Blood Purification 14(2):170-176. 1996
20. Deuber, H. Kidney International 40(3):496-500. 1991
21. Ding, X. Mineral & Electrolyte Metabolism 23(3-6):194-197. 1997
22. Druml, W. Kidney International- Suppl 16:s139-142. 1983
23. Elisaf, M. American J. Nephrology 17(2):153-157. 1997
24. England, B. Blood Purification 13(3-4):147-152. 1995
25. Fazekas, G. J. Neurological Sciences 134(1-2):83-88. 1995
26. Fenves, A. American J. Kidney Diseases 7(2):130-134. 1986
27. Fieren, M. Blood Purification 14(2):179-187. 1996
28. Fox, E. Renal Failure 15(2):211-214. 1993
29. Franz, M. Mineral & Electrolyte Metabolism 23(3-6):189-193. 1997
30. Gilli, P. Clinical Nephrology 19(4):188-192. 1983
31. Goldwasser, P. J. American Society of Nephrology 3(9):1613-1622. 1993
32. Gouin- Charnet, A. Biochemical & Biophysical Research Communications 231(1):48-51. 1997
33. Gries, E. Life Support Systems 3 Suppl 1:125-130. 1985
34. Guarnieri, G. Kidney International- Suppl 62:s41-44. 1997
35. Hachache, T. Nephrologie 17(2):117-121. 1996
36. Horkko, S. Annals of Medicine 26(4):271-282. 1994
37. Hurst, N. Annals of the Rheumatic Diseases 48(5):409-420. 1989
38. Ikizler, T. American J. Kidney Diseases 26(1):256-265. 1995
39. Ikizler, T. Kidney International- Suppl 57:s53-56. 1996
40. Iseki, K. Kidney International 44(5):1086-1090. 1993
41. Jaeger, B. Circulation 96(9 Suppl):II-154-8. 1997
42. Kagan, A. Peritoneal Dialysis International 17(3):243-249. 1997
43. Kawaguchi, Y. Peritoneal Dialysis International 16 Suppl 1:s223-230. 1996
44. Kindler, J. Proceedings of the European Dialysis & Transplant Association 19:168-174. 1983
45. Koster, V. ROFO: Fortschritte auf dem Gebiete der Rontgenstrahlen und der Nuklearmedizin 150(5):598-601. 1989
46. Lai, K. American J. Kidney Diseases 28(5):721-726. 1996

47. Lees, R. J. Clinical Apheresis 11(3):132-137. 1996

48. Leu, J. J. Formosan Medical Association 97(1):49-54. 1998

49. Lin, Y. American J. Nephrology 16(4):293-299. 1996

50. Lockwood, A. Neurologic Clinics 7(3):617-627. 1989

51. Lupien, P. Lancet 1(7972):1261-1265. 1976

52. Lupien, P. Pediatric Research 14(2):113-117. 1980

53. Mitch, W. American J. Clinical Nutrition 67(3):359-366. 1998

54. Miyata, T. Current Opinion in Nephrology & Hypertension 4(6):493-497. 1995

55. Monteagudo, F. Medical Toxicology & Adverse Drug Experience 4(1):1-16. 1989

56. Morita, T. Archives of Pathology & Laboratory Medicine 109(11):1029-1032. 1985

57. Mourad, G. J. American Society of Nephrology 7(5):798-804. 1996

58. Mudher, A. Neuroscience 89(2):329-333. 1999

59. Murphey, M. Radiographics 13(2):357-379. 1993

60. Ogawa, H. ASAIO Transactions 35(3):317-319. 1989

61. Okada, M. Clinica Chimica Acta 220(2):135-144. 1993

62. Onoyama, K. Japanese Heart J. 27(5):685-691. 1986

63. Park, J. Atherosclerosis 115(1):1-8. 1995

64. Pereira, B. Blood Purification 13(3-4):135-146. 1995

65. Reusche, E. Acta Neuropathologica 86(3):249-258. 1993

66. Ritz, E. Mineral & Electrolyte Metabolism 22(1-3):9-12. 1996

67. Roccatello, D. Nephrology, Dialysis, Transplantation 12(2):292-297. 1997

68. Rosati, G. J. Neurology 223(4):251-257. 1980

69. Rysz, J. Kidney International 51(1):294-300. 1997

70. Savazzi, G. Clinical Nephrology 23(2):89-95. 1985

71. Savazzi, G. Nephron 49(2):94-103. 1988

72. Savazzi, G. Nephron 69(1):29-33. 1995

73. Schlatter, C. Medicina del Lavoro 83(5):470-474. 1992

74. Schnaper, H. American J. Kidney Diseases 2(6):645-650. 1983

75. Schneider, H. Klinische Wochenschrift 69(16):749-756. 1991

76. Scholtz, C. Clinical Neuropathology 6(3):93-97. 1987

77. Schuff-Werner, P. European J. Clinical Investigation 24(11):724-732, 1994

78. Sehgal, A. American J. Kidney Diseases 30(1):41-49. 1997

79. Seidel, D. Artificial Organs 20(4):303-310. 1996

80. Sivri, A. Scandinavian J. Rheumatology 23(5):287-290. 1994

81. Sole, M. Applied Pathology 7(6):350-360. 1989

82. Steinberg, A. International J. Pediatric Nephrology 6(2):121-126. 1985

83. Sutherland, W. Clinical Nephrology 43(6):392-398. 1995

84. Takada, K. Clinical Chemistry 43(7):1188-1195. 1997

85. Tan, S. Amyloidosis Histopathology 25(5):403-414. 1994

86. Trappler, B. General Hospital Psychiatry 8(1):57-60. 1986

87. Ward, R. Advances in Renal Replacement Therapy 2(4):362-370. 1995

88. Wisniewski, H. Ciba Foundation Symposium 169:142-154. 1992

89. Ylinen, K. Nephrology, Dialysis, Transplantation 7(9):908-912. 1992

90. Yokokawa, K. Annals of Internal Medicine 123(1):35-37. 1995

91. Ziesat, H. Perceptual & Motor Skills 50(1):311-318. 1980

13-4

1. Achord, J. American J. Gastroenterology 82(1):1-7. 1987

2. Alldredge, B. Epilepsia 34(6):1033-1037. 1993

3. Alling, C. Substance & Alcohol Actions/Misuse 4(2-3):67-72. 1983

4. Anonymous Missouri Medicine 87(12):875-876. 1990

5. Armbrecht, H. J. Pharmacology & Experimental Therapeutics 226(2):387-391. 1983

6. Baraona, E. J. Lipid Research 20(3):289-315. 1979

7. Baumhackl, U. European Neurology 34 Suppl 1:71-73. 1994

8. Blansjaar, B. Clinical Neurology & Neurosurgery 94(3):197-203. 1992

9. Blau, J. Headache 30(11):701-704. 1990

10. Butters, N. J. Clinical & Experimental Neuropsychology 7(2):181-210. 1985

11. Carlen, P. Neurology 31(4):377-385. 1981

12. Carlen, P. Substance & Alcohol Actions/Misuse 4(2-3):191-197. 1983

13. Carlen, P. Canadian J. Neurological Sciences 11(4):441-446. 1984

14. Carlen, P. Alcoholism, Clinical & Experimental Research 10(3):226-232. 1986

15. Carlen, P. Acta Medica Scandinavica- Suppl 717:19-26. 1987

16. Cheung, R. Bone 16(1):143-147. 1995

17. Chin, J. Advances in Experimental Medicine & Biology 85a:111-122. 1977

18. Chin, J. Biochimica et Biophysica Acta 513(3):358-363. 1978

19. Chin, J. Lipids 19(12):929-935. 1984

20. Clark, K. Western J. Nursing Research 19(1):32-45. 1997

21. Claus, D. Klinische Wochenschrift 65(4):185-193. 1987

22. Colles, S. Biochemistry 34(17):5945-5959. 1995

23. De la Monte, S. Archives of Neurology 45(9):990-992. 1988

24. Devetag, F. Italian J. Neurological Sciences 4(3):275-284. 1983

25. Egbert, A. Geriatrics 48(7):63-66. 1993

26. Emsley, R. Alcohol & Alcoholism 31(5):479-486. 1996

27. Fink, A. Archives of Internal Medicine 156(11):1150-1156. 1996

28. Freund, G. Alcohol 9(3):233-240. 1992

29. Gallucci, M. J. Computer Assisted Tomography 13(3):395-398. 1989

30. Goldstein, D. Annals of Emergency Medicine 15(9):1013-1018. 1986

31. Grove, J. Hepatology 26(1):143-146. 1997

32. Gustavsson, L. Upsala J. Medical Sciences, Suppl 48:245-266. 1990

33. Harding, A. Hippocampus 7(1):78-87. 1997

34. Harris, R. Currents in Alcoholism 8:461-468. 1981

35. Hayakawa, K. Acta Radiologica 33(3):201-206. 1992

36. Kato, A. Japanese J. Psychiatry & Neurology 45(1):27-35. 1991

37. Kimble, R. Alcoholism, Clinical & Experimental Research 21(3):385-391. 1997

38. Kroll, P. J. Clinical Psychiatry 41(12 Pt 1):417-421. 1980

39. Lusins, J. Alcoholism, Clinical & Experimental Research 4(4):406-411. 1980

40. Marchesi, C. Progress in Neuro-Psychopharmacology & Biological Psychiatry 18(3):519-535. 1994

41. Meldgaard, B. Acta Neurologica Scandinavica 70(5):336-344. 1984

42. Menzano, E. Alcoholism, Clinical & Experimental Research 18(4):895-901. 1994

43. Moscatelli, E. Biochimica et Biophysica Acta 596(3):331-337. 1980

44. Nanji, A. Hepatology 26(1):90-97. 1997

45. Nicolas, J. Annals of Neurology 41:590-598. 1997

46. Palencia, G. J. Studies on Alcohol 56(2):140-146. 1995

47. Pieninkeroinen, I. Alcoholism, Clinical & Experimental Research 16(5):955-959. 1992

48. Preedy, V. FASEB J. 8(14):1146-1151. 1994

49. Ron, M. Brain 105(Pt 3):497-514. 1982

50. Salmon, D. Recent Developments in Alcoholism 5:27-58. 1987

51. Sampson, H. Alcoholism, Clinical & Experimental Research 21(3):400-403. 1997

52. Schafer, C. Zeitschrift fur Gastroenterologie 33(9):503-508. 1995

53. Seeman, E. Australian Family Physician 26(2):135-143. 1997

54. Skullerud, K. Acta Neurologica Scandinavica. Suppl 102:1-94. 1985

55. Smith, T. Life Sciences 31(14):1419-1425. 1982

56. Sullivan, E. Alcoholism, Clinical & Experimental Research 20(2):348-354. 1996

57. Sun, G. Currents in Alcoholism 7:83-91. 1979

58. Sun, G. Alcoholism, Clinical & Experimental Research 9(2):164-180. 1985

59. Teichman, M. American J. Drug & Alcohol Abuse 13(3):357-363. 1987

60. Trabert, W. Acta Psychiatrica Scandinavica 92(2):87-90. 1995

61. Urbano-Marquez, A. New England J. Medicine 320(7):409-415. 1989

62. Walker, D. Science 209(4457):711-713. 1980

63. Wiggins, R. Metabolic Brain Disease 3(1):67-80. 1988

64. Wilkinson, D. J. Studies on Alcohol 41(1):129-139. 1980

13-5

1. Endo, Y. Neuroscience 79(3):745-752. 1997

2. Heinz, E. J. Computer Assisted Tomography 1(4):415-418. 1977

3. Mandal, S. Indian J. Physiology & Pharmacology 29(4):255-258. 1985

4. Mauri, M. Acta Neurologica Scandinavica 87(1):52-55. 1993

5. McEwen, B. Molecular Psychiatry 2(3):255-262. 1997

6. Momose, K. Radiology 99(2):341-348. 1971

7. Raccah, D. Revue de Medecine Interne 13(4):302-304. 1992

8. Starkman, M. Biological Psychiatry 32(9):756-765. 1992

9. Stokes, P. European Neuropsychopharmacology 5 Suppl:77-82. 1995

10. Taskinen, M. J. Clinical Endocrinology & Metabolism 57(3):619-626. 1983

11. Uthman, I. J. Rheumatology 22(10):1964-1966. 1995

12. Yakushiji, F. Endocrine J. 42(2):219-223. 1995

13. Yanovski, J. Endocrinology & Metabolism Clinics of North America 23(3):487-509. 1994

13-6

1. Abbott, M. J. Infection 31(1):1-4. 1995
2. Adamson, D. Science 274(5294):1917-1921. 1996
3. Adle-Biassette, H, Archives d Anatomie et de Cytologie Pathologiques 45(2-3):86-93. 1997
4. Aloia, R. Proceedings/America 90(11):5181-5185. 1993
5. An, S. J. Neuropathology & Experimental Neurology 56(11):1262-1268. 1997
6. Antonian, L. Neuroscience & Biobehavioral Reviews 11(4):399-413. 1987
7. Arbiser, J. J. American Academy of Dermatology 34(3):486-497. 1996
8. Aylward, E. American J. Psychiatry 152(7):987-994. 1995
9. Barbaro, G. Cardiologia 41(12):1199-1207. 1996
10. Bartolomei, F. Presse Medicale 20(42):2135-2138. 1991
11. Benhamou, Y. Digestive Diseases & Sciences 39(10:2163-2169. 1994
12. Berman, A. J. Rheumatology 18(10):1564-1567. 1991
13. Bjugstad, K. Brain Research 795(1-2):349-357. 1998
14. Brew, B. Annals of Neurology 38(4):563-570. 1995
15. Broderick, D. American J. Roentgenology 161(1):177-181. 1993
16. Brody, D. American J. Psychiatry 148(2):248-250. 1991
17. Brugieres, P. J. Neuroradiology 22(3):163-168. 1995
18. Bukrinsky, M. Molecular Medicine 2(4):460-468. 1996
19. Buskila, D. Clinical & Experimental Rheumatology 8(6):567-573. 1990
20. Chiesi, A. J. Neurological Sciences 144(1-2):107-113. 1996
21. Chlebowski, R. Nutrition & Cancer 7(1-2):85-91. 1985
22. Chlebowski, R. J. American Dietetic Association 95(4):428-432. 1995
23. Christeff, N. Annales de Medecine Interne 146(7):490-495. 1995
24. Christeff, N. Psychoneuroendocrinology 22 Suppl 1:s11-8. 1997
25. Chui, D. J. Gastroenterology & Hepatology 9(3):291-303. 1994
26. Clerici, M. Psychoneuroendocrinology 22 Suppl 1:s27-31. 1997
27. Cohen, J. J. Acquired Immune Deficiency Syndromes 4(1):31-33. 1991
28. Colman, N. Seminars in Oncology 14(2 Suppl 3):54-62. 1987
29. Connor, R. Biochemical & Biophysical Research Communications 176(2):852-859. 1991
30. Constans, J. European J. Clinical Investigation 24(6):416-420. 1994
31. Coodley, G. J. Acquired Immune Deficiency Syndromes 7(1):46-51. 1994
32. Cozzi, P. Clinical Infectious Diseases 14(1):189-191. 1992
33. Crinelli, R. European J. Biochemistry 247(1):91-97. 1997
34. Cupler, E. Brain 119(Pt 6):1887-1893. 1996
35. Dal Pan, G. Neurology 42(11):2125-2130. 1992
36. DeCarli, C. Annals of Neurology 34(2):198-205. 1993
37. Di Sclafani, V. J. International Neuropsychological Society 3(3):276-287. 1997
38. Duvic, M. J. Investigative Dermatology 105(1 Suppl):117s-121s. 1995
39. Edwards, P. Australian & New Zealand J. Medicine 20(2):141-148. 1990

40. Enwonwu, C. European J. Oral Sciences 104(3):322-324. 1996

41. Esiri, M. AIDS 5(9):1081-1088. 1991

42. Esiri, M. J. Neurology, Neurosurgery & Psychiatry 65(1):29-33. 1998

43. Espinoza, L. Rheumatic Diseases Clinics of North America 18(1):257-266. 1992

44. Eustace, S. Radiologic Clinics of North America 34(2):450-453. 1996

45. Feingold, K. J. Clinical Endocrinology & Metabolism 76(6):1423-1427. 1993

46. Foli, A. AIDS Research & Human Retroviruses 13(10):829-839. 1997

47. Francis, C. Current Problems in Cardiology 15(10):569-639. 1990

48. Freeman, R. Neurology 40(4):575-580. 1990

49. Fujimura, R. J. Virological Methods 55(3):309-325. 1995

50. Giometto, B. Annals of Neurology 42(1):34-40. 1997

51. Glass, J. Annals of Neurology 38(5):755-762. 1995

52. Gordon, L. Biochimica et Biophysica Acta 943(2):331-342. 1988

53. Graef, A. Clinical Immunology & Immunopathology 72(3):390-393. 1994

54. Groeneveld, P. Scandinavian J. Infectious Diseases 28(4):341-345. 1996

55. Grunfeld, C. J. Clinical Endocrinology & Metabolism 74(5):1045-1052. 1992

56. Guenter, P. J. Acquired Immune Deficiency Syndromes 6(10):1130-1138. 1993

57. Guillamon Toran, L. Revista Espanola de Cardiologia 50(10):721-728. 1997

58. Haug, C. J. Infectious Diseases 169(4):889-893. 1994

59. Haug, C. J. Clinical Endocrinology & Metabolism 83(11):3832-3838. 1998

60. Herskowitz, A. Current Opinion in Cardiology 11(3):325-331. 1996

61. Hestad, K. Acta Neurologica Scandinavica 88(2):112-118. 1993

62. Husebekk, A. Scandinavian J. Infectious Diseases 18(5):389-394. 1986

63. Janier, M. Annales de Dermatologie et de Venereologie 114(2):185-202. 1987

64. Jernigan, T. Archives of Neurology 50(3):250-255. 1993

65. Kereveur, A. Annales de Medecine Interne 147(5):333-343. 1996

66. Khoo, S. AIDS 11(4):423-428. 1997

67. Kieburtz, K. Archives of Neurology 53(2):155-158. 1996

68. Lacey, C. International J. STD & AIDS 7(7):485-489. 1996

69. Launay, J. Nouvelle Revue Francaise d Hematologie 31(2):159-161. 1989

70. Lazarini, F. J. Neurovirology 3(4):299-303. 1997

71. Liebowitz, D. J. Clinical Gastroenterology 8(1):66-68. 1986

72. Luginbuhl, L. JAMA 269(22):2869-2875. 1993

73. Mahoney, S. J. Clinical Investigation 88(1):174-185. 1991

74. Manji, H. J. Neurology, Neurosurgery & Psychiatry 57(2):144-149. 1994

75. Mankertz, J. Biochimica et Biophysica Acta 1317(3):233-237. 1996

76. Marks, C. World J. Surgery 19(1):127-132. 1995

77. Masood, R. AIDS Research & Human Retroviruses 9(8):741-746. 1993

78. Maziere, J. Biomedicine & Pharmacotherapy 48(2):63-67. 1994

79. McKenzie, R. Medicine 70(5):326-343. 1991

80. Medina-Rodriguez, F. J. Rheumatology 20(11):1880-1884. 1993

81. Miro, O. J. Neurological Sciences 150(2):153-159. 1997

82. Mizusawa, H. Acta Neuropathologica 76(5):451-457. 1988

83. Montazeri, A. International J. Dermatology 35(7):475-479. 1996

84. Montero, A. Neurological Research 20(1):2-4. 1998

85. Moseson, M. J. Acquired Immune Deficiency Syndromes 2(3):235-247. 1989

86. Myskowski, P. Medical Clinics of North America 80(6):1415-1435. 1996

87. Norbiato, G. J. Clinical Endocrinology & Metabolism 74(3):608-613. 1992

88. Nordstrom, D. Arthritis & Rheumatism 32(4):475-479. 1989

89. Oberfield, S. J. Acquired Immune Deficiency Syndromes 7(1):57-62. 1994

90. Obuch, M. J. American Academy of Dermatology 27(5 Pt 1):667-673. 1992

91. Ornstein, M. Arthritis & Rheumatism 38(11):1701-1706. 1995

92. Ott, D. J. Virology 72(4):2962-2968. 1998

93. Ott, M. Zeitschritte fur Gastroenterologie 31(11):661-665. 1993

94. Pauza, C. J. Leukocyte Biology 53(2):157-164. 1993

95. Pereira, F. AIDS Research & Human Retroviruses 13(14):1203-1211. 1997

96. Poutiainen, E. Acta Neurologica Scandinavica 87(2):88-94. 1993

97. Qureshi, A. Archives of Neurology 54(9):1150-1153. 1997

98. Raininko, R. Neuroradiology 34(3):190-196. 1992

99. Raja, F. Acta Neuropathologica 93(2):184-189. 1997

100. Razani, J. Physiology & Behavior 59(4-5):877881. 1996

101. Reyes, E. Archives of Pathology & Laboratory Medicine 118(11):1130-1134. 1994

102. Rondanelli, M. AIDS Research & Human Retroviruses 13(14):1243-1249. 1997

103. Roth, W. International J. Cancer 42(5):767-773. 1988

104. Rovira, E. Revista Clinica Espanola 195(455-458. 1995

105. Rowe, I. Quarterly J. Medicine 73(272):1167-1184. 1989

106. Rubsamen-Waigmann, H. Infection 19 Suppl 2:s77-82. 1991

107. Salazar-Gonzales, J. Clinical Immunology & Immunopathology 84(1):36-45. 1997

108. Schlesinger, M. Immunology Letters 22(4):307-311. 1989

109. Schnaudigel, O. Ophthalmologe 91(5):668-670. 1994

110. Schneebaum, C. Gastroenterology 92(5 Pt 1):1127-1132. 1987

111. Schubert, U. J. Virology 72(3):2280-2288. 1998

112. Seilhean, D. Acta Neuropathologica 93(5):508-517. 1997

113. Sempere, A. Acta Neurologica Scandinavica 86(2):134-138. 1992

114. Shapiro, D. J. Rheumatology 23(10):1818-1820. 1996

115. Shor-Posner, G. American J. Medicine 94(5):515-519. 1993

116. Singer, P. Nutrition 13(2):104-109. 1997

117. Sqalli-Houssaini, H. Biotechnology Therapeutics 5(1-2):69-85. 1994

118. Stanley, L. J. Neuropathology & Experimental Neurology 53(3):231-238. 1994

119. Stein, C. J. Rheumatology 23(3):506-511. 1996

120. Subbiah, P. J. Neuropathology & Experimental Neurology 55(10):1032-1037. 1996

121. Suttmann, U. J. Acquired Immune Deficiency Syndromes & Human Retrovirology 8(3):239-246. 1995

122. Tomasselli, A. J. Biological Chemistry 266(22):14548-14553. 1991

123. Torre, D. Clinical Infectious Diseases 22(4):650-653. 1996

124. Vago, L. Acta Neurologica 12(1):32-35. 1990

125. Van Paesschen, W. Epilepsia 36(2):146-150. 1995

126. Weitzul, S. Seminars in Cutaneous Medicine & Surgery 16(3):213-218.1997

127. Wiley, C. Brain Pathology 8(2):277-284. 1998

128. Wilson, L. Metabolism: Clinical & Experimental 45(6):738-746. 1996

129. Winchester, R. Dermatologic Clinics 13(4):779-792. 1995

130. Zangerle, R. J. Acquired Immune Deficiency Syndromes 7(11):1149-1156. 1994

131. Zangerle, R. Immunobiology 193(1):59-70. 1995

13-7

1.   Dusart, I. Neuroscience 51(1):137-148. 1992

2.   Kawarabayashi, T. Brain Research 563(1-2):334-338. 1991

3.   Kulmala, H. Experimental Aging Research 13(1-2):67-72. 1987

4.   Ong, W. J. fur Hirnforschung 38(3):353-361. 1997

5.   Shoham, S. Experimental Neurology 147(2):361-376. 1997

6.   Sola, C. Brain Research. Molecular Brain Research 17(1-2):41-52. 1993

7.   Ueda, Y. Epilepsy Research 26(2):329-333. 1997

13-8   —None

Chapter 14

14-1

1.   Akiyama, H. Tohoku J. Experimental Medicine 174(3):295-303. 1994

2.   Frecker, M. Canadian J. Neurological Sciences 21(2):112-119. 1994

3.   Leblhuber, F. Deutsche Medizinische Wochenschrift 123(25-26):787-791. 1998

4.   Veerhuis, R. Acta Neuropathologica 91(1):53-60. 1996

14-2

1.   Jara, L. Seminars in Arthritis & Rheumatism 20(5):273-284. 1991

2.   Kalman, J. Acta Neurologica Scandinavica 96(4):236-240. 1997

3.   McGeer, P. Alzheimer Disease & Associated Disorders 8(3):149-158. 1994

4.   Molta, C. Clinical & Experimental Rheumatology 7(3):229-236. 1989

5.   Neidhart, M. J. Neuroimmunology 26(2):97-105. 1990

6.   Sels, F. J. Rheumatology 24(5):856-859. 1997

14-3

1.   Blumenthal, H. J. Pathology 151(4):305-314. 1987

2.   Engelbrecht, F. South African Medical J. 62(18):648-651. 1982

3.   Hoshii, Y. American J. Pathology 151(4):911-917. 1997

4.   Kunitomo, M. Japanese J. Pharmacology 44(1):15-22. 1987

5.   Laufer, A. Acta Pathologica Microbiologica Scandinavia, Sect A. 80, Suppl 233:183-188. 1972

6.   Livni, N. J. Pathology 132(4):343-348. 1980

7.   Mizisin, A. J. Neuroimmunology 16(3):381-395. 1987

8.   Polliack, A. British J. Experimental Pathology 54(6):6-12. 1973

9. Ram, J. Proceedings of the Society for Experimental Biology & Medicine 127(3):854-856. 1968

10. Selgas, L. Chronobiology International 14(3):253-265. 1997

11. Stenstad, T. Biochemical J. 303(Pt 2):663-670. 1994

12. Suzuki, T. Acta Pathologica Japonica 30(4):557-564. 1980

13. Taranova, N. Neurochemical Research 10(11):1483-1497. 1985

14. Yamaguchi, Y. Japanese J. Pharmacology 50(4):377-386. 1989

14-4   —None

14-5

1. Ali, A. General Pharmacology 18(2):153-157. 1987

2. Andersen, K. Neurology 45(8):1441-1445. 1995

3. Beard, C. Mayo Clinic Proceedings 73(10):951-955. 1998

4. Bjornsson, O. J. Lipid Research 33(7):1017-1027. 1992

5. Breitner, J. Neurobiology of Aging 16(4):523-530. 1995

6. Breitner, J. Annual Review of Medicine 47:401-411. 1996

7. Dash, P. Biochemical & biophysical Research Communications 208(2):542-548. 1995

8. De Bittencourt Junior, P. Biochemistry & Molecular Biology International 33(3):463-475. 1994

9. Hasan, M. Gerontology 41(4):212-219. 1995

10. Fagarasan, M. Brain Research 723(1-2):231-234. 1996

11. Jelic-Ivanovic, Z. Clinical Chemistry 31(7):1141-1143. 1985

12. Korhonen, T. European J. Clinical Pharmacology 48(2):97-102. 1995

13. Krone, W. J. Lipid Research 29(12):1663-1669. 1988

14. Leibovitz, A. J. American Geriatrics Society 44:216. 1996

15. Mackenzie, I. Neurology 50(4):986-990. 1998

16. McGeer, P. Neurology 47(2):425-432. 1996

17. Nanji, A. Hepatology 26(1):90-97. 1997

18. Pasinetti, G. Neuroscience 87(2):319-324. 1998

19. Pate, J. J. Reproduction & Fertility 87(2):439-446. 1989

20. Pomerantz, K. Biochemistry 32(49):13624-13635. 1993

21. Rich, J. Neurology 45(1):51-55. 1995

22. Rogers, J. Neurology 43(8):1609-1611. 1993

23. Rogers, J. Neurobiology of Aging 17(5):681-686. 1996

24. Schwartz, K. Atherosclerosis 71(1):9-16. 1988

25. Silverstein, F. Digestive Diseases & Sciences 43(3):447-458. 1998

26. Sinzinger, H. British J. Pharmacology 103(3):1626-1628. 1991

27. Smalheiser,N. Neurology 46(2)583. 1996

28. Spangler, R. Seminars in Arthritis & Rheumatism 26(1):435-446. 1996

29. Stewart, W. Neurology 48(3):626-632. 1997

30. Stoller, D. J. Surgical Research 54(1):7-11. 1993

31. Stratman, N. Brain Research. Molecular Brain Research 50(1-2):107-112. 1997

32. Vane, J. Seminars in Arthritis & Rheumatism 26(6 Suppl 1):2-10. 1997

33. Vane, J. Annual Review of Pharmacology & Toxicology 38:97-120. 1998

14-6

1. Chandra, R. American J. Clinical Nutrition 66(2):460s-463s. 1997
2. Krenitsky, J. AACN Clinical Issues 7(3):359-369. 1996
3. Lesourd, B. American J. Clinical Nutrition 66(2):478s-484s. 1997
4. Leme-Brasil, M. Agents & Actions 10(5):445-450. 1980
5. Lipschitz, D. Clinics in Geriatric Medicine 3(2):319-328. 1987
6. Nohr, C. Surgery 98(4):769-776. 1985

14-7

1. Bondeson, J. Biochemical Pharmacology 50(11):1753-1759. 1995
2. Bruckle, W. Clinical Rheumatology 13(2):209-216. 1994
3. Burmester, G. Zeitschrift fur Rheumatologie 55(5):299-306. 1996
4. Dawes, P. Annals of the Rheumatic Diseases 45(11):945-949. 1986
5. Dequeker, J. Clinical Rheumatology 3 Suppl 1:67-74. 1984
6. Havekes, L. Atherosclerosis 56(1):81-92. 1985
7. Herman Hernandes, C. Clinical & Experimental Rheumatology 4(4):347-350. 1986
8. Jones, G. British J. Rheumatology 35(11):1154-1158. 1996
9. Kambouris, A. FEBS Letters 230(1-2):176-180. 1988
10. Lewandowicz, J. Archivum Immunologiae et Therapiae Experimentalis 43(3-4):195-198. 1995
11. Lorber, M. British J. Rheumatology 24(3):250-255. 1985
12. Malassine, A. Histochemistry 87(5):457-464. 1987
13. Malassine, A. Placenta 11(2):191-204. 1990
14. Munro, R. Annals of the Rheumatic Diseases 57(2):88-93. 1998
15. Myllykangas-Luosujarvi, R. J. Rheumatology 22(12):2214-2217. 1995
16. Palit, J. British J. Rheumatology 29(4):280-283. 1990
17. Patel, N. Annals of Clinical Biochemistry 29(Pt 3):283-286. 1992
18. Robenek, H. J. Ultrastructure Research 82(2)>143-155. 1983
19. Shapiro, D. J. Rheumatology 23(10):1818-1820. 1996

Chapter 15
15-1

1. Aarsland, D. Archives of Neurology 53(6):538-542. 1996
2. Abbott, R. European J. Clinical Nutrition 46(12):879-884. 1992
3. Arai, H. Neurology 42(7):1315-1322. 1992
4. Bellomo, G. J. Neurology 238(1):19-22. 1991
5. Bennett, D. Lancet 351:1631. 1998
6. Beyer, P. J. American Dietetic Association 95(9):979-983. 1995
7. Blum-Degen, D. Neuroscience Letters 202(1-2):17-20. 1995
8. Boka, G. Neuroscience Letters 172(1-2):151-154. 1994
9. Braak, H. J. Neural Transmission- Parkinson's Disease & Dementia Section 2(1):45-57. 1990

10. Braak, H. J. Neural Transmission 103:455-490. 1996
11. Breteler, M. American J. Epidemiology 142(12):1300-1305. 1995
12. Brevetti, G. Clinical Cardiology 13(7):474-478. 1990
13. Buee-Scherrer, V. Annals of Neurology 42(3):356-359. 1997
14. Burn, D. Neurology 42(10):1894-1900. 1992
15. Churchyard, A. Neurology 49(6):1570-1576. 1997
16. Corthesy, D. Schweizer Archiv fur Neurologie und Psychiatrie 136(1):75-85. 1985
17. Crino, P. Annals of Otology, Rhinology & Laryngology 104(8):655-661. 1995
18. De Angelis, G. Revue Neurologique 140(6-7):440-442. 1984
19. De Rijk, M. Archives of Neurology 54(6):762-765. 1997
20. Dexter, D. Movement Disorders 9(1):92-97. 1994
21. Dexter, D. Annals of Neurology 35(3):298-303. 1994
22. Double, K. Dementia 7(6):304-313. 1996
23. Durif, F. European Neurology 32(1):32-36. 1992
24. Durrieu, G. Clinical Autonomic Research 2(3):153-157. 1992
25. Duvoisin, R. Advances in Neurology 45:307-312. 1987
26. Filoteo, J. J. Clinical & Experimental Neuropsychology 19(6):878-888. 1997
27. Frigyesi, T. Advances in Experimental Medicine & Biology 90:63-107. 1977
28. Fujiyama, J. Japanese J. Medicine 30(2):189-192. 1991
29. Fukui, T. European Neurology 35(2):86-92. 1995
30. Gearing, M. Neurology 45(11):1985-1990. 1995
31. Gray, F. Revue Neurologique 144(4):229-248. 1988
32. Hartmann, A. Neurobiology of Aging 18(3):285-289. 1997
33. Hawkes, C. Annals of the New York Academy of Sciences 855:608-615. 1998
34. Hillen, M. Archives of Physical Medicine & Rehabilitation 77(7):710-712. 1996
35. Holthoff, V. Annals of Neurology 36(2):176-182. 1994
36. Jankovic, J. Annals of Neurology 19(4):405-408. 1986
37. Jellinger, K. Annals of the New York Academy of Sciences 640:203-209. 1991
38. Jimenez-Jimenez, F. Revue Neuroligique 147(3):244-245. 1991
39. Johnson, W. Movement Disorders 5(3):187-194. 1990
40. Kao, C. Nuclear Medicine Communications 15(3):173-177. 1994
41. Kitani, M. Gerontology 36(5-6):361-368. 1990
42. Laakso, M. Neurology 46(3):678-681. 1996
43. Lawton, N. J. Neurology, Neurosurgery & Psychiatry 43(11):1012-1015. 1980
44. Levine, R. Stroke 23(6):839-842. 1992
45. Mahler, M. Alzheimer Disease & Associated Disorders 4(3):133-149. 1990
46. Mann, D. Neuroscience Letters 109(1-2):68-75. 1990
47. Markus, H. Clinical Science 83(2):199-204. 1992
48. Markus, H. J. Neural Transmission- Parkinson's Disease & Dementia Section 5(2):117-125. 1993
49. Marschall, I. J. Neural Transmission. Suppl 33:81-92. 1991
50. Marttila, R. Neurology 38(8):1217-1219. 1988

51. Mastaglia, F. Progress in Clinical & Biological Research 317:475-484. 1989

52. Mesholam, R. Archives of Neurology 55(1):84-90. 1998

53. Mogi, M. Neuroscience Letters 1651-2):208-210. 1994

54. Mogi, M. J. Neural Transmission- Parkinson's Disease & Dementia Section 9(1):87-92. 1995

55. Morano, A. Acta Neurologica Scandinavica 89(3):164-170. 1994

56. Musanti, R. Biochemical Medicine & Metabolic Biology 49(2):133-142. 1993

57. Nussbaum, R. Human Molecular Genetics 6(10):1687-1691. 1997

58. Nussbaum, R. New England J. Medicine 348(14):1356-1364. 2003

59. Otake, K. Acta Medica Hungarica 50(1-2):3-13. 1994

60. Peppard, R. J. Neuroscience Research 27(4):561-568. 1990

61. Perl, D. Annals of Neurology 44(3 Suppl 1):s19-31. 1998

62. Pranzatelli, M. Pediatric Neurology 10(2):131-140. 1994

63. Qureshi, G. Neuroreport 6(12):1642-1644. 1995

64. Reyes, M. Panminerva Medica 38(1):8-14. 1996

65. Schapiro, M. J. Neurology, Neurosurgery & Psychiatry 56(8):859-864. 1993

66. Schneider, E. J. Neurology 217(1):11-16. 1977

67. Shergill, J. Biochemical & Biophysical Research Communications 228(2):298-305. 1996

68. Shibata, N. Rinsho Shinkeigaku- Clinical Neurology 30(9):978-984. 1990

69. Starkstein, S. Movement Disorders 8(1):51-55. 1993

70. Stern, M. Archives of Neurology 48(9):903-907. 1991

71. Struck, L. Stroke 21(10):1395-1399. 1990

72. Tarczy, M. Acta Bio-Medica de l Ateneo Parmense 66(3-4):93-97. 1995

73. Toth, M. Neurology 48(1):88-91. 1997

74. Vander Borght, T. J. Nuclear Medicine 38(5):797-802. 1997

75. Vieregge, P. Neurology 42(8):1453-1461. 1992

76. Yamada, T. Japanese J. Geriatrics 32(10):637-640. 1995

77. Zareparsi, S. Annals of Neurology 42(4):655-658. 1997

15-2

1. Blanc, E. J. Neurochemistry 68(5):1870-1881. 1997

2. Buee, L. Acta Neuropathologica 87(5):469-480. 1994

3. Buee, L. Annals of the New York Academy of Sciences 826:7-24. 1997

4. Chu, C. J. Neuropathology & Experimental Neurology 57(1):30-38. 1998

5. Hachinski, V. Annals of the New York Academy of Sciences 826:1-6. 1997

6. Kalaria, R. Annals of the New York Academy of Sciences 826:263-271. 1997

7. Mandybur, T. Neurology 29(10):1336-1340. 1979

8. Zarow, C. Annals of the New York Academy of Sciences 826:147-160. 1997

15-3

1. Cross, C. J. Laboratory & Clinical Medicine 115(4):396-404. 1990

2. Davidson, K. American J. Physiology 272(1 Pt 1):L106-114. 1997

3. Hine, L. American J. Gastroenterology 83(10):1128-1131. 1988

4. Kurygin, G. Biulleten Eksperimentalnoi Biologii I Meditsiny 105(2):152-154. 1988
5. Kyle, R. Medicine 54(4):271-299. 1975
6. Renvall, M. J. American Dietetic Association 93(1):47-52. 1993

15-4

1. Antonucci, A. Ultrastructural Pathology 21(5):449-452. 1997
2. Burke, J. Biochemical Medicine & Metabolic Biology 37(2):148-156. 1987
3. Bush, A. J. Biological Chemistry 269(16):12152-12158. 1994
4. Constantinidis, J. Medical Hypotheses 35(4):319-323. 1991
5. Cuajungco, M. Brain Research-Brain Research Reviews 23(3):219-236. 1997
6. Cunnane, S. Progress in Food & Nutrition Science 12(2):151-188. 1988
7. Hiller, R. Annals of Epidemiology 5(6):490-496. 1995
8. Ripa, S. Minerva Medica 85(12):647-654. 1994
9. Shankar, S. International J. Vitamin & Nutrition Research 56(4):329-337. 1986
10. Laitinen, R. J. American College of Nutrition 8(5):400-406. 1989
11. Napolitano, G. American J. Medical Genetics- Suppl 7:63-65. 1990
12. Prasad, A. Progress in Clinical & Biological Research 165:49-58. 1984
13. Tully, C. Neuroreport 6(16):2105-2108. 1995

15-5

1. Choi, J. J. Pharmacology & Experimental Therapeutics 289(1):572-579. 1999
2. Iimura, O. Kidney International 52(4):962-972. 1997
3. Padayatty, S. J. Clinical Endocrinology & Metabolism 82(5):1434-1439. 1997
4. Rubins, J. American J. Respiratory & Critical Care Medicine 157(5 Pt 1):1616-1622. 1998

Chapter 16
None

Chapter 17

17-1

1. Alessandri, C. Clinica Terapeutica 141(8):109-114. 1992
2. Anonymous JAMA 269(23):3-15-3023. 1993
3. Castelli, W. American J. Kidney Diseases 16(4 Suppl 1):41-46. 1990
4. Castelli, W. Atherosclerosis 124 Suppl:s1-9. 1996
5. Corti, M. Annals of Internal Medicine 126(10):753-760. 1997
6. Corti, M. JAMA 274(7):539-544. 1995
7. Denke, M. Archives of Internal Medicine 153(9):1093-1103. 1993
8. Denke, M. Archives of Internal Medicine 154(4):401-410. 1994
9. Dietschy, J. J. Lipid Research 34(10):1637-1659. 1993
10. Fallest-Strobl, P. American Family Physician 56(6):1607-1612, 1615-1616. 1997
11. Garber, A. American J. Medicine 102(2a):26-30. 1997
12. Garrison, R. Annals of Internal Medicine 103(6(Pt 2)):1006-1009. 1985
13. Ginsberg, H. Arteriosclerosis 1(6):463-470. 1981

14. Goldbourt, U. British Medical J. Clinical Research Ed. 290(6477):1239-1243. 1985

15. Goldstein, D. International J. Obesity & Related Metabolic Disorders 16(6):397-415. 1992

16. Gordon, T. American J. Medicine 62(5):707-714. 1977

17. Harris, T. JAMA 259(10):1520-1524. 1988

18. Herzum, M. Herz 23(3):193-196. 1998

19. Hooper, P. J. American College of Nutrition 1(4):337-343. 1982

20. Hubert, H. Circulation 67(5):968-977. 1983

21. Hulley, S. JAMA 272(17):1372-1374. 1994

22. Hulley, S. Jama 269(11):1416-1419. 1993

23. Imai, H. Science 207(4431):651-653. 1980

24. Imeson, J. J. Epidemiology & Community Health 43(3):223-227. 1989

25. James, T. Circulation 96(5):1696-1700. 1997

26. Jenner, J. Circulation 87(4):1135-1141. 1993

27. Kaltenbach, M. Versicherungsmedizin 47(4):112-116. 1995

28. Kannel, W. American J. Cardiology 76(9):69c-77c. 1995

29. Keys, A. J. Epidemiology & Community Health 42(1):60-65. 1988

30. Klor, H. European J. Medical Research 2(6):243-257. 1997

31. Kmietowicz, Z. BMJ 316(7133):725. 1998

32. Knuiman, J. American J. Epidemiology 116(4):631-642. 1982

33. Krumholz, H. JAMA 272(17):1335-1340. 1994

34. Lamon-Fava, S. Arteriosclerosis, Thrombosis & Vascular Biology 16(12):1509-1515. 1996

35. Lehto, S. J. Internal Medicine 233(2):179-185. 1993

36. Lippi, U. Clinica Chimica Acta 130(3):283-289. 1983

37. Martin, M. Lancet 2(8513):933-936. 1986

38. McNamara, D. Canadian J. Cardiology 11 Suppl G:123g-126g. 1995

39. McNamara, D. J. Clinical Investigation 79(6):1729-1739. 1987

40. Millen, B. J. Clinical Epidemiology 49(6):657-663. 1996

41. Mistry, P. J. Clinical Investigation 67(2):493-502. 1981

42. Mosca, L. American J. Cardiology 80(7):825-830. 1997

43. Newbold, H. Southern Medical J. 81(1):61-63. 1988

44. Nichols, A. JAMA 236(17):1948-1953. 1976

45. Ravnskov, U. BMJ 305(6844):15-19. 1992

46. Salonen, J. Circulation 95(4):840-845. 1997

47. Schaefer, E. American J. Clinical Nutrition 65(3):823-830. 1997

48. Schaefer, E. Metabolism: Clinical & Experimental 38(4):293-296. 1989

49. Tzonou, A. Epidemiology 4(6):511-516. 1993

50. Verschuren, W. JAMA 274(2):131-136. 1995

51. Walsh, J. JAMA 274(14):1152-1158. 1995

52. Wilson, P. American J. Hypertension 7(7 Pt 2):7s-12s. 1994

17-2

1. Anonymous, Circulation 97(15):1440-1445. 1998
2. Anonymous, New England J. Medicine 339(19):1349-1357. 1998
3. Anonymous, Lancet 344(8934):1383-1389. 1994
4. Anonymous, Lancet 348(9038):1339-1342. 1996
5. Corti, M. Current Opinion in Lipidology 8(4):236-241. 1997
6. Freemantle, N. BMJ 316(7139):1241-1242. 1998
7. Grundy, S. New England J. Medicine 335(1239-1240. 1996
8. Lewis, S. Annals of Internal Medicine 129(9):681-689. 1998
9. Lewis, S. J. American College of Cardiology 32(1):140_146. 1998
10. Pedersen, T. Circulation 97(15):1453-1460. 1998
11. Pharoah, P. BMJ 316(7139):1241-1242. 1998
12. Rogers, S. New England J. Medicine 334(20):1333. 1996
13. Sacks, F. New England J. Medicine 335(14):1001-1009. 1996
14. Sacks, F. Circulation 97(15):1446-1452. 1998
15. Shepherd, J. New England J. Medicine 333(20):1301-1307. 1995
16. Smith, G. BMJ 306(6889):1367-1373. 1993

17-3

1. Arnold, A. Cleveland Clinic J. Medicine 60(5):393-398. 1993
2. Benfante, R. J. Chronic Diseases 38(5):385-395. 1985
3. Berceli, S. J. Vascular Surgery 13(2):336-347. 1991
4. Campeau, L. New England J. Medicine 311(21):1329-1332. 1984
5. Chobanian, A. Archives of Internal Medicine 156(17):1952-1956. 1996
6. Davis, P. Atherosclerosis 56(1):27-37. 1985
7. Dilley, R. Australian & New Zealand J. Surgery 62(4):297-303. 1992
8. Glueck, C. American J. Industrial Medicine 30(3):331-340. 1996
9. Hagen, P. Artery 9(4):275-284. 1981
10. Levy, D. Clinical & Experimental Hypertension- Part A, Theory & Practice 14(1-2):85-97. 1992
11. Shaper, A. J. Human Hypertension 8(1):3-10. 1994
12. Van der Wal, A. European J. Cardio-Thoracic Surgery 6(9):469-473. 1992

17-4

1. De Faire, U. Cardiovascular Drugs & Therapy 11 Suppl 1:257-263. 1997
2. Donner, M. European J. Medical Research 2(6):270-274. 1997
3. Gould, K. Circulation 89(4):1530-1538. 1994
4. Hadjiisky, P. Archives des Maladies du Coeur et des Vaisseaux 81(11):1411-1417. 1988
5. Niebauer, J. Circulation 96(8):2534-2541. 1997
6. Spacil, J. Angiology 48(9):761-767. 1997
7. Wendelhag I. Atherosclerosis 117(2):225-236. 1995
8. Williams, R. JAMA 255(2):219-224. 1986

17-5

1. Clifton, P. American J. Clinical Nutrition 64(3):361-367. 1996
2. Dawber, T. American J. Clinical Nutrition 36(4):617-625. 1982

3. Dougherty, R. American J. Clinical Nutrition 48(4):970-979. 1988
4. Edington, J. British Medical J. Clinical Research Ed. 294(6568):333-336. 1987
5. Edington, J. American J. Clinical Nutrition 50(1):58-62. 1989
6. Flynn, M. American J. Clinical Nutrition 32(5):1051-1057. 1979
7. Garwin, J. J. Nutrition 122(11):2153-2160. 1992
8. Hirshowitz, B. British J. Plastic Surgery 28(3):185-188. 1975
9. Kummerow, F. American J. Clinical Nutrition 30(5):664-673. 1977
10. Liebman, M. American J. Clinical Nutrition 38(4):612-619. 1983
11. Oh, S. American J. Clinical Nutrition 42(3):421-431. 1985
12. Sacks, F. Hypertension 6(2 Pt 1):193-198. 1984
13. Schnohr, P. J. Internal Medicine 235(3):249-251. 1994
14. Vorster, H. American J. Clinical Nutrition 55(2):400-410. 1992
15. Vorster, H. American J. Clinical Nutrition 46(1):52-57. 1987

17-6

1. Ilowite, N. Current Opinion in Rheumatology 8(5):455-458. 1996
2. Levy, P. American J. Gastroenterology 92(3):494-497. 1997
3. Manzi, S. American J. Epidemiology 145(5):408-415. 1997
4. Maxwell, S. Postgraduate Medical J. 70(830):863-870. 1994
5. Nashel, D. American J. Medicine 80(5):925-929. 1986
6. Petri, M. American J. Medicine 93(5):513-519. 1992
7. Stiller, M. J. American Academy of Dermatology 27(3):434-438. 1992

17-7   —None

Chapter 18

1. Durrington, P. Scandinavian J. Clinical & Laboratory Investigation- Suppl. 198:86-91. 1990
2. Harris, T. J. Clinical Epidemiology 45(6):595-601. 1992
3. Hulley, S. Circulation 86(3):1026-1029. 1992
4. Jacobs, D. Circulation 86(3):1046-1060. 1992
5. Kannel, W. American J. Cardiology 76(9):69c-77c. 1995
6. Menotti, A. European J. Epidemiology 13(4):379-386. 1997
7. Notkola, I. Neuroepidemiology 17(1):14-20. 1998
8. Pekkanen, J. American J. Epidemiology 139(2):155-165. 1994
9. Robbins, J. J. American Geriatrics Society 43:855-859. 1995
10. Rudman, D. J. Parenteral & Enteral Nutrition 12(2):155-158. 1988
11. Schaefer, E. American J. Clinical Nutrition 65(3):823-830. 1997
12. Simes, R. Australian & New Zealand J. Medicine 24(1):113-119. 1994
13. Smith, S. Clinical Chemistry 39(6):1012-1022. 1993

Chapter 19

19-1

1. Bucht, G. J. American Geriatrics Society 32(7):491-498. 1984

2. Chandra, V. Neurology 36(2):209-211. 1986

3. Charletta, D. Neurology 45(8):1456-1461. 1995

4. Corey-Bloom, J. J. American Geriatrics Society 41(1):31-37. 1993

5. De la Torre, J. Gerontology 43(1-2):26-43. 1997

6. Garbarino, K. American J. Medicine 86:734-735. 1989

7. Gorelick, P. Neurology 44(8):1391-1396. 1994

8. Hebert, R. Neuroepidemiology 14(5):240-257. 1995

9. Hofman, A. Lancet 349(9046):151-154. 1997

10. Hontela, S. J. American Geriatrics Society 27(3):104-106. 1979

11. Hulette, C. Neurology 48(3):668-672. 1997

12. Irina, A. Stroke 30(3):613-618. 1999

13. Juby, A. Clinical & Investigative Medicine- Medecini Clinique et Experimentale 21(1):4-11. 1998

14. Kalaria, R. Pharmacology & Therapeutics 72(3):193-214. 1996

15. Kivipelto, M. BMJ 322(7300):1447-1451. 2001

16. Kivipelto, M. Annals Internal Medicine 137(3):149-155. 2002

17. Koopmans, R. Nederlands Tijdschrift voor Geneeskunde 136(45):2223-2227. 1992

18. Kosunen, O. Stroke 26(5):743-748. 1995

19. Langer, R. American J. Epidemiology 134(1):29-38. 1991

20. Mortel, K. Angiology 44(8):599-605. 1993

21. Muckle, T. Lancet 1(8439)1191-1193. 1985

22. Natte, R. Stroke 29(8):1588-1594. 1998

23. Nielsen, H. Acta Psychiatrica Scandinavica 84(3):277-282. 1991

24. Notkola, I. Neuroepidemiology 17(1):14-20. 1998

25. St. Clair, D. British J. Psychiatry 143:274-276. 1983

26. Sparks, D. Neurobiology Aging 17(2):291-299. 1996

27. Thal, L. Neurology 38(7):1083-1090. 1988

28. Thorpe, J. Aging 6(3):159-166. 1994

29. Tomimoto, H. Acta Neuropathologica 90(6):608-614. 1995

30. Tresch, D. J. American Geriatrics Society 33(8):530-537. 1985

31. Urakami, K. Japanese J. Psychiatry & Neurology 41(4):743-748. 1987

32. Wolf-Klein, G. J. American Geriatrics Society 36(3):219-224. 1988

19-2

1. Aronow, W. Angiology 39(7 Pt 1):563-566. 1988

2. Gatchev, O. Annals of Epidemiology 3(4):403-409. 1993

3. Iribarren, C. JAMA 273(24):1926-1932. 1995

4. Iso, H. New England J. Medicine 320(14):904-910. 1989

5. Itoh, Y. J. Neurological Sciences 116(2):135-141. 1993

6. Kaste, M. Stroke 19(9):1097-1100. 1988

7. Koziak, M. Neurologia i Neurochirurgia Polska 12(2):121-128. 1978

8. Menotti, A. European J. Epidemiology 13(4):379-386. 1997

9. Reed, D. American J. Epidemiology 131(4):579-588. 1990

10. Seino, F. J. Nutritional Science & Vitaminology 43(1):83-99. 1997
11. Shimamoto, T. J. Epidemiology 6(3 Suppl):s43-47. 1996

19-3

1. Beard, C. Annals of Epidemiology 6(3):195-200. 1996
2. Ewbank, D. American J. Public Health 89(1):90-92. 1999
3. Olichney, J. J. American Geriatrics Society 43(8):890-893. 1995
4. Parker, J. Southern Medical J. 78(12):1411-1413. 1985
5. Thomas, B. Age & Aging 26(5):401-406. 1997

19-4

1. Berlinger, W. J. of the American Geriatrics Society 39(10):973-978. 1991

Chapter 20

20-1

1. Arai, H. Gerontology 43 Suppl 1:2-10. 1997
2. Blacker, D. Neurology 48(1):139-147. 1997
3. Blacker, D. Archives of Neurology 55:294-296. 1998
4. Cruts, M. Annals of Medicine 39(6):560-565. 1998
5. De Jonghe, C. Neurobiology of Disease 6(4):280-287. 1999
6. Gomez-Isla, T. Brain 122(Pt 9):1709-1719. 1999
7. Hutton, M. Essays in Biochemistry 33:117-131. 1998
8. Mayeux, R. Annals of Neurology 46(3):412-416. 1999
9. Urmoneit, B. Prostaglandins & Other Lipid Mediators 55(5-6):331-343. 1998
10. Wavrant- De Vrieze, F. Neuroscience Letters 269(2):67-70. 1999

20-2

1. Breitner, J. Archives of Neurology 52(8):763-771. 1995
2. Lai, F. Neurology 53(2):331-336. 1999
3. Lannfelt, L. Alzheimer Disease & Associated Disorders 9(3):166-169. 1995
4. Van Gool, W. Annals of Neurology 38(2):225-230. 1995
5. Wisniewski, T. Annals of Neurology 37(1):136-138. 1995

20-3

1. Asada, T. J. of the American Geriatrics Society 44(2):151-155. 1996
2. Bader, G. Gerontology 44(5):293-299.1998
3. Evans, D. JAMA 277(10):822-824. 1997
4. Henderson, A. Lancet 346(8987):1387-1390. 1995
5. Hyman, B. Annals of Neurology 40(1):55-66. 1996
6. Rebeck, G. Neurology 44(8):1513-1516. 1994
7. Sobel, E. Neurology 45(5):903-907. 1995

20-4

1. Barber, R. Archives of Neurology 56(8):961-965. 1999
2. Corcer, E. Archives of Neurology 54(3):273-277. 1997
3. Gomer-Isla, T. Annals of Neurology 41(1):17-24. 1997
4. Haas, C. Biochemical J. 325(Pt 1):169-175. 1997

5. Hirono, N. Alzheimer Disease & Associated Disorders 12(4):362-367. 1998
6. Murphy, G. Jr. American J. of Psychiatry 154(5):603-608. 1997
7. Pirttila, T. Neurobiology of Aging 18(1):121-127. 1997
8. Skoog, I. Neurodegeneration 4(4):433-442. 1995
9. Slooter, A. J. of Neurology 246(4):304-308. 1999

20-5

1. Bertrand, P. Brain Research. Molecular Brain Research 33(1):174-178. 1995
2. Campos, H. Arteriosclerosis, Thrombosis & Vascular Biology 16(6):794-801. 1996
3. Eichner, J. American J. of Cardiology 71(2):160-165. 1993
4. Guillaume, D. J. of Neurochemistry 66(6):2410-2418. 1996
5. Ji, Z. J. of Biological Chemistry 273(22):13452-13460. 1998
6. Lehtinen, S. Atherosclerosis 114(1):83-91. 1995
7. Mulder, M. Alzheimer Disease & Associated Disorders 12(3):198-203. 1998
8. Schaefer, E. Arteriosclerosis & Thrombosis 14(7):1105-1113. 1994
9. Steinmetz, A. Arteriosclerosis 9(3):405-411. 1989
10. Wilson, P. JAMA 272(21):1666-1671. 1994

Chapter 21
21-1

1. Filley, C. American J. of Obstetrics & Gynecology 176(1 Pt 1):1-7. 1997
2. Fratiglioni, L. Neurology 48(1):132-138. 1997
3. Lobo, R. American J. of Obstetrics & Gynecology 173(3 Pt 2):982-989. 1995
4. Paganini-Hill, A. International J. of Fertility & Menopausal Studies 40 Suppl 1:54-62. 1995
5. Ribot, C. Current Opinion in Rheumatology 9(4):362-369. 1997

21-2

1. Haslam, S. Endocrinology 122(3):860-867. 1988
2. Lewko, W. Life Sciences 39(13):1201-1206. 1986
3. Mukku, V. Endocrinology 111(2):480-487. 1982
4. Sabbah, M. Proceedings/America 96(2):11217-11222. 1999
5. Usuki, S. Gynecology Endocrinology 2(4):283-291. 1988
6. Vanderboom, R. J. Cellular Physiology 156(2):367-372. 1993

21-3

1. Akahoshi, M. Circulation 94(1):61-66. 1996
2. Arca, M. JAMA 271(6):453-459. 1994
3. Bruschi, F. Obstetrics & Gynecology 88(6):950-954. 1996
4. Brussaard, H. Arteriosclerosis, Thrombosis & Vascular Biology 17(2):324-330. 1997
5. Campos, H. Metabolism: Clinical & Experimental 39(10):1033-1038. 1990
6. Denke, M. American J. Medicine 99(1):29-35. 1995
7. Desoye, G. J. Clinical Endocrinology & Metabolism 64(4):704-712. 1987
8. Egeland, G. Obstetrics & Gynecology 76(5 Pt 1):776-782. 1990
9. Erickson, S. J. Lipid Research 30(11):1763-1771. 1989

10. Ma, P. Proceedings/America 83(3):792-796. 1986

11. O'Brien, T. Mayo Clinic Proceedings 72(3):235-244. 1997

12. Perrone, G. International J. Fertility & Menopausal Studies 41(6):509-515. 1996

13. Stevenson, J. Atherosclerosis 98(1):83-90. 1993

14. Van Beresteijn, E. American J. Epidemiology 137(4):383-392. 1993

15. Vaziri, S. Archives of Internal Medicine 153(19):2200-2206. 1993

21-4

1. Ayres, S. J. Laboratory & Clinical Medicine 128(4):367-375. 1996

2. Rifici, V. Metabolism: Clinical & Experimental 41(10):1110-1114. 1992

3. Shwaery, G. Circulation 95(6):1378-1385. 1997

21-5

1. Barrett-Connor, E. JAMA 269(20):2637-2641. 1993

2. Behl, C. Molecular Pharmacology 51(4):535-541. 1997

3. Birge, S. Neurology 48(5 Suppl 7):s36-41. 1997

4. Brenner, D. American J. Epidemiology 140(3):262-267. 1994

5. Drake, E. Neurology 2000; 54:599-603. 2000

6. Gollapudi, L. J. Neuroscience Research 56(1):99-108. 1999

7. Goodman, Y. J. Neurochemistry 66(5):1836-1844. 1996

8. Henderson, V. Psychoneuroendocrinology 21(4):421-430. 1996

9. Henderson, V. Neurology 2000; 54:295-301. 2000

10. Honjo, H. J. Steroid Biochemistry & Molecular Biology 41(3-8):633-635. 1992

11. Kawas, C. Neurology 48(6):1517-1521. 1997

12. Keller, J. J. Neuroscience Research 50(4):522-530. 1997

13. Manly, J. Neurology 2000; 54:833-837. 2000

14. Mook-Jung, I. Neuroscience Letters 235(3):101-104. 1997

15. Mortel, K. J. Neuropsychiatry & Clinical Neurosciences 7(3):334-337. 1995

16. Ohkura, T. Endocrine J. 41(4):361-371. 1994

17. Ohkura, T. Dementia 6(2):99-107. 1995

18. Paganini-Hill, A. Archives of Internal Medicine 156(19):2213-2217. 1996

19. Rapp, S. JAMA 289(20):2663-2672. 2003

20. Resnick, S. Neurology 49(6):1491-1497. 1997

21. Shumaker, S. JAMA 289(20):2651-2662. 2003

22. Smith, J.D. J. Molecular Neuroscience 20(3):277-282. 2003

23. Sohrabji, F. Proceedings/America 92(24):11110-11114. 1995

24. Srivastava, R. Biochemistry & Molecular Biology International 38(1):91-101. 1996

25. Stone, D. Experimental Neurology 143(2):313-318. 1997

26. Tang, M. Lancet 348(9025):429-432. 1996

27. Teter, B. Neuroscience 91(3):1009-1016. 1999

28. Yaffe, K. JAMA 289(20):2717-2719. 2003

21-6

1. Barrett-Connor, E. J. Clinical Endocrinology & Metabolism 84(6):1848-1853. 1999

2. Cauley, J. Archives of Internal Medicine 157(19):2181-2187. 1997

3. Dallongeville, J. Atherosclerosis 118(1):123-133. 1995
4. Grady, G. Controlled Clinical Trials 19(4):314-335. 1998
5. Grodstein, F. Epidemiology 10(5):476-480. 1999
6. Heckbert, S. Archives of Internal Medicine 157(12):1330-1336. 1997
7. Herrington, D. Annals of Internal Medicine 131(6):463-466. 1999
8. Hulley, S. JAMA 280(7):605-613. 1998
9. Kannel, W. Archives of Internal Medicine 155(1):57-61. 1995
10. Lee, H. J. Molecular & Cellular Cardiology 30(7):1359-1368. 1998
11. Schenck-Gustafsson, K. European Heart J. 17 Suppl D:2-8. 1996
12. Schrott, H. JAMA 277(16):1281-1286. 1997
13. Subbiah, M. Proceedings of the Society for Experimental Biology & Medicine 217(1):23-29. 1998
14. Sullivan, J. Cardiology Clinics 14(1):105-116. 1996

21-7

1. Biswas, D. Molecular Medicine 4(7):454-467. 1998
2. Castagnetta, L. Endocrinology 136(5):2309-2319. 1995
3. Chalbos, D. J. Clinical Endocrinology & Metabolism 55(2):276-283. 1982
4. Edwards, D. Advances in Experimental Medicine & Biology 138:133-149. 1981
5. Galtier-Dereure, F. J. Clinical Endocrinology & Metabolism 75(6):1497-1502. 1992
6. Gapstur, S. JAMA 281(22):2091-2097. 1999
7. Garnier, M. J. Neuroscience 17(12):4591-4599. 1997
8. Geisinger, K. Cancer 63(2):280-288. 1989
9. Holli, K. J. Clinical Oncology 16(9):3115-3120. 1998
10. Korenaga, D. Hepato-Gastroenterology 44(13):78-83. 1997
11. Kyprianou, N. Cancer Research 51(1):162-166. 1991
12. Schairer, C. Epidemiology 8(1):59-65. 1997
13. Shi, Y. Cancer Research 49(13):3574-3580. 1989

21-8

1. Flaisler, F. Revue Du Rhumatisme, English Ed. 62(9):549-554. 1995
2. Latman, N. American J. Medicine 74(6):957-960. 1983
3. McNeill, M. American J. Obstetrics & Gynecology 159(4):896-897. 1988
4. Ushiyama, T. J. Rheumatology 22(3):421-426. 1995
5. Van Vollenhoven, R. Cleveland Clinic J. Medicine 61(4):276-284. 1994
6. Wilder, R. J. Rheumatology- Suppl 44:10-12. 1996

21-9

1. Dunn, L. Archives of Dermatology 133(3):339-342. 1997
2. Grodstein, F. Epidemiology 10(5):476-480. 1999
3. Keeting, P. J. of Bone & Mineral Research 6(3):297-304. 1991
4. Pierard, G. J. of the American Geriatrics Society 43(6):662-665. 1995

21-10

1. Hughes, S. Endocrinology 138(9):3711-3718. 1997
2. Love-Schimenti, C. Cancer Research 56(12):2789-2794. 1996

3. Simboli-Campbell, M. Breast Cancer Research & Treatment 42(1):31-41. 1997
4. Stio, M. Mehanisms of Ageing & Development 91(1):23-36. 1996

Chapter 22

1. Arnelo, U. Scandinavian J. of Gastroenterology 31(1):83-89. 1996
2. Batterham, R. Annals N Y Academy Sciences 994:162-168. 2003
3. Batterham, R. J. Clinical Endocrinological Metabolism 88(8):3989-3992. 2003
4. Charge, S. J. of Pathology 179(4):443-447. 1996
5. Clark, A. Diabetologia 33(5):285-289. 1990
6. Kazuho, A. Brain Research 762:285-288. 1997
7. Lorenzo, A. Nature 368(6473):756-760. 1994
8. Lorenzo, A. Annals of the New York Academy of Sciences 777:89-95. 1996
9. Ludvik, B. Diabetic Medicine 14 Suppl 2:S9-13. 1997
10. Morley, J. American J. of Physiology 267(1 Pt 2):R178-184. 1994
11. Morley, J. Canadian J. of Physiology & Pharmacology 73(7):1042-1046. 1995
12. Raber, J. J. of Biological Chemistry 272(24):15057-15060. 1997
13. Solin, M. Clinical Science 93(6):581-584. 1997
14. Tan, S. Histopathology 25(5):403-414. 1994
15. Tomita, T. Pathology 35(1):34-36. 2003

Chapter 23

23-1

1. Ackerman-Liebrich, U. Sozial- und Praventivmedizin 25(4):180-181. 1980
2. Barness, L. American J. of Medical Genetics 50(4):353-354. 1994
3. Vaughn, M. Scientific American 232(1):100-109. 1975
4. Haenel, H. Nahrung 33(9):867-887. 1989
5. Kaplan, R. Preventive Medicine 21(1):33-52. 1992
6. McHenry, H. Science 190(4213):425-431. 1975
7. Moore, J. Digestive Diseases & Sciences 29(10):907-911. 1984
8. Partenyi, Z. Medical Hypotheses 5:1113-1116. 1979
9. Pirke, K. Fertility & Sterility 46(6):1083-1088. 1986
10. Roshanai, F. Human Nutrition—Applied Nutrition 38(5):345-354. 1984

23-2

1. Lalueza, C. American J. of Physical Anthropology 100(3):367-387. 1996
2. Pellicciotta, E. Annali dell Ospedale Maria Vittoria di Torino 27(7-12):271-281. 1984
3. Walker, A. Philosophical Transactions of the Royal Society of London—Series B: Biological Sciences 292(1057):57-64. 1981

23-3   —None

23-4

1. Clarkson, T. Archives of Pathology 92:37-45. 1971
2. Hopkins, P. American J. of Clinical Nutrition 55(6):1060-1070. 1992

3. Ho, K. Proceedings of the Society for Experimental Biology & Medicine 150(2):271-277. 1975
4. Kovanen, P. J. of Lipid Research 16(3):211-223. 1975
5. Miller, J. Diabetologia 37(12):1280-1286. 1994
6. Nervi, F. J. of Biological Chemistry 250(11):4145-4151. 1975
7. Newbold, H. Southern Medical J. 81(1):61-63. 1988
8. Overturf, M. J. of Lipid Research 30(2):263-273. 1989
9. Parker, T. Proceedings/America 79(9):3037-3041. 1982
10. Spady, D. Annual Review of Nutrition 13:355-381. 1993
11. Van Zutphen, L. Laboratory Animals 15(1):61-67. 1981

Chapter 24

4-1   —None

4-2

1. Andreasen, N. Neuroscience Letters 273(1):5-8. 1999
2. Botti, R. Clinical Neuropharmacology 14(3):256-261. 1991
3. Bracco, L. Alzheimer Disease & Associated Disorders 13(3):157-164. 1999
4. Buch, K. Nervenarzt 69(5):379-385. 1998
5. Galasko, D. J. of Neural Transmission Suppl 53:209-221. 1998
6. Gerson, R. Fundamental & Applied Toxicology 16(2):320-329. 1991
7. Golebiowski, M. Dementia & Geriatric Cognitive Disorders 10(4):284-288. 1999
8. Guillot, R. J. of Cardiovascular Pharmacology 21(2):339-346. 1993
9. Hulstaert, F. Neurology 52(8):1555-1662. 1999
10. Ishiguro, K. Neuroscience Letters 270(2):91-94. 1999
11. Kanai, M. Annals of Neurology 44(1):17-26. 1998
12. Krasovec, M. Dermatology 186(4):248-252. 1993
13. Kurz, A. Alzheimer Disease & Associated Disorders 12(4):372-377. 1998
14. Lifshitz, F. American J. of Diseases of Children 143(5):537-542. 1989
15. Martins, R. Neuroreport 4(6):757-759. 1993
16. Mosley, S. J. of Lipid Research 30(9):1411-1420. 1989
17. Owen, K. Human & Experimental Toxicology 13(5):357-368. 1994
18. Pavlov, O. Neurotoxicology & Teratology 17(1):31-39. 1995
19. Proksch, E. British J. of Dermatology 128(5):473-482. 1993
20. Proksch, E. Hautarzt 46(2):76-80. 1995
21. Quiec, D. Biochemical J. 310(Pt 1):305-309. 1995
22. Rossor, M. Alzheimer Disease & Assoicated Disorders 11 Suppl 5:S6-9. 1997
23. Saheki, A. Pharmaceutical Research 11(2):305-311. 1994
24. Scheltens. P. Alzheimer Disease & Associated Disorders 11(2):63-70. 1997
25. Vgontzas, A. Clinical Pharmacology & Therapeutics 50(6):730-737. 1991
26. Walsh, K. Toxicologic Pathology 24(4):468-476. 1996
27. Whyte, S. Annals of Neurology 41(1):121-124. 1997
28. Williams, M. Archives of Dermatology 123(11):1535-1538. 1987

Chapter 25

25-1

1. Aarsland, D. American J. of Psychiatry 153(2):243-247. 1996
2. Chen, P. Archives of General Psychiatry 56(3):261-266. 1999
3. Eastley, R. International J. of Geriatric Psychiatry 12(4):484-487. 1997
4. Greenwald, B. Psychological Medicine 27(2):421-431. 1997
5. Hock, C. European Neurology 39(2):111-118. 1998
6. Lyketsos, C. J. of Neuropsychiatry & Clinical Neurosciences 9(4):556-561. 1997
7. Taragano, F. Psychosomatics 38(3):246-252. 1997
8. Tsai, S. Alzheimer Disease & Associated Disorders 10(2):82-85. 1996
9. Tune, L. Depression & Anxiety 8 Suppl 1:91-95. 1998
10. Wetherell, J. Alzheimer Disease & Associated Disorders 13(1):47-52. 1999

25-2

1. Cadeddu, G. Minerva Medica 86(6):251-256. 1995
2. Davidson, K. Behavioral Medicine 22(2):82-84. 1996
3. Golier, J. American J. of Psychiatry 152(3):419-423. 1995
4. Horsten, M. Psychosomatic Medicine 59(5):521-528. 1997
5. Maes, M. Acta Psychiatrica Scandinavica 95(3):212-221. 1997
6. Modai, I. J. Clinical Psychiatry 55(6):252-254. 1994
7. Morgan, R. Lancet 341(8837):75-79. 1993
8. Olusi, S. Biological Psychiatry 40(11):1128-1131. 1996
9. Papassotiropoulas, A. Pharmacopsychiatry 32(1):1-4. 1999
10. Partonen, T. British J. Psychiatry 175:259-262. 1999
11. Suarez, E. Psychosomatic Medicine 61(3):273-279. 1999
12. Sullivan, P. Biological Psychiatry 36(7):472-477. 1994

25-3

1. Bruera, E. Cancer Treatment Reports 68(6):873-876. 1984
2. Casper, R. Depression & Anxiety 8 Suppl 1:96-104. 1998
3. Fishman, P. Geriatrics 49(10):39-42. 1994
4. Herpertz-Dahlmann, B. Acta Psychiatrica Scandinavica 91(2):114-119. 1995
5. Kennedy, S. J. Psychosomatic Research 38(7):773-782. 1994
6. Kerstetter, J. J. American Dietetic Association 92(9):1109-1116. 1992
7. Laessle, R. Biological Psychiatry 23(7):719-725. 1988
8. Morley, J. Drugs & Aging 8(2):134-155. 1996
9. Pollice, C. International J. Eating Disorders 21(4):367-376. 1997
10. Smith, C. J. American Academy of Child & Adolescent Psychiatry 31(5):841-843. 1992
11. Von Zerssen, D. Psychiatric Developments 4(3):237-256. 1986
12. Westin, T. Archives of Otolaryngology- Head & Neck Surgery 114(12):1449-1453. 1988

25-4

1. Albouz, S. Life Sciences 31(23):2549-2554. 1982

2. Beg, Z. J. of Biological Chemistry 260(3):1682-1687. 1985
3. Beg, Z. Metabolism: Clinical & Experimental 36(9):900-917. 1987
4. Kaye, W. J. of Clinical Psychiatry 52(11):464-471. 1991
5. Kumar, R. Neurochemical Research 22(1):1-10. 1997
6. Mann, C. British J. of Pharmacology 115(4):595-600. 1995
7. Miller, S. Advances in Enzyme Regulation 28:65-77. 1989
8. Silver, P. European J. of Pharmacology 121(1):65-71. 1986
9. Vaitla, R. Skin Pharmacology 10(4):191-199. 1997

Chapter 26 —None

END OF REFERENCES

24908076R00185

Made in the USA
Lexington, KY
10 August 2013